Guides to Clinical
Aspiration Biopsy

Head and Neck

Guides to Clinical Aspiration Biopsy

Series Editor: Tilde S. Kline, M.D.

Prostate
Tilde S. Kline, M.D.

Retroperitoneum and Intestine
Kenneth C. Suen, M.B., B.S., F.R.C.P.(C)

Thyroid
Sudha R. Kini, M.D.

Lung, Pleura and Mediastinum
Liang-Che Tao, M.D., F.C.A.P., F.R.C.P.(C)

Head and Neck
Ali H. Qizilbash, M.B., B.S., F.R.C.P.(C)
J. Edward M. Young, B.Sc., M.D., F.R.C.S.(C), F.A.C.S.

Liver and Pancreas
Denise Frias-Hidvegi, M.D.

Guides to Clinical Aspiration Biopsy

Head and Neck

Ali H. Qizilbash, M.B., B.S., F.R.C.P.(C)

Pathologist
Henderson General Hospital

Professor of Pathology
McMaster University
Hamilton, Ontario, Canada

J. Edward M. Young, B.Sc., M.D., F.R.C.S.(C), F.A.C.S.

Head, Head and Neck Service
St. Joseph's Hospital

Clinical Professor of Surgery
McMaster University
Hamilton, Ontario, Canada

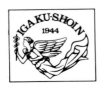

IGAKU-SHOIN   New York • Tokyo

Typesetting by Achorn Graphic Services, Inc. in Garamond
Printing and Binding by Arcata Graphics/Halliday

Published and distributed by

IGAKU-SHOIN Medical Publishers, Inc.
1140 Avenue of the Americas, New York, N.Y. 10036

IGAKU-SHOIN Ltd.,
5-24-3 Hongo, Bunkyo-ku, Tokyo

Library of Congress Cataloging-in-Publication Data

Qizilbash, Ali H.
  Head and neck.

  (Guides to clinical aspiration biopsy)
  Includes index.
  1. Head—Biopsy, Needle. 2. Neck—Biopsy, Needle.
3. Head—Cytopathology. 4. Neck—Cytopathology.
5. Head—Tumors—Diagnosis. 6. Neck—Tumors—Diagnosis.
I. Young, J. Edward M. II. Title. III. Series.
[DNLM: 1. Biopsy, Needle. 2. Cytodiagnosis—methods.
3. Head and Neck Neoplasms—diagnosis. WE 707 Q13h]
RC936.Q59 1988   617'.5107582   87-36207

ISBN: 0-89640-143-X (New York)
ISBN: 4-260-14143-0 (Tokyo)

Printed and bound in USA

10 9 8 7 6 5 4 3 2 1

After the long and irritable hours, weeks and months that have gone into the final publication of this book, it would be unseemly to dedicate this book to anyone but the two persons to whom we have been the greatest trial. Accordingly, we gratefully dedicate this volume to our wives, Batool and Linda.

Preface

We have tried to present in this monograph an overview of the application of needle aspiration biopsy in various benign and malignant lesions involving the many structures in the head and neck. This book is a joint endeavor of the two authors and reflects our accumulated experience.

When we first began to apply this technique to the head and neck approximately a decade ago, it was not popular. Without the help of the clinicians and pathologists who were prepared to accept the challenge this technique offered, we would not have been able to gain the experience and develop the expertise necessary to undertake this task. Needle aspiration biopsy truly is a technique that requires close cooperation between the clinician and the cytopathologist, and working with others has allowed us to learn together and from each other. This point is well emphasized in the text.

The first chapter briefly reviews the clinical application, biopsy and laboratory methods and terminology used in reporting results. Later chapters review the clinical and histologic features of common lesions and describe their cytologic appearances. Attempts have been made to correlate the histologic and cytologic images because needle aspiration biopsy, like surgical pathology, depends in part on recognition of patterns and the usual cytologic features. Pitfalls and complications are stressed. It is our hope that clinicians, especially head and neck surgeons and oncologists, and pathologists will find this text valuable in their respective practices.

Ali H. Qizilbash
J. Edward M. Young

Acknowledgments

We wish to acknowledge the cooperation and contributions of the many people who helped in the preparation of this book. Our colleagues and friends have provided material, given helpful advice and support and substituted for us in a professional capacity when necessary.

At St. Joseph's Hospital, we thank Drs. Michael Kay and Vicky Chen, Department of Pathology, for their support. Mr. Kurt Krakauer and the other cytotechnologists deserve special thanks. We are grateful to Ms. Alice Chou for compiling the data and preparing the Tables 2.14 and 2.15. We are greatly indebted to members of the Head and Neck Service, especially Dr. Stuart D. Archibald, who generously allowed us to use two clinical photographs. We also express our appreciation and gratitude to the audiovisual department, especially to Mr. Tom Daly for preparation of prints. We also are indebted to Dr. G. Alan Lane of the Head and Neck Service and to Dr. Karl Shier, formerly Head of the Cytology Service, who were prepared to accept the challenge needle aspiration offered.

At Henderson General Hospital, thanks are due to all members of the Department of Pathology, particularly Drs. James Thornley, Director of Laboratories, and George Frank, Head of Anatomical Pathology, for their assistance and support. The technical staff of the Cytology Laboratory, particularly Ms. Linda Turner-Smith, who was always ready for assistance and advice on technical matters, deserves our special thanks and gratitude. We also acknowledge the endless hours of work provided by Mr. Gerald Farrell, the medical artist, and Mr. Roy Cooke, Chief of the Audiovisual Department, Hamilton Civic hospitals, and his staff for the artwork and printing of the photomicrographs.

Special thanks are also due to Dr. Khanh Nguyen, Associate Professor of Pathology, University of Alberta, who kindly provided several photographs used in Chapter 4. We are grateful to Dr. Harvey Baker, Clinical Professor of Surgery, University of Oregon Medical School, Portland, for permission to use Dr. Hayes Martin's picture in Chapter 1. All clinical photographs (except as noted) are taken by J. E. M. Young and the cytology and pathology photomicrographs (except as noted) by A. H. Qizilbash.

This book would have been impossible without the hard work and patience of our secretaries, Kim Whicher and Betty Bradley, and without the constant support and perseverance of Dr. Tilde Kline, series editor, and George Schall and Lila Maron of Igaku-Shoin.

Ali H. Qizilbash
J. Edward M. Young

Contents

Preface   vii

1. **Introduction, Clinical Application, Biopsy and Laboratory Techniques   1**

   Introduction   1
   Clinical application   2
   Aspiration biopsy technique   4
   Fixation and staining   10
   Principles of interpretation   11
   Method of reporting   13

2. **Salivary Glands   15**

   Introduction   15
   Normal salivary glands   20
   Cysts   26
   Inflammatory lesions   28
       Acute sialadenitis   29
       Chronic sialadenitis   31
       Granulomatous sialadenitis   32
       Chronic lymphadenitis or hyperplasia of intraparotid lymph nodes   36
   Autoimmune disorders   38
       Benign lymphoepithelial lesion and related conditions
           (Mikulicz's disease and Sjögren's syndrome)   38
   Benign neoplasms   43
       Pleomorphic adenoma (benign mixed tumor)   44
       Monomorphic adenoma   54
   Malignant tumors   71
       Adenoid cystic carcinoma   71
       Mucoepidermoid carcinoma   79
       Acinic cell carcinoma   86
       Carcinoma ex pleomorphic adenoma   92
       Malignant mixed tumor   94
       Primary squamous cell carcinoma   94
       Undifferentiated carcinoma   96

            Adenocarcinoma   98
            Clear-cell carcinoma   99
            Sebaceous carcinoma   100
            Malignant lymphoma   102
            Mesenchymal tumors   103
            Metastatic neoplasms   103
        Diagnostic pitfalls   105
            Neoplasms that simulate cysts   105
            Cellular atypia in cytology preparations   105
            Basaloid tumors   106
            Mucoepidermoid tumors   106
            Lymphocytes in smears   106
        Complications of aspiration biopsy cytology   107
        Results of aspiration biopsy cytology   107

3. Lymph Nodes   117

        Introduction   117
        Indications for needle aspiration biopsy   117
        Normal lymph nodes   119
            Lymphocytes   122
            Histiocytes   123
            Other cell types   123
        Benign enlargement of lymph nodes   123
            Reactive lymphoid hyperplasia   123
            Granulomatous lymphadenopathy   129
            Acute or chronic lymphadenitis   134
            Generalized persistent lymphadenopathy and acquired immune
                deficiency syndrome   134
        Lymphoma   135
            Non-Hodgkin's lymphoma   135
            Hodgkin's lymphoma   150
        Diagnostic pitfalls in lymphoma   155
        Results of aspiration biopsy cytology in lymphoma   156
        Metastatic neoplasms   157
            Squamous cell carcinoma   160
            Adenocarcinoma   166
            Undifferentiated carcinoma   177
            Nasopharyngeal carcinoma   179
            Small-cell undifferentiated carcinoma   180
            Large-cell undifferentiated carcinoma   182
            Merkel cell tumor   182
            Giant-cell and spindle cell variants of undifferentiated carcinoma   183
            Malignant melanoma   186
            Seminoma   196
        Diagnostic pitfalls in metastatic neoplasms   196
        Results of aspiration biopsy cytology in metastatic neoplasms   198
        Complications of needle aspiration biopsy of lymph nodes   199

4. Soft-Tissue Tumors   205

        Introduction   205
            Pathologic classification   206
            General cytologic features of needle aspirates   206
        Tumors of adipose tissue   206
            Lipoma   206
            Liposarcoma   210

Tumors and tumor-like lesions of fibrous tissue 214
   Nodular fasciitis 214
   Fibromatosis 215
   Fibrosarcoma 216
Fibrous histiocytic tumors 219
   Benign fibrous histiocytoma 219
   Malignant fibrous histiocytoma 219
Tumors of smooth muscle 223
   Leiomyoma 223
   Leiomyosarcoma 223
Tumors of striated muscle 225
   Rhabdomyoma 225
   Rhabdomyosarcoma 226
Tumors of peripheral nerves 230
   Neurilemoma (schwannoma) 230
   Neurofibroma 231
   Neurofibrosarcoma 233
Tumors of the sympathetic nervous system 235
   Ganglioneuroma, neuroblastoma and ganglioneuroblastoma 235
   Olfactory neuroblastoma 238
Tumors of blood and lymphatic vessels 238
   Lymphangioma 238
   Hemangioma 239
   Hemangiopericytoma 239
   Angiosarcoma 245
Tumors of synovium 248
   Synovial sarcoma 248
Miscellaneous tumors 249
   Granular cell tumor 249
   Myxoma 249
   Alveolar soft-part sarcoma 250
   Epithelioid sarcoma 251
   Extraskeletal chrondosarcoma 251
   Extraskeletal Ewing's sarcoma 254
   Chordoma 256

5. **Congenital and Other Cystic Lesions of the Neck**   265
Introduction 265
Thyroglossal duct cysts 265
Branchial cleft cysts 266
Thymic cysts 267
Dermoid and epidermoid cysts 271
Cytologic features 271
Differential diagnosis 274
Pitfalls 276
Results 276

6. **Carotid Body Tumors and Other Paragangliomas**   279
Introduction 279
Clinical features 280
Histologic features 282

Cytologic features 283
Differential diagnosis 286
Complications 287
Results 287

7. Miscellaneous Lesions 291

Superficial structures 291
    Merkel cell tumor 291
    Malignant melanoma 292
    Tumors of the epidermal appendages 293
    Kaposi's sarcoma 294
Oral cavity 295
    Lesions of the minor salivary glands 295
    Miscellaneous polypoid lesions 297
Maxillary antrum 298
Orbits and periorbital region 299

8. Ancillary Techniques 303

Cytochemical methods 303
Immunoperoxidase methods 303
    Direct-smear technique 304
    Cytocentrifuge technique 304
    Cell-Block technique 304
Electron microscopy 306

Index 311

1

Introduction, Clinical Application, Biopsy and Laboratory Techniques

INTRODUCTION

Of the many areas of controversy in head and neck surgery, no topic in the past decade has provided as much discussion and disagreement as needle aspiration biopsy. On the one hand are clinicians who are not even prepared to consider its use and cytopathologists who refuse to report needle aspirations. On the other are those who have extensively investigated and used the technique and are convinced not only of its usefulness but also of its tremendous advantages in regard to cost effectiveness, speed of diagnosis and patient acceptability. Between these two extremes are clinicians and pathologists who are still trying to determine the place in their practice of this well-established but underused technique. We have written this book in an attempt to provide a reference text for the numerous practitioners who are familiar with the principles of needle aspiration biopsy but lack firsthand experience with the technique and its interpretation. It is also hoped that this text will facilitate the useful communication between clinicians and pathologists. Certainly in some areas of the world, such as Scandinavia, most or all aspirations are done by a group of interested and highly trained cytopathologists to whom patients with diagnostic problems are referred. In large clinical settings, patients are assessed and aspirated and the reports interpreted by the same person. However, in most other centers and especially in regard to head and neck problems, patients with masses who present for aspiration usually have their method of investigation decided by the clinician to whom they are first referred. For most patients with head and neck masses, this clinician is a head and neck surgeon (whose initial training is in general surgery, otolaryngology or plastic surgery). For those enlightened clinicians to whom needle aspiration is an early part of their investigation, an interested and trained pathologist is essential and the communication between the two becomes mandatory. As we will emphasize, there are areas of difficulty in the cytologic

1

interpretation of needle aspirates for which communication between aspirator and interpreter is essential. The communication required is akin to that necessary between the operating surgeon and the pathologist who interprets a frozen section intraoperatively. In the latter situation, the pathologist needs all possible information to give the most accurate diagnosis. Similarly, the cytopathologist is most valuable to the clinician when he or she is aware not only of the site of the lesion aspirated but also of the clinical picture, particularly when there is previous or concurrent abnormality in the head or neck. Although metastatic squamous cell carcinoma in lymph nodes provides an aspirate that can be easily diagnosed correctly by even the most inexperienced cytologist, such lesions as carotid body tumor, schwannoma, lymphoma, adenoid cystic carcinoma and metastatic hypernephroma provide a challenge to even the most experienced cytologist. In the latter situations, discussion, reassessment and occasional reaspiration can lead to further appropriate investigation and a correct preoperative diagnosis in most cases. It has become exceedingly rare on most head and neck services where needle aspiration biopsy is used appropriately for a patient to go to the operating room without a preoperative diagnosis being established. In most centers, this situation is in marked contrast to what occurred even a decade ago. Formerly, women would routinely be anesthetized unaware as to whether they would awaken with or without a breast (because a definitive diagnosis of a breast lump had not been established preoperatively). This practice has largely been replaced by a premastectomy needle (aspiration or Tru-cut) or even open biopsy done under local anesthesia on an outpatient basis several days before planned surgical intervention. Similarly, until recently, most head and neck patients were routinely required to give preoperative consent for an operation to include a neck mass biopsy, possible neck dissection, possible total thyroidectomy, possible parotidectomy and possible oropharyngeal resection. This practice clearly is no longer acceptable, not only because there is increased patient litigation but also because available methodology can avoid this diagnostic problem. With frequent use of needle aspiration biopsy, lesions 1 centimeter or smaller can easily be aspirated accurately and interpreted correctly. We hope that this book will stimulate clinicians who infrequently use needle aspiration to perform it more often and will assist in the interpretation of the apirates thus obtained. It is our recommendation that no patient with a palpable mass in the head and neck should undergo extensive investigation or operation before having needle aspiration biopsy. We hope that this book facilitates that goal.

CLINICAL APPLICATION

Patients who present with abnormal swellings in the head or neck have been diagnostic dilemmas for clinicians for centuries. The differential diagnosis for such lesions includes such diverse conditions as benign and malignant neoplasms, acute or chronic inflammatory lesions, vascular, neurogenic, muscular and other soft-tissue processes (e.g., degenerative, inflammatory or neoplastic), developmental anomalies relating to the branchial clefts or thyroglossal tract, benign or malignant cystic lesions in the salivary glands and thyroid, traumatic swellings and reactive lymph nodes. The large number of diagnostic possibilities has resulted in a well-

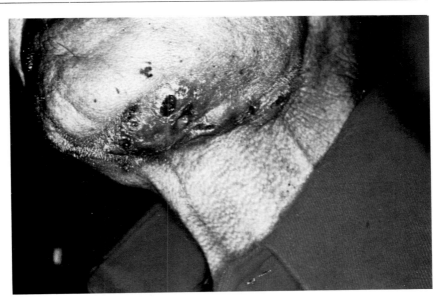

Fig. 1.1. A patient referred to us because of local spread of tumor in the neck after an open biopsy. Biopsy had revealed squamous cell carcinoma. Such cases are better investigated by needle aspiration biopsy.

defined approach to a patient who presents with an abnormal swelling in the head or neck. Several generations of head and neck surgeons have delineated the steps necessary to establish a definitive diagnosis before starting therapy. Unfortunately, many physicians who evaluate patients with lumps in the neck mistakenly recommend, or proceed with, an open biopsy of the lesion in an attempt to determine the diagnosis. In inflammatory, traumatic or other reactive lesions, a benign needle aspiration biopsy allows observation and followup until resolution, thus avoiding unnecessary operation. In some cases, an open biopsy is clearly contraindicated, (Fig. 1.1); for example, in cases of primary or metastatic malignant lesions, in which ill-advised early biopsy may make subsequent treatment more difficult (e.g., if the incision is inappropriately placed for subsequent surgical incisions). In many cases, open biopsy probably adversely affects the patient's chance for curative treatment. In this regard, tumors spread through the planes of an open incisional or excisional biopsy have an increased risk for local recurrence at that site because the tumor cells are difficult to identify at subsequent radical surgical resection, and because they have been rendered relatively anoxic and are more difficult to sterilize with radical radiotherapy. For these reasons, a careful and appropriate evaluation of the patient includes examination for a primary malignant tumor elsewhere in the head or neck, and assessment for a history of a previous malignant lesion anywhere or previous irradiation of the head or neck. Before surgical biopsy, needle aspiration biopsy (Fig. 1.2) provides the most useful evaluation of a mass in the head or neck since this technique permits a cytologic diagnosis and directs further investigation and/or treatment as indicated.

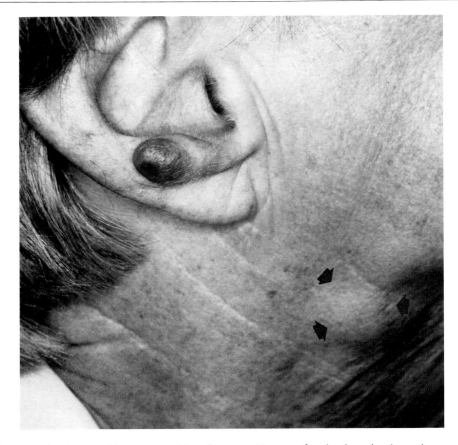

Fig. 1.2. A 73-year-old woman, with a five-year history of a slowly enlarging, pigmented lesion on the right pinna. Over the past four months, a swelling developed in the right submandibular triangle (arrows). Clinical diagnosis was malignant melanoma with nodal metastases. Aspiration biopsy of the lesion in the ear was not diagnostic, consisting of amorphous cellular debris and a few anucleate squames. The submandibular aspirate revealed features of a pleomorphic adenoma. At surgical intervention for pleomorphic adenoma, the ear lesion was removed and pathologic examination revealed it to be a pilar cyst.

ASPIRATION BIOPSY TECHNIQUE

In the 1930s, Dr. Hayes Martin (Fig. 1.3), a renowned head and neck surgeon at Memorial Hospital, New York, advocated the use of needle aspiration biopsy to evaluate masses in the head and neck area.[1] Martin and his trainees over the subsequent years proved that this procedure was easy to perform and extremely accurate. Unfortunately, the technique did not gain general acceptance because of the fear of tumor implantation along the needle tract. Martin recommended the use of an 18-gauge needle.[1,2] There have been rare instances of tumor implantation with larger-bore needles, supporting the concern of clinicians who considered this phenomenon

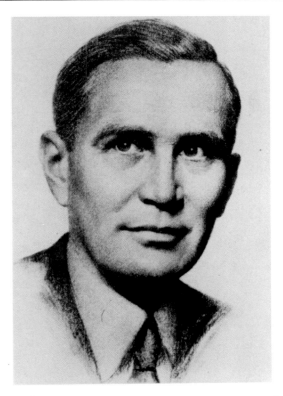

Fig. 1.3. Dr. Hayes Martin (courtesy of Dr. H. W. Baker).

a risk of the procedure.[3-5] However, even with an 18-gauge needle, tumor implantation is an exceedingly rare complication and when aspiration is done with a 22-gauge needle, tumor implantation does not seem to occur. We have used 22-gauge needles to aspirate more than 5000 head and neck lesions and have not experienced tumor implantation. The technique that we recommend is simple and rapid, taking only a few minutes in a clinic, an office or in a hospital.

A variety of syringe holders have been devised and are available commercially. They are not essential in obtaining an adequate aspirate. We use a standard, disposable, 10-milliliter syringe and a 22-gauge needle. The lesion is stabilized with one hand and the needle, mounted on the syringe, is inserted into the lesion (Fig. 1.4). When the tip of the needle is in the lesion, suction is applied to the syringe and the tip of the needle is moved within the confines of the lesion, maintaining maximal suction (6 to 8 milliliters) on the syringe (Fig. 1.5). As the tip of the needle moves through various portions of the lesion, it samples each area, collecting material within the needle. If the lesion has a cystic component, fluid appears in the syringe. Suction is then released on the syringe before the tip of the needle is removed from the patient. This maneuver prevents the sample in the needle from being sucked up into the barrel, where it would be more difficult to retrieve, and also, at least theoretically, prevents tumor cells from being sucked along the needle tract. Gauze is applied to the puncture site and the patient is asked to apply pressure to the site

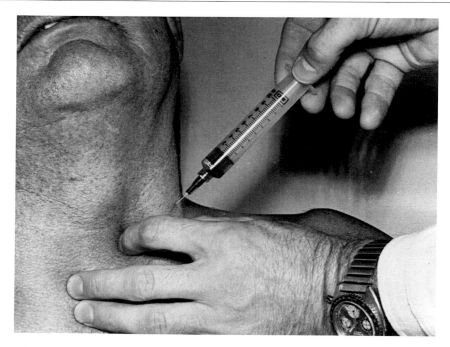

Fig. 1.4. A 22-gauge needle mounted on a 10-milliliter syringe is inserted into the lesion to be biopsied while the lesion is steadied with the opposite hand.

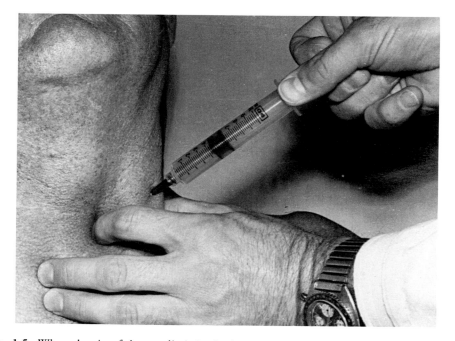

Fig. 1.5. When the tip of the needle is in the lesion, suction is applied to the syringe while the tip of the needle is moved within the confines of the lesion in several directions. Suction is then released and the needle is removed.

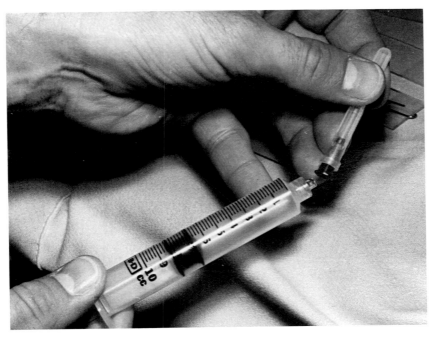

Fig. 1.6. The syringe is disconnected from the needle and filled with air. The needle is then reconnected.

for several minutes. If the syringe contains fluid, several drops are placed on glass slides and the remainder is placed in 50 percent ethanol or in balanced electrolyte solution and the solution is used to rinse out the syringe and needle. In most cases, there is no fluid in the syringe and the sample is within the needle. In this situation, when the needle is withdrawn, the needle and syringe are disconnected, the syringe is filled with air (Fig. 1.6), the needle is reapplied to the syringe, and the air is used to express a small amount of the specimen directly onto a slide (Fig. 1.7). A second slide is dipped in 95 percent ethanol and placed on top of the slide that contains the sample (Fig. 1.8) and the two slides are pulled apart in a longitudinal direction (Fig. 1.9). This technique smears the specimen and prevents drying of the cells. Both slides are then placed into the bottle of 95 percent ethanol (Fig. 1.10). Before smearing, alternate slides are prepared with a paper clip on the frosted end to prevent the slides from adhering to each other when they are placed in the alcohol bottle. Two to six slides can usually be prepared from each aspirate.

For clinicians who do not wish to prepare their own slides, the aspirated sample can be expressed directly into balanced electrolyte solution and the solution then used to rinse the needle and syringe. The solution that contains the aspirated sample is sent immediately to the cytology laboratory, where it is spun down and slides subsequently prepared. If the specimen cannot be sent to the cytology laboratory without delay, it should be collected in 50 percent ethanol. We have found that either of the techniques described above produces excellent cytology specimens, but we believe that immediately prepared slides yield slightly superior results.

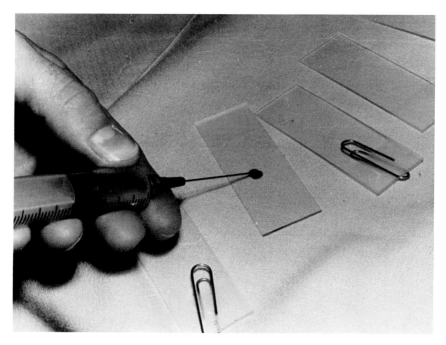

Fig. 1.7. Air in the syringe is used to express the specimen (which is primarily in the needle) onto a glass slide.

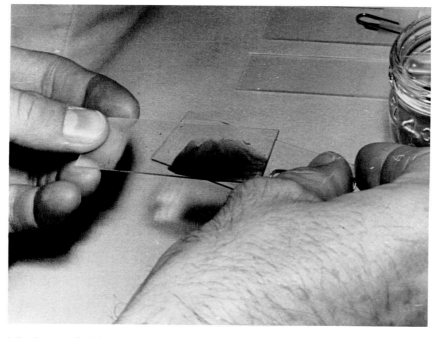

Fig. 1.8. A second slide is dipped in 95 percent alcohol and placed on top of the specimen.

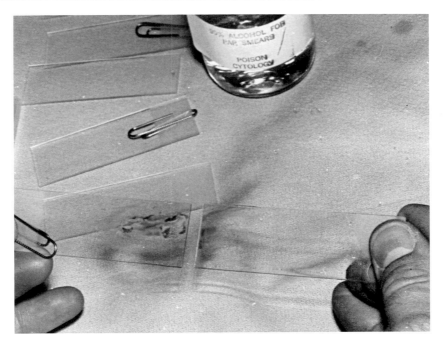

Fig. 1.9. Light pressure is used to pull the two slides apart (this maneuver spreads the specimen and prevents drying).

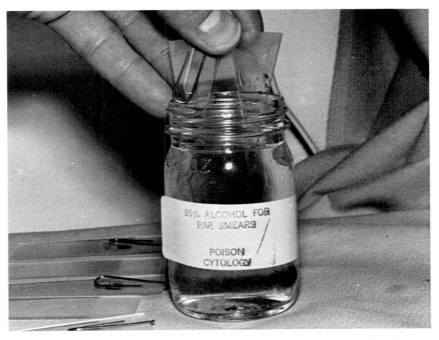

Fig. 1.10. The slides are immediately placed in a jar of 95 percent alcohol and sent to the cytology laboratory for staining and interpretation.

When a lesion is aspirated, the clinician occasionally obtains a dry tap, or an aspirate that contains virtually no material for subsequent preparation. In such instances, we immediately repeat the aspiration to obtain better material. On the rare occasions when a second aspirate (obtained simultaneously or subsequently) fails to yield adequate material, we perform aspiration with an 18-gauge needle in an attempt to obtain a more adequate sample. It is worthwhile to emphasize here that nondiagnostic aspirates, whether obtained with a 22- or an 18-gauge needle, must be carefully assessed in the light of the clinical situation, particularly if a malignant process is suspected. In such situations, more invasive biopsies should be considered, either Tru-cut or even open biopsy, to assure that a malignant lesion is not missed.

Occasionally, aspiration of a congenital cystic lesion (e.g., branchial or thyroglossal) or an inflammatory lesion (a walled-off or sterilized abscess) with a 22-gauge needle yields thick material, suggesting incomplete evacuation of the lesion. On such occasions, aspiration should be repeated immediately or within a few days with an 18-gauge needle in an attempt to completely evacuate the lesion. Complete evacuation may prevent recurrence and obviate surgical intervention.

Aspiration biopsy performed with a 22-gauge needle is one of the simplest, best tolerated diagnostic procedures available to clinicians. It requires no local anesthesia and is often painless and rarely uncomfortable. Patients have greater tolerance for aspiration biopsy than they have for sigmoidoscopy, rectal examination or even indirect laryngoscopy. The method that we have described can be used to teach aspiration biopsy to residents, interns and medical students. Two, three or more lesions can be aspirated on the same occasion and questionable aspirates can easily be repeated.

FIXATION AND STAINING

We recommend fixation of aspirates in 95 percent ethanol and have found the cytologic results satisfactory. As an alternate method, slides can be prepared and immediately sprayed with a fixative. We have found, however, that most clinicians simply cannot resist the opportunity to admire their smears before spraying and this results in air drying and leads to poor or inadequate specimens. We routinely use the Papanicolaou or hematoxylin and eosin staining method and choose the air-dried May-Grünwald Giemsa technique only when a lymphoproliferative process is suspected. In wet-fixed smears, there is minimal distortion of cells and tissue fragments maintain their architectural patterns, a definite advantage for tissue pathologists. The nuclear detail is also well preserved in wet-fixed material stained by the Papanicolaou or hematoxylin and eosin method. Cytoplasmic granules, secretions and background material, such as colloid and mucus, however, are better visualized with the May-Grünwald-Giemsa technique.

For special studies, such as immunocytochemistry and electron microscopy, the cytocentrifuge and cell-block method of preparation are recommended and are described in detail in Chapter 8.

All slides in our laboratory are routinely stained with the Papanicolaou technique, as outlined in Table 1.1. Hematoxylin and eosin and other special stains are also

TABLE 1.1. Papanicolaou Stain for Needle Aspirates

1. Running water bath	10 seconds
2. Hematoxylin*	2 minutes
3. Running water bath	2 minutes
4. 2% Lithium carbonate	2 minutes
5. Running water bath	10 seconds
6. 95% Alcohol	10 dips
7. 95% Alcohol	10 dips
8. IG-6 Stain-Ortho	2 minutes
9. 95% Ethanol	10 dips
10. 95% Ethanol	10 dips
11. 95% Ethanol	10 dips
12. EA Stain-Ortho	1½ minutes
13. 95% Ethanol	10 dips
14. 95% Ethanol	10 dips
15. 95% Ethanol	10 dips
16. 100% Ethanol	10 dips
17. 100% Ethanol	2 minutes
18. Xylene until coverslipping	(At least 5 minutes)

*Half-oxidized hematoxylin solution.

employed as indicated. Examples of properly prepared and stained smears are shown in Figure 1.11.

PRINCIPLES OF INTERPRETATION

A knowledge of normal histologic features and surgical pathology are essential to develop expertise in needle biopsy cytology. Pathologists therefore have an excellent opportunity to develop the skills necessary for interpretation. These are acquired largely through experience. A good way to develop expertise is through

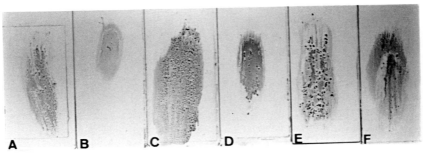

Fig. 1.11. Examples of well-prepared smears. (a) pleomorphic adenoma, salivary gland; (b) medullary carcinoma, breast; (c) metastatic adenocarcinoma, cervical lymph node; (d) follicular hyperplasia, cervical lymph node; (e) sebaceous carcinoma, eyelid; (f) metastatic squamous cell carcinoma, submandibular gland.

exposure to a large volume of material and working closely with clinicians. Continuing education courses, workshops and seminars are helpful and give one an idea of what is being accomplished by other clinicians working with similar material. However, one of the best ways to develop interpretative skills is to correlate cytologic findings with histopathologic features. This can be done by the subsequent histologic review of surgical pathology material in patients who initially underwent needle aspiration biopsy. We, however, recommend that the novice pathologist practice correlation by means of examination of imprints and needle aspiration smears prepared on specimens sent for frozen section and the fresh surgical pathology material that one receives daily in the pathology laboratory. This gives instant correlation when images are still fresh in ones memory. We use this method in our department on a daily basis and recommend it for teaching needle aspiration biopsy interpretation to our resident staff.

One of the other prerequisites of a successful needle biopsy is the quality of the aspirate. This largely depends on the experience and skills of the aspirator. The cytopathologist cannot be of much help to the clinician if the smear is unsatisfactory. Scanty, dried and improperly smeared material are the usual causes of unsatisfactory smears. In most cases, an experienced aspirator knows that he or she has a satisfactory specimen if small tissue fragments are in the smears. In the superficial head and neck masses, we have not routinely used immediate microscopic assessment of the aspirated material to judge adequacy of the aspirate because reaspiration is easily accomplished, although we routinely make such an assessment on deep needle biopsy specimens from the lungs, pancreas, liver, retroperitoneum and other structures. In such situations, staining by the rapid hematoxylin and eosin method usually provides the answer within 10 to 15 minutes at the bedside.

Like histopathology, needle aspiration biopsy depends on pattern recognition and to be effective should not only provide diagnosis of malignant processes but also accurately predict the cell type. Expressed differently, like surgical biopsy, needle aspiration biopsy is a diagnostic technique. With experience, this can be achieved in a vast majority of cases. Criteria for interpretation on needle biopsy are somewhat different from those of cervicovaginal cytology, where cells are spontaneously exfoliated. Unlike cervical cytology, low-power evaluation of the needle aspirate smear is important and sheds light on the cellularity of the aspirate; generally, aspirates from malignant processes are cellular, usually ascribed to the poor intercellular cohesion. On the other hand, aspirates of a benign lesion tend to be poor in cells due to good cellular adhesiveness. Exceptions are not, however, uncommon and scirrhous carcinomas are notorious in yielding poor cellular samples. Architectural patterns are easily recognizable on low-power examination and are helpful in diagnosing different lesions. A cellular smear generally contains numerous tissue fragments. Cells in flat, monolayer sheets or irregular, three-dimensional, multilayer clusters are frequent. Other arrangements include a glandlike configuration, microacinar and papillary formations, a rosette-like appearance, a trabecular pattern, loose fascicles, a single-file pattern and dispersed cells. Mixed patterns are not uncommon. High-power examination is necessary to study the nuclear features in more detail. The usual criteria of malignancy used in exfoliative cytology are also applicable in needle aspiration biopsy. These criteria include cellular and nuclear size, nuclear to cytoplasmic ratio, hyperchromasia, irregularity of nuclear membrane and presence, number and size of nucleoli. The background of the aspirate is helpful at times in suggesting the correct diagnosis. The presence of a large amount of blood and few tumor cells is in keeping with a vascular neoplasm. On the other hand, necrosis is frequent both in rapidly growing tumors and in infectious processes. The presence of a large amount of mucus in the background along with scanty glandular elements in an aspirate from an enlarged lymph node should suggest the diagnosis of metastatic colloid or mucinous carcinoma.

METHOD OF REPORTING

Because needle aspiration is a diagnostic procedure, attempts should be made to give the clinician a diagnosis similar to the histopathologic diagnosis on excised tissue. Specific diagnostic terms should be used. For example, reporting an aspirate as "negative for malignancy" may be meaningless in a patient with a mass in the parotid gland. The clinician would like to know if there is evidence of chronic inflammation, a benign lymphoepithelial lesion, hyperplasia of an intraparotid lymph node, Warthin's tumor or a pleomorphic adenoma. One should state that the smear shows changes consistent with or diagnostic of, for example, reactive hyperplasia of an intraparotid lymph node or a pleomorphic adenoma. Similarly, it is not sufficient to state that the aspirate of a lymph node is positive for metastatic carcinoma. Attempts should be made to state the exact cell type and degree of differentiation of the lesion. For example, the reports should read as follows:

Malignant cells present, diagnostic of metastatic mucus-secreting adenocarcinoma, consistent with a primary tumor in the gastrointestinal tract; or Monotonous population of small lymphocytes present, consistent with a diagnosis of small, cleaved-cell lymphoma.

If the smear is not diagnostic, it should be so stated and the clinician then has to decide whether to follow the patient, repeat the aspiration or subject the patient to a Tru-cut or open surgical biopsy. For example, a nondiagnostic report of a needle aspirate of a mass in the submandibular triangle may be worded as follows:

Nondiagnostic smear, consisting of a few atypical ductal cells, no definite evidence of malignancy present, suggest repeat or consider biopsy.

Many times discussion of a case with the clinician may clarify a situation and suggest the etiologic basis of the changes seen in the cells. In the preceding example, the atypical ductal cells in the aspirate from the submandibular gland would be a normal finding in a patient who has received irradiation for metastatic squamous cell carcinoma in the neck. In this situation, a malignant process is ruled out and the swelling of the submandibular gland reflects chronic inflammation secondary to irradiation.

Dried, improperly made smears or smears with scanty cellular material are the usual causes of unsatisfactory specimens. This should be indicated to the clinician so that the aspiration can be repeated.

REFERENCES

1. Martin HE, Ellis EB: Biopsy by needle puncture and aspiration. *Anal Surg* 92:169–181, 1930.

2. Baker HW: Needle aspiration biopsy: An introduction. *Ca* 36:69–70, 1986.

3. Sinner WN, Zajicek J: Implantation metastasis after percutaneous transthoracic needle aspiration biopsy. *Acta Radiol Diagn* 17:473, 1976.

4. Koss LG, Woyke S, Olszewski W: *Aspiration Biopsy. Cytologic Interpretation and Histologic Bases.* New York, Igaku-Shoin, 1984, p 289.

5. Zajicek J: Aspiration biopsy cytology. Part I. Cytology of supradiaphragmatic organs. *Monogr Clin Cytol* 4:21–23, 1974.

2

Salivary Glands

INTRODUCTION

The salivary glands may become enlarged as the result of a local or systemic process, and enlargement can occur secondary to cystic disease, acute or chronic infection, nonspecific inflammatory or degenerative processes and benign or malignant neoplasms. These processes can involve one or more salivary glands (Table 2.1). The nature of the lesion often cannot be determined on clinical examination alone and in the past most cases required histologic study for a definitive diagnosis. Today, needle aspiration biopsy has emerged as an effective and sensitive technique for the diagnosis of lesions that involve the salivary glands. Scandinavian workers first demonstrated the usefulness of this technique in the investigation of salivary gland masses.[1-3] Similar results have been reported in England,[4] the United States[5-8] and Canada.[9] Aspiration biopsy is a helpful adjunct to careful physical examination of patients with masses in the salivary glands. It not only provides the clinician with a definitive preoperative diagnosis but also prevents unnecessary surgical intervention in many patients. We have recently shown that approximately one-third of all patients undergoing needle aspiration biopsy are spared subsequent operative procedures.[9]

To clinicians who employ needle aspiration biopsy selectively and with reluctance, its use in patients with salivary gland lesions has been anathema. Their reasons are based on statistics (approximately 75 percent of parotid tumors are benign mixed lesions, and therefore cytopathologists would simply have to call all aspirates from the parotid "benign mixed" to be correct 75 percent of the time) and on the risk of tumor implantation. Their concern is based on the realization that benign mixed tumors implant at a surgical site with great frequency if the tumor margin is transgressed at the time of operation. Skeptical clinicians further maintain that the result of needle aspiration will not affect either the decision to proceed with surgical intervention or the extent of operation necessary.

In our initial experience with needle aspiration biopsy, we similarly did not aspirate parotid lesions or submandibular triangle lesions that were salivary gland tumors on the basis of clinical criteria. However, we began to see patients who had

TABLE 2.1. Causes of Salivary Gland Enlargement

Cysts	Malignant neoplasms
True simple cyst	Adenoid cystic carcinoma
Mucocele	Mucoepidermoid carcinoma
Epidermal inclusion cyst	Acinic cell carcinoma
Branchial cleft cyst	Carcinoma ex pleomorphic adenoma
Inflammatory disorders	Malignant mixed tumor
Acute sialadenitis (viral, bacterial)	Squamous cell carcinoma
Chronic sialadenitis (sialolithiasis)	Undifferentiated carcinoma
Granulomatous sialadenitis (sarcoid,	Adenocarcinoma
tuberculosis)	Sebaceous carcinoma
Hyperplasia of intraparotid lymph	Malignant lymphoma
nodes	Sarcoma
Autoimmune disorders	Metastatic carcinoma
Benign lymphoepithelial lesion	
Sjögren's syndrome	
Benign neoplasms	
Pleomorphic adenoma	
Monomorphic adenoma	
Papillary cystadenoma lymphomatosum	
Oncocytoma	
Basal cell adenoma	
Sebaceous adenoma	
Clear-cell adenoma	

been successfully treated for malignant intraoral lesions present months or years later with a swelling in the submandibular triangle that clearly could be an obstructed submandibular salivary gland or a primary neoplasm in the submandibular gland. Although in some cases the diagnosis appeared obvious, in others the differentiation among alternative diagnoses was difficult, even for experienced radiation oncologists and head and neck surgeons. In these situations, needle aspiration biopsy provided helpful information that could be used to guide subsequent investigation and treatment (Fig. 2.1). Not surprisingly, some patients in whom the diagnosis seemed most obvious were those in whom needle aspiration provided a diagnosis that differed most radically from the presumed diagnosis suspected by the clinician. These results led us to be more aggressive in our use of needle aspiration biopsy in lesions in the submandibular triangle, whether they were obstructive, infective or of neoplastic origin. The useful information obtained by that approach prompted us to use needle aspiration biopsy in parotid lesions. Because of the concern that a benign mixed tumor might be implanted along the needle tract (although the Scandinavian series suggests that implantation does not occur when a 22-gauge needle is used), we tattoo the needle puncture site with India ink following aspiration and subsequently excise an ellipse of skin, and underlying tissue in continuity with the parotidectomy specimen (Fig. 2.2).

We were pleasantly surprised at the usefulness of needle aspiration biopsy for salivary swellings. For example, some lesions that were tumors on clinical grounds were found to be cystic on needle aspiration, benign cytologically, and in long-term follow-up have not recurred. Localized areas of sialadenitis that appeared identical

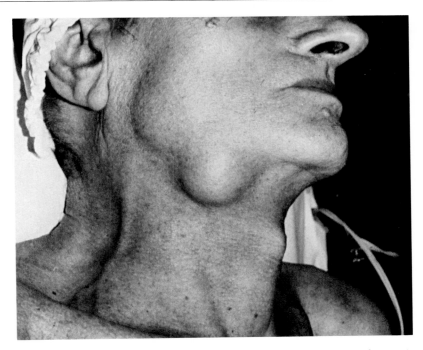

Fig. 2.1. Obstruction of the right submandibular gland with secondary infection in an immunocompromised patient with leukemia. Aspiration biopsy yielded an inflammatory exudate, followed by drainage within 24 hours.

to tumors yielded a benign inflammatory aspirate and almost always responded to antibiotic therapy, thus avoiding unnecessary exploration. In tumors, the advantage of knowing the likely pathologic diagnosis preoperatively cannot be underestimated. The difference between the surgical approach used for benign and that used for malignant parotid tumors may be minimal in the hands of some head and neck surgeons, but even they will admit that the knowledge that a lesion is definitely malignant alters the extent of their surgical intervention to include sampling of upper jugular lymph nodes as an early part of the surgical procedure and preparation for total parotidectomy rather than a lesser procedure. Those surgeons would make no attempt to preserve the sensory great auricular nerve in cases of malignant parotid tumors, whereas its sacrifice is usually not indicated for benign lesions. It should be emphasized that in all areas of medicine, the more information that is available to the clinician, the more likely his or her treatment will be beneficial to the patient with minimal morbidity.

Inflammatory intraparotid lymph nodes can be indistinguishable on a clinical basis from primary or secondary parotid neoplasms. An aspiration biopsy specimen that contains a mixture of lymphocytes compatible with inflammation suggests the need for a conservative approach, with a period of observation before excision is contemplated. A monotonous field of one type of lymphocyte suggests lymphoma, which can be diagnosed directly by excisional nodal biopsy rather than full lateral parotid lobectomy. Metastatic squamous cell carcinoma in an intraparotid lymph node (Fig.

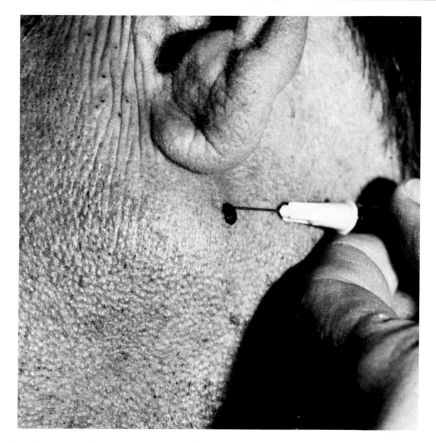

Fig. 2.2. Any aspiration tract can easily be tattooed for subsequent excision by puncturing the adjacent skin with a 25-gauge needle through a tiny drop of India ink.

2.3) from a previous or coexistent skin or upper aerodigestive tract primary tumor may be managed more appropriately with radiotherapy than with parotidectomy or, if surgical intervention is indicated, by a more extensive operation than is indicated for a benign parotid tumor and even for most malignant parotid lesions. Metastatic melanoma in an intraparotid lymph node was encountered in our series in a patient who had no apparent primary tumor at presentation or in subsequent follow-up over several years. A head and neck surgeon who sends a superficial parotid lobe to a pathologist and gets a frozen-section diagnosis of metastatic melanoma might be less than happy with his initial investigation (did he do funduscopic examination? check every inch of the scalp for lesions?) and, in particular, will be unlikely to have prepared the patient for the extensiveness of the operation that may be necessary at the time. Given the availability and accuracy of needle aspiration biopsy, it seems ludicrous to consider subjecting a patient (or a surgeon) to a parotid operation without obtaining a cytologic diagnosis preoperatively.

In comparison to needle aspiration biopsy, sialograms for solitary parotid lesions are nearly useless (they will usually only confirm that there is an abnormality in the

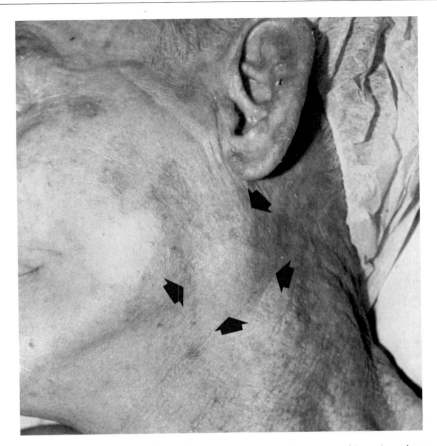

Fig. 2.3. Metastatic squamous cell carcinoma (arrows) in an intraparotid lymph node presenting as a primary tumor of parotid gland.

salivary parenchyma and are probably indicated only as an investigative procedure in cases of diffuse salivary gland swelling compatible with obstruction with or without secondary infection) and computed tomograms are of limited utility (they can show the extent of large lesions of the deep lobe or help define the relationship of a nonparotid lesion to the salivary parenchyma and adjacent structures). We have seen one young woman who presented with a firm, superficial mass in the parotid area with some associated tenderness (Fig. 2.4). To all the clinicians who examined her, the mass was apparently a parotid tumor, possibly malignant. Needle aspiration and subsequent computed tomography suggested and subsequently confirmed the diagnosis of paraganglioma (glomus intravagale), a lesion that requires specific operative management, including sacrifice of the vagus nerve. No clinician could possibly object to having that diagnosis established preoperatively.

It is for these reasons that we recommend routine needle aspiration of all salivary gland lesions no matter how obvious the diagnosis appears when the patient first presents. No other method of investigation provides as much useful information as rapidly and accurately.

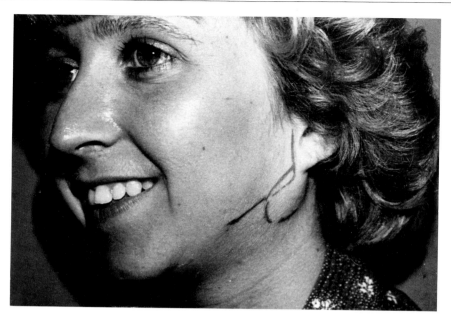

Fig. 2.4. A young woman with a mass in the left parotid space (angle of mandible marked and tumor mass circled). The clinical diagnosis was parotid tumor, possibly malignant. Aspiration biopsy suggested a diagnosis of paraganglioma, which was confirmed by histopathologic examination of the excised tumor.

Because of the variety of tumors that occur in the salivary glands, experience in the interpretation of needle biopsy aspirates is essential if errors are to be kept to a minimum.[7] Moreover, cytopathologists should be familiar with the complete histories and clinical findings of patients before making reports on aspirates. It is also important that personnel who make reports on smears be familiar with the normal structure of the salivary glands before interpreting pathologic changes.

NORMAL SALIVARY GLANDS

ANATOMIC STRUCTURES. A large number of salivary glands deliver a serous or mucous fluid into the oral cavity. These glands are classified as major or minor. The major glands are the paired parotid, submandibular and sublingual glands (Fig. 2.5). Minor glands are widely distributed under the mucosal lining of the oral cavity and upper aerodigestive tracts to include the nasopharynx, sinuses and trachea.

The major salivary glands are encapsulated, lobulated structures. The parotid gland lies in front of and below the ear, covering the angle of the mandible. It is the largest of the major salivary glands, weighing approximately 25 grams. Its secretion is primarily serous and drains through Stensen's duct, which leaves the gland along its anterior border and opens into the oral cavity on the buccal surface of the cheek opposite the second upper molar tooth.

The submandibular gland is about the size of a small walnut, weighing approximately 10 grams. It lies below the body of the mandible in the digastric triangle. Its

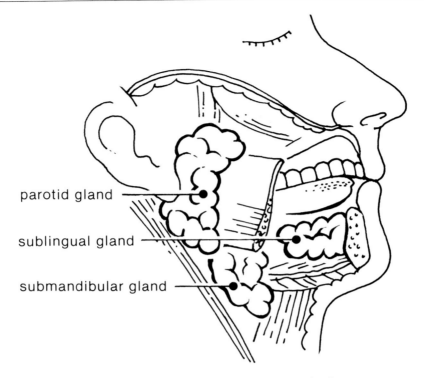

Fig. 2.5. Diagram of the major salivary glands.

secretion is mixed but predominantly serous and drains via Warthin's duct into the oral cavity at the summit of the sublingual caruncle close to the frenulum of the tongue.

The sublingual gland is shaped like an almond and weighs about 3 grams. It lies in the floor of the mouth close to the symphysis adjacent to the midline. It secretes a mixed, primarily mucous secretion through a number of small ducts on its superior surface. These ducts communicate directly with the oral cavity through the overlying mucosa.

The minor salivary glands are located submucosally throughout the upper aerodigestive tract and are nonencapsulated aggregates of serous, mucous or mixed seromucous acini.

HISTOLOGIC FEATURES. Microscopy demonstrates that the salivary glands are compound, tubuloalveolar glands. From the fibrous capsule, thin, fibrous septa extend into the gland, dividing it into lobes and smaller lobules. Fat cells are present in the fibrous septa. Each lobule is made up of ducts and secretory units called alveoli or acini (Fig. 2.6). The parotid acini are lined by pyramid-shaped cells that have round nuclei toward the base. The cytoplasm is finely granular and appears basophilic with hematoxylin and eosin stain. The acini are enclosed in a basal lamina with myoepithelial cells in between the acinar lining cells and the basal lamina. The acini of the submandibular gland are similar. However, because this gland is a mixed gland, there are also mucinous acini with serous crescents (Fig. 2.7). The mucous cells have

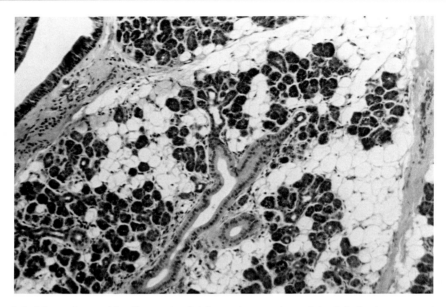

Fig. 2.6. Normal parotid salivary gland. The major portion of the lobule shown consists of acini and intercalated and striated ducts. A portion of a large excretory duct is in the top left-hand corner of the photomicrograph. Hematoxylin and eosin preparation. × 150.

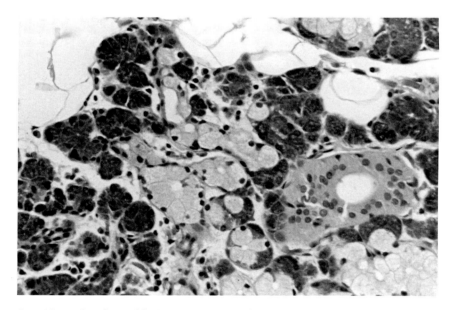

Fig. 2.7. Normal submandibular salivary gland. Mucus and serous acini are visible. Hematoxylin and eosin preparation. × 390.

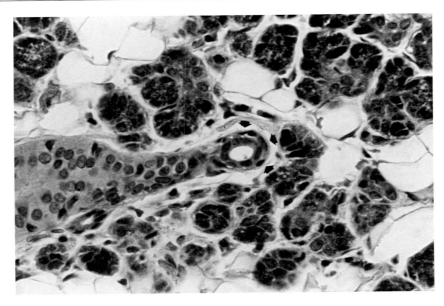

Fig. 2.8. Normal parotid salivary gland. The intercalated duct is in the center. Note the outer layer of flattened, elongated myoepithelial cells (arrows). Hematoxylin and eosin preparation. ×625.

pale vacuolated cytoplasm with round nucleus. The sublingual gland, unlike the other major salivary glands, lacks a definite capsule, although it is divided, like the others, into lobes and lobules by thin septa.

The duct systems of the three major salivary glands are essentially similar. The secretion from the gland passes via the intercalated duct into the striated and excretory ducts. The cells that line the intercalated ducts are cuboidal, whereas those that line the striated ducts are tall and columnar and have basal striations in the cytoplasm. The excretory ducts are lined by stratified, columnar epithelium.

Oncocytic cells are occasionally seen in histologic sections of normal salivary glands. An oncocytic cell is a large epithelial cell that has eosinophilic, finely granular cytoplasm and a round nucleus. Its cell borders are distinct. Oncocytic cells can be seen lining acini and ducts. Another type of cell, the myoepithelial cell, occurs between the basal lamina surrounding the acini and the lining epithelial cells (Fig. 2.8). These cells are flattened and have elongated nuclei, as demonstrated by light and electron microscopy in histologic sections.

CYTOLOGIC FEATURES. Because most salivary gland tumors occur in the major salivary glands, aspirates from the parotid and submandibular glands comprise the majority of specimens. However, abnormal salivary tissue in any area of the upper aerodigestive tract can be aspirated for diagnosis and the technique is particularly helpful in cases of intraoral lesions at any site (see Chapter 7). Aspirates from normal parotid glands consist of intralobular ducts with attached acini (Fig. 2.9). Intact lobules are aspirated and dissociated cells are uncommon. The acini are composed of serous cells that have vacuolated cytoplasm and small, round, uniform,

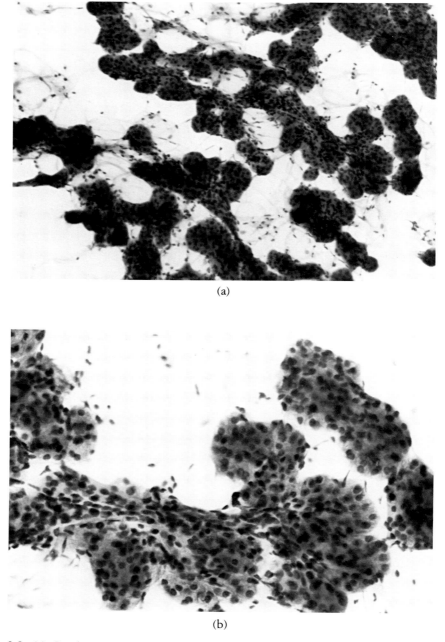

(a)

(b)

Fig. 2.9. (a) Cytology specimen contains intact lobules of normal serous acini and ducts. Fat cells separate small, round masses of acinar tissue. Papanicolaou preparation. ×150. (b) ×390.

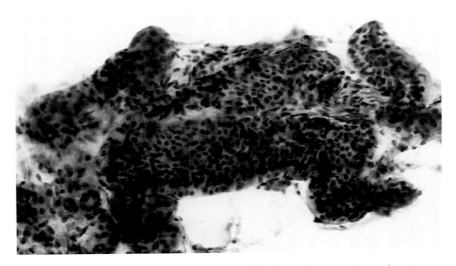

Fig. 2.10. Cytology specimen contains ductal epithelium. Hematoxylin and eosin preparation. ×390.

peripherally located nuclei. Fat cells may be present and easily identifiable. Ductal structures may be aspirated intact, or strips and sheets of ductal epithelium may be seen (Fig. 2.10). The ductal lining cells have scanty cytoplasm and round, uniform nuclei. With Papanicolaou's stain, the acinar cells assume a pale, basophilic color, whereas the ductal cells appear pink to orangeophilic. A honeycomb appearance may be observed when cells are seen "en face" (Fig. 2.11). Aspirates from normal

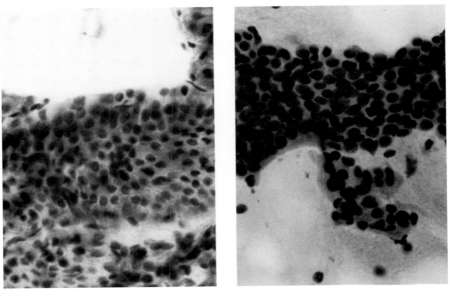

Fig. 2.11. Cytology specimen contains ductal epithelium. Hematoxylin and eosin preparation. ×625.

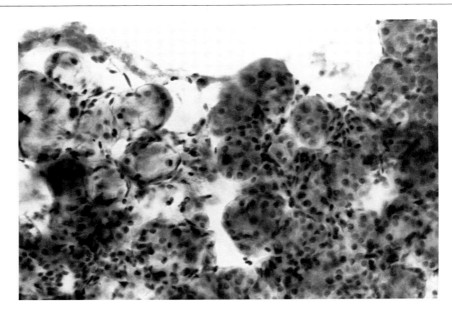

Fig. 2.12. Cytology specimen from a submandibular gland contains a mixture of serous (*right*) and mucinous (*left*) acini. Papanicolaou preparation. × 390.

submandibular glands are similar to those from the parotid gland; however, in addition, mucinous cells lining the acini are frequently observed (Fig. 2.12). Smears obtained from sublingual glands are composed predominantly of mucous-lined acini.

Oncocytes are difficult to find in aspirates from normal glands. It should be noted that similar cells occur in other organs, particularly the thyroid gland, where they are known as Hürthle cells, and they can appear in aspirates from this area. Electron microscopy has shown that oncocytes are rich in mitochondria, which give the cells their distinctive histologic and cytologic appearances. Myoepithelial cells are also difficult to identify cytologically in an aspirate from a normal gland. The myoepithelial cells are thought to play an important part in the histogenesis of pleomorphic adenoma and adenoid cystic carcinoma.

CYSTS

Nonneoplastic salivary gland cysts are relatively rare at any site but are commonest in the parotid gland. They are easily mistaken for tumors because they tend to be confined under the tough parotid capsule. They can be accurately diagnosed by fine-needle aspiration biopsy—sometimes therapeutically, thus in many cases obviating surgical intervention. Most salivary gland cysts are retention cysts or mucoceles. Figure 2.13 shows a minor salivary gland cyst that presented as a mass in the submental triangle.

Retention cysts are true cysts, having an epithelial lining (Fig. 2.14). They may be lined by cuboidal, columnar or mucus-secreting epithelium with or without areas of

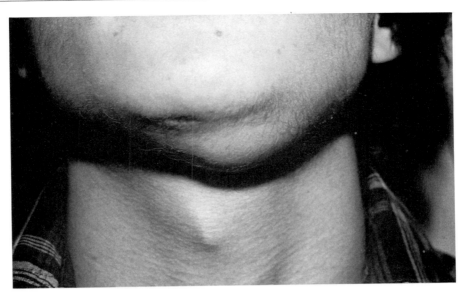

Fig. 2.13. Cyst of a minor salivary gland presenting as a mass in the submental triangle.

squamous metaplasia. They usually result from intermittent rather than complete obstruction of the ducts.[8,9] Mucoceles may evolve from mucous cysts, but they are different from such cysts in that they are devoid of an epithelial lining (Fig. 2.15). They usually occur in the floor of the mouth secondary to obstruction of the minor salivary glands.[8] A variety of other cystic lesions can occur within or adjacent to salivary gland tissue. Branchial cleft cysts (Fig. 2.16) occasionally present as parotid

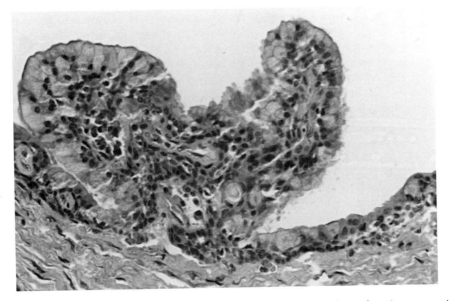

Fig. 2.14. Retention cyst lined by columnar epithelium. Hematoxylin and eosin preparation. ×390.

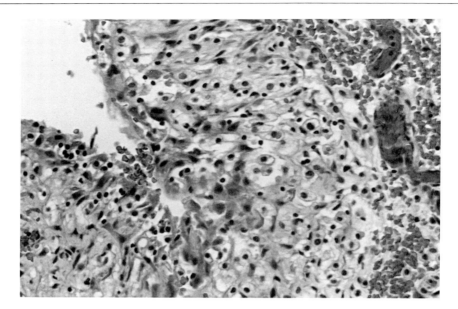

Fig. 2.15. Mucocele lacking a true epithelial lining. The wall consists of foamy histiocytes. Hematoxylin and eosin preparation. ×390.

space lesions[10] and epidermal inclusion cysts can occur adjacent to salivary glands. Branchial cleft cysts are further discussed in Chapter 5.

CYTOLOGIC FEATURES. Aspiration of cystic lesions yields clear or cloudy fluid that may be watery or viscid. Microscopy reveals that aspirates contain only a few histiocytes (Fig. 2.17). When secondary infection occurs, inflammatory cells are seen. In true cysts, a few epithelial lining cells may be visible (Fig. 2.18) and some normal salivary gland elements may also be seen because of aspiration of tissue surrounding the cyst. The cytologic features of cystic lesions are summarized in Table 2.2. After aspiration, cystic salivary gland lesions usually resolve, but they may recur within hours, weeks, months or, occasionally, even years. If a lesion recurs, it should be reaspirated to attempt cure by aspiration and to obtain a further sample for cytologic examination. Reaspiration is necessary because some neoplasms can have a cystic component and it has been our practice to manage all cystic lesions surgically if they recur after a second or third aspiration or if an aspirate has a suspicious cytologic appearance. Similarly, a cystic lesion that does not completely resolve with aspiration should be managed surgically. The various types of cystic tumor that may occur in the salivary glands are summarized in Table 2.3.

INFLAMMATORY LESIONS

Acute or chronic inflammation, either specific or nonspecific, may present as salivary gland enlargement.

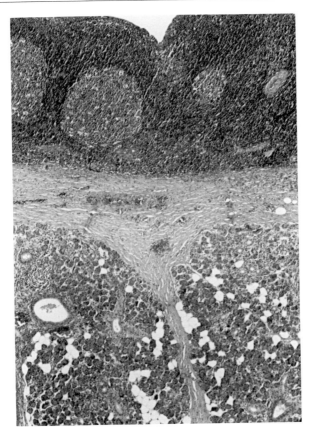

Fig. 2.16. Branchial cleft cyst arising within a parotid gland. Note the abundance of lymphoid tissue, characteristic of the cyst wall. Hematoxylin and eosin preparation. ×50.

Acute Sialadenitis

A variety of viral infections have a predilection for involving the parotid gland rather than other salivary gland tissue. The parotid gland becomes swollen and tender. The infectious agents usually responsible include mumps virus, coxsacki A virus, echovirus and the virus of lymphocytic choriomeningitis. In children, the diagnosis is usually obvious and the likelihood of a neoplasm is so small that needle aspiration is generally not necessary.

Acute bacterial infections occur primarily in the parotid and submandibular salivary glands in association with either obstruction of the duct due to sialolithiasis or trauma to the duct or its orifice or poor oral care in conjunction with dehydration and an altered immune defense system. The parotid gland is most commonly involved and the patient presents with a diffusely swollen gland with purulent discharge from the duct. Occasionally, however, localized areas of inflammation with or without a small abscess can mimic a tumor and in such cases aspiration biopsy can be invaluable. Patients with bacterial sialadenitis usually have a low-grade fever with leukocytosis and, except in cases in which the infection is localized, needle aspira-

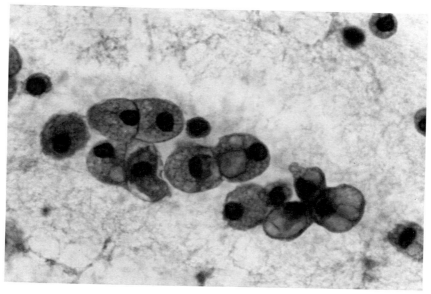

Fig. 2.17. Cytology specimen from an aspirate of a mucocele. Note the foamy histiocytes. No epithelial cells were seen. Papanicolaou preparation. ×625.

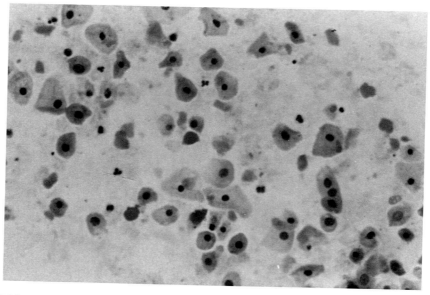

Fig. 2.18. Cytology specimen consists of benign squamous cells from an aspirate of a branchial cleft cyst of a parotid gland. Papanicolaou preparation. ×150.

TABLE 2.2. Nonneoplastic Cysts: Summary of Cytologic Features

Watery or viscid contents
Mucus, histiocytes and inflammatory cells
Benign cuboidal or flattened epithelial cells in true cysts

tion is usually unnecessary. *Streptococcus viridans* and *Staphylococcus aureus* account for most cases and histologic studies show that the gland is infiltrated by acute and chronic inflammatory cells.

CYTOLOGIC FEATURES. Aspirates from glands with acute inflammation consist of large numbers of neutrophils, a few lymphocytes and histiocytes (Fig. 2.19). Epithelial cells are also present and necrotic cellular debris is visible in the background.

Chronic Sialadenitis

Chronic, nonspecific inflammation is usually the result of sialolithiasis or postsurgical scarring and is more common in the submandibular salivary gland than in the parotid gland.[11] Calculi most commonly occur in middle-age patients and are rare in children. The signs and symptoms of chronic sialadenitis are characteristic, with recurring pain and swelling of the gland occurring on eating and gradual resolution of symptoms taking place an hour or so after meals. The diagnosis is usually made on the basis of the clinical features in combination with radiographic findings obtained with a simple occlusal film of the floor of the mouth demonstrating a calculus or with a sialogram. Again, needle aspiration is usually not necessary, although in cases in which a malignant lesion was diagnosed previously, particularly in the anterior floor of the mouth, it is reassuring to get a benign needle aspirate from a persistent swelling in the submandibular triangle. Similarly, needle aspiration of the localized swelling can help exclude a primary neoplasm of the salivary glands. Chronic sialadenitis can occur in the absence of calculi or trauma to the duct and may in these situations be due to decreased salivary gland secretion with stasis and retrograde infection. This type of sialadenitis seems to involve the parotid gland more frequently than other glands.

In chronic sialadenitis, histologic studies demonstrate chronic inflammation with loss of acini and fibrosis. The ductal epithelium may have mucous or squamous metaplasia.

TABLE 2.3. Salivary Gland Neoplasms That May Have a Cystic Component

Pleomorphic adenoma
Warthin's tumor
Low-grade mucoepidermoid carcinoma
Papillary-cystic acinic cell carcinoma*
Papillary-cystic carcinoma*
Metastatic keratinizing squamous cell carcinoma

*Rare.

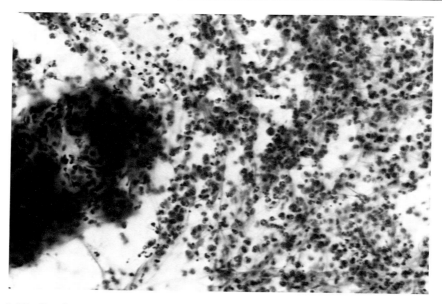

Fig. 2.19. Cytology specimen from a case of acute sialadenitis. Papanicolaou preparation. ×390.

CYTOLOGIC FEATURES. Aspirates from patients with chronic sialadenitis usually contain lymphocytes, macrophages and few neutrophils. Spindle-shaped fibroblasts may also be observed (Fig. 2.20). Due to chronic inflammation and atrophy, acinar elements are usually lacking, although ductal cells are seen. The cytologic features are summarized in Table 2.4.

Atypical changes in ductal cells may be observed and should not be construed as evidence of a malignant process. We have seen a few cases of postradiation atrophy and fibrosis involving the parotid and submandibular glands. Smears from such cases consist of sparse cellular elements with a few groupings of atypical duct cells. Clinically, differentiation between irradiation fibrosis and a recurrent malignant process may at times be difficult and needle aspiration is helpful in excluding a malignant lesion. Caution however is advised because irradiation may result in marked atypical changes in the ductal lining cells and such features should not be regarded as malignant.

Granulomatous Sialadenitis

Tuberculosis, sarcoidosis and other granulomatous processes, such as cat-scratch fever, may involve the lymph nodes in the vicinity of the salivary glands or the salivary glands by direct extension. In tuberculosis, the parotid gland is most commonly involved.[12] The disease may be primary or, more likely, the result of extension from a lesion in the oral cavity. Secondary involvement in generalized tuberculosis also occurs.

Similarly, sarcoidosis may also involve the salivary glands.[7,13-15] Uveoparotid fever (Heerfordt's syndrome) is a form of sarcoidosis in which parotid enlargement,

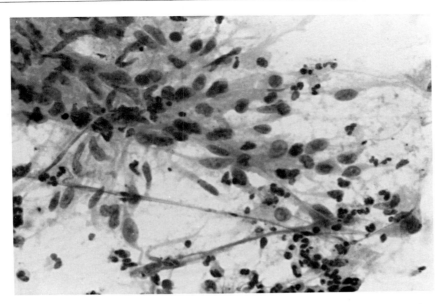

Fig. 2.20. Cytology specimen from a case of chronic sialadenitis contains elongated fibroblasts and inflammatory cells. Papanicolaou preparation. ×625.

uveitis and facial paralysis occur. The disease is bilateral in 50 percent of cases. The glands are not painful, but they are firm and nodular. Occasionally, a localized swelling, simulating a neoplasm, may be the presenting feature and needle aspiration in such a situation provides the correct diagnosis.

HISTOLOGIC FEATURES. Granulomatous disease is characterized by focal aggregates of elongated, epithelioid histiocytes, lymphocytes, plasma cells and few neutrophils and eosinophils (Figs. 2.21 and 2.22). Multinucleated giant cells are also observed. In sarcoidosis, the granulomas have no evidence of necrosis, whereas necrotizing granulomas are seen in tuberculosis, cat-scratch fever and certain fungal infections.

CYTOLOGIC FEATURES. The smears contain a mixture of acute and chronic inflammatory cells along with small aggregates of elongated epithelioid cells and multinucleated giant cells (Fig. 2.23). In tuberculosis and cat-scratch fever, amorphous, granular, necrotic debris may be seen in the background (Fig. 2.24). This material stains pink with hematoxylin and eosin and pale green with Papanicolaou's method. Acid-fast stains can be used to make a definitive diagnosis of tuberculosis if un-

TABLE 2.4. Chronic Sialadenitis: Summary of Cytologic Features

Scanty cellular material
Lymphocytes, macrophages and few neutrophils
Spindle-shaped fibroblasts in some cases
Scanty acinar elements due to atrophy; ductal epithelium

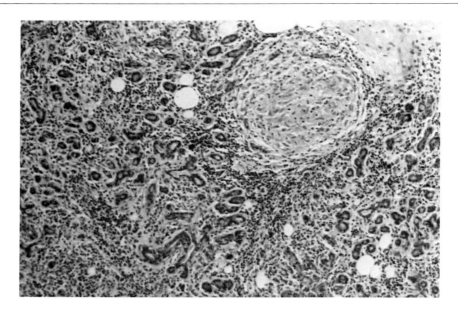

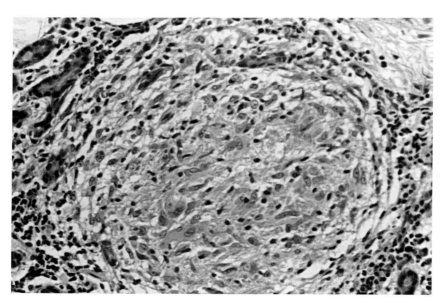

Figs. 2.21 and 2.22. Granulomatous sialadenitis. Nonspecific chronic inflammation coexists with small, well-circumscribed, noncaseating granuloma, consistent with sarcoid. Hematoxylin and eosin preparations. ×150 and ×390.

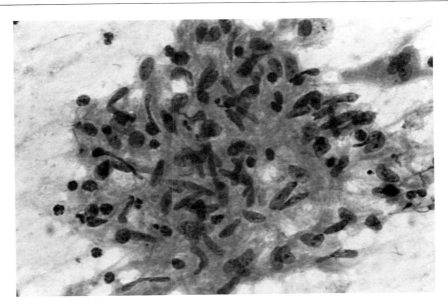

Fig. 2.23. Cytology specimen consists of loose groupings of elongated, histiocytic (epithelioid) cells. No necrosis is evident. Papanicolaou preparation. ×625.

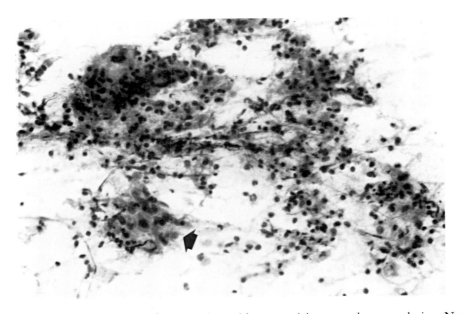

Fig. 2.24. Cytology specimen from a patient with a necrotizing, granulomatous lesion. Note the necrotic debris. The epithelioid (arrow) and giant cells on such background material suggest a diagnosis of tuberculosis or cat-scratch fever. Hematoxylin and eosin preparation. ×390.

TABLE 2.5. Granulomatous Sialadenitis: Summary of Cytologic Features

Mixed inflammatory cells
Loose aggregates of elongated, epithelioid cells
Multinucleated giant cells
In tuberculosis and other necrotizing lesions, amorphous, granular, cellular debris in
  background

stained slides are also prepared. If granulomatous disease is suspected on needle
aspiration or on clinical grounds, reaspiration should be done and material submitted for microbiologic studies. The cytologic features of granulomatous
sialadenitis are summarized in Table 2.5.

Chronic Lymphadenitis or Hyperplasia of Intraparotid Lymph Nodes

Small lymph nodes are normally found in and around the parotid glands. Nodes
within the parotid gland are the result of late encapsulation, which the gland undergoes during fetal life.[3] Lymph nodes are not found within the substance of other
major salivary glands. Enlargement of lymph nodes from any cause cannot be differentiated from a neoplasm of the parotid gland by clinical examination alone. However, needle aspiration biopsy is a reliable method of differentiating between hyperplasia, lymphoma, metastatic carcinoma involving the intraparotid lymph nodes or
primary parotid gland neoplasms.[7]

HISTOLOGIC FEATURES. In reactive follicular hyperplasia, histologic studies demonstrate large follicles with prominent germinal centers (Fig. 2.25). Within the germinal centers, one sees small and large lymphocytes and macrophages that contain
ingested cell debris, the so-called tingible-body macrophages (Fig. 2.26). Mitotic
activity is also increased.

CYTOLOGIC FEATURES. Cytologic examination reveals that the aspirates reflect the
histologic appearance of the lymph node. The smears are generally cellular and
consist of a mixed population of cells. Large follicular-center cells are mixed with
small lymphocytes. Immunoblasts are also seen. The nuclei of the lymphocytes are
cleaved or round and contain one or more nucleoli. Histiocytes with abundant
cytoplasm that contain phagocytosed cellular debris are usually numerous in such
aspirates (Fig. 2.27). The appearance is characteristic of reactive follicular hyperplasia and substantially different from a malignant lymphoma, in which a monotonous cellular pattern is the rule.[16] The cytologic features of lymph node hyperplasia
are summarized in Table 2.6. Lymph node disorders are further discussed in
Chapter 3.

DIFFERENTIAL DIAGNOSIS. Distinction between a lymphoepithelial lesion and reactive hyperplasia may at times be difficult. Aspirates from lesions of salivary glands
that contain lymphocytes are listed in Table 2.7, and differential diagnosis discussed
on page 41.

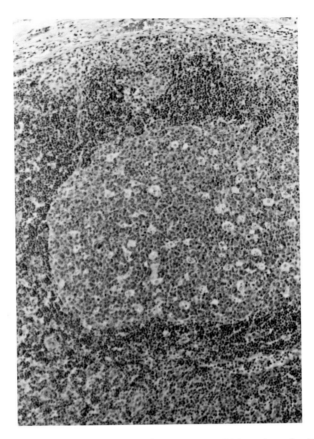

Fig. 2.25. Reactive follicular hyperplasia of an intraparotid lymph node. Hematoxylin and eosin preparation. ×150.

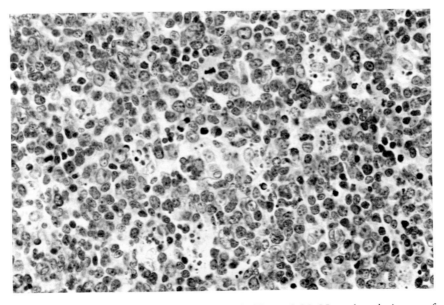

Fig. 2.26. High-power view of the lesion shown in Figure 2.25. Note the admixture of cells with numerous tingible-body macrophages. Hematoxylin and eosin preparation. ×390.

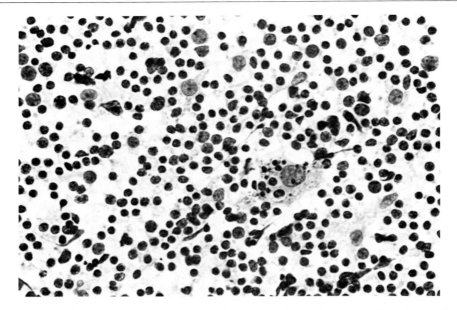

Fig. 2.27. Cytology specimen consists of a mixture of small and large cells. Note the tingible-body macrophages. Papanicolaou preparation. ×625.

AUTOIMMUNE DISORDERS

Benign Lymphoepithelial Lesion and Related Conditions (Mikulicz's Disease and Sjögren's Syndrome)

This term was originally coined by Godwin in 1952 to describe a lesion that involved the salivary and lacrimal glands.[17] The disease may present as unilateral or bilateral successive enlargement of salivary and/or lacrimal glands. Most cases occur in women in the fifth and sixth decades. When there is a single discrete mass, differentiation from a neoplasm may be extremely difficult (Fig. 2.28).

In 1888, Mikulicz described a similar condition in which there was symmetric enlargement of the salivary and lacrimal glands with no apparent underlying cause.[18] Mikulicz's disease and benign lymphoepithelial lesion are terms that are now considered synonymous and Mikulicz's syndrome is the term used to denote enlargement of the salivary and lacrimal glands usually secondary to a systemic disease.[19] The term Sjögren's syndrome is reserved for a disease characterized by keratoconjunc-

TABLE 2.6. Hyperplasia of Intraparotid Lymph Nodes: Summary of Cytologic Features

Cellular aspirate in most cases
Mixed cell population of small and large lymphocytes, immunoblasts, plasma cells and few neutrophils and eosinophils
Histiocytes with ingested cellular debris in cytoplasm

TABLE 2.7. Salivary Gland Aspirates That Contain Lymphocytes

Chronic sialadenitis
Lymphoepithelial lesion
Warthin's tumor
Acinic cell carcinoma (follicular variant)
Malignant lymphoma
Intraparotid lymph nodes
    Hyperplasia
    Malignant lymphoma

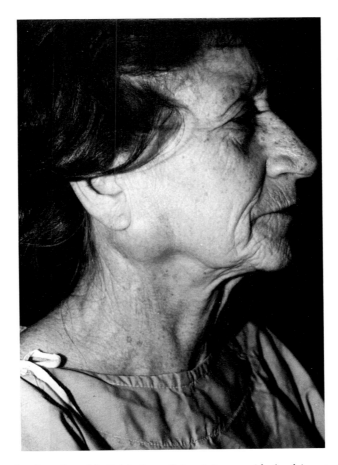

Fig. 2.28. Benign lymphoepithelial lesion of the right parotid gland in a patient with Sjögren's syndrome. Parotidectomy was done to relieve pain and swelling. The subsequent involvement of bilateral submandibular glands was confirmed by needle aspiration.

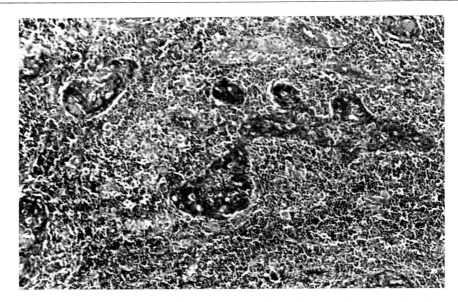

Fig. 2.29. Benign lymphoepithelial lesion. Note the acinar atrophy, a result of severe, chronic inflammation. There is proliferation of the epithelial lining of the ducts. Hematoxylin and eosin preparation. × 150.

tivitis sicca (dry eyes), xerostomia (dry mouth) and a connective tissue disorder, usually rheumatoid arthritis. The histologic and cytologic features of all these lesions are similar. Involvement of the minor salivary glands is an important component of Sjögren's syndrome and the diagnosis can usually be made by biopsy of the lip.[20]

The salivary glands usually are diffusely enlarged and have a fleshy, grayish white appearance. Localized masses tend to have circumscribed borders and a smooth, grayish pink cut surface, resembling lymph nodes.

HISTOLOGIC FEATURES. Histologic examination shows acinar atrophy with infiltration by lymphocytes, plasma cells, neutrophils, eosinophils and histiocytic cells (Fig. 2.29). Lymphoid follicles with reactive germinal centers are usually encountered. In addition, there is proliferation of the epithelial cells that line the ducts, causing obstruction of their lumina (Fig. 2.30). These areas of proliferation usually appear as epithelial islands on a background of a dense, lymphocytic infiltrate.

CYTOLOGIC FEATURES. The aspirates consist of lymphoreticular elements and salivary gland tissue in variable proportions (Figs. 2.31, 2.32 and 2.33). The lymphoid elements consist of a mixed cell population, with small and large lymphocytes. Plasma cells and histiocytes may also be seen. In some cases, small loose groupings of elongated, histiocytic cells are encountered, similar to those commonly seen in granulomatous lesions (Fig. 2.33). The ductal epithelium is sparse or nonexistent and found only by a careful search. Acinar elements are usually lacking. The ductal cells are in the form of monolayer sheets or small, cohesive, ductlike structures (Figs. 2.31 and 2.32) surrounded by lymphoreticular elements, a picture similar to

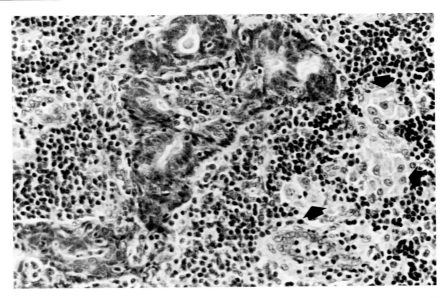

Fig. 2.30. Benign lymphoepithelial lesion. High-power view of the lesion shown in Figure 2.29. Larger histiocytic cells (*arrows*) are visible in this photomicrograph. Hematoxylin and eosin. × 390.

that seen on histologic examination. The cytologic features of such lesions are summarized in Table 2.8.

The development of malignant lymphoma is a well-recognized complication in patients with benign lymphoepithelial lesion and related conditions.[21-23] Undifferentiated carcinoma has also been encountered in the salivary glands of such patients.[24,25]

DIFFERENTIAL DIAGNOSIS. In the differential diagnosis, the lesions listed in Table 2.7 have to be considered. If mixed lymphoreticular elements and ductal epithelial cells are seen in the aspirate, the diagnosis of benign lymphoepithelial lesion is simple. However, if ductal epithelial cells are not found in the smears, differentiation from lymphoma and hyperplasia may be difficult. In malignant lymphoma, a monotonous lymphoid cell population is usually seen, whereas in reactive lymphoid hyperplasia and benign lymphoepithelial lesion the infiltrate is of a mixed type. In nonspecific chronic sialadenitis, the lymphoid elements are not as numerous and the inflammatory infiltrate consists of a mixture of lymphocytes, plasma cells and few neutrophils and eosinophils. Elongated, spindle-shaped cells, probably fibroblasts, are also observed. Scanty salivary gland elements are also seen, but in severe lesions, the acinar elements are difficult to find.

By contrast, the aspirate from Warthin's tumor consists of sheets of polyhedral, oncocytic cells with dense to granular, eosinophilic cytoplasm on a background of cellular debris and lymphoreticular cells. Moreover, because Warthin's tumor tends to be cystic, the aspirate may contain one or more milliliters of turbid fluid, unlike the aspirates from other lesions in the differential diagnosis discussed previously.

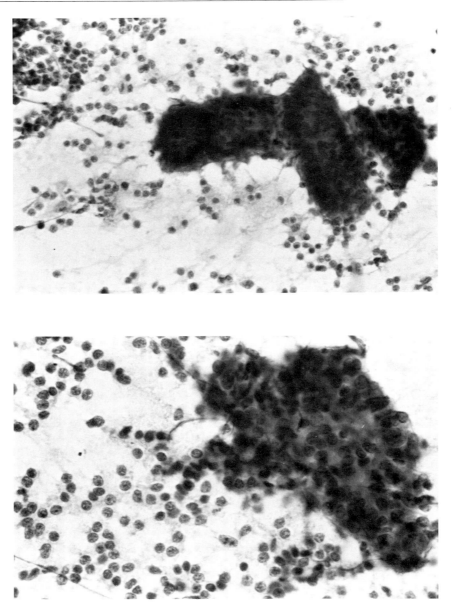

Figs. 2.31 and 2.32. Cytology specimen from a patient with a benign lymphoepithelial lesion contains ductal cells on a background of inflammatory cells. Papanicolaou preparation. × 390 and × 625. (Figure 2.31 from Qizilbash et al: *Acta Cytol* 29:503–512, 1985, with permission.)

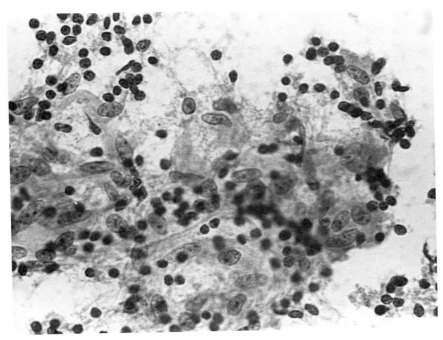

Fig. 2.33. Aspirate from a patient with Sjögren's syndrome contains a loose collection of histiocytes. Papanicolaou preparation. ×625.

BENIGN NEOPLASMS

A diverse group of tumors arise in the salivary glands. Neoplasms of the salivary glands constitute less than 3 percent of all tumors that develop in the head or neck.[26] Data from the literature suggest an incidence of approximately 2 per 100,000 population.[27] Tumors occur more often in the parotid gland than in the submandibular or minor salivary glands. In comparison, neoplasms that arise in the sublingual gland are rare. For every tumor that develops in the sublingual gland, 10 arise in the submandibular gland, 10 in the minor salivary glands and 100 in the parotid gland.[28] For many years, it has been accepted that all tumors arise from the reserve cells of the intercalated and excretory ducts rather than from the acini.[29,30] Current data suggest a common stem-cell origin for acinar or ductal epithelial cells and for myoepithelial cells.

TABLE 2.8. Lymphoepithelial Lesion: Summary of Cytologic Features

Mixed lymphocytic infiltrate with small, loose aggregates of histiocytes
Monolayer sheets and cohesive groupings of ductal epithelium
Acinar elements lacking in most cases

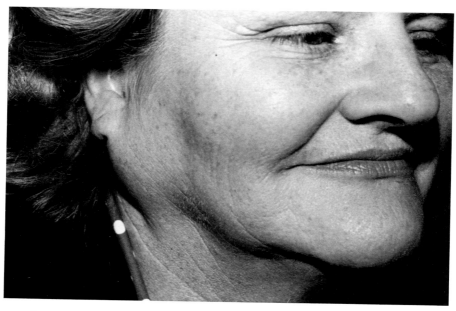

Fig. 2.34. Large, benign tumor of the deep lobe of a parotid gland (pleomorphic adenoma) in a patient with normal facial nerve function.

Pleomorphic Adenoma (benign mixed tumor)

This neoplasm is the most common salivary gland tumor. It comprises about 75 percent of all tumors that occur in the parotid gland.[31] The tumor is more common in women and can occur at any age. Some authors have suggested that ductal epithelial cells are the cells of origin of such tumors,[32,33] other investigators have suggested the myoepithelial cells.[34,35] In addition, some authors have maintained both epithelial cells and myoepithelial cells are responsible for the development of such neoplasms.[36] On the basis of ultrastructural studies, Dardick and colleagues[37] have recently suggested that pleomorphic adenomas are the result of neoplastic transformation of the complete ductal-acinar unit and not the neoplastic product of any particular ductal reserve cell. On the basis of immunohistochemical staining, we have found that myoepithelial cells or their precursor cells play an important role in the development of pleomorphic adenoma. Pleomorphic adenomas are solitary, well-circumscribed, painless, slowly growing tumors (Fig. 2.34). The overlying skin is not involved, but it may be markedly thinned in large lesions (Fig. 2.35). Multiple tumors are rare. Malignant change rarely occurs and is discussed on page 92. Pleomorphic adenomas have a tendency to recur unless adequately excised.

These tumors are poorly encapsulated and have smooth or bosselated external surfaces. Nodularity is observed in recurrent tumors because inadequate resection (lumpectomy) results in seeding of the tumor throughout the surgical site. Most such tumors measure 2 to 6 centimeters in diameter at the time of diagnosis. The cut surface is solid and grayish white and there are semitranslucent, cartilage-like areas. Mucoid areas may be observed and cystic degeneration is not uncommon.

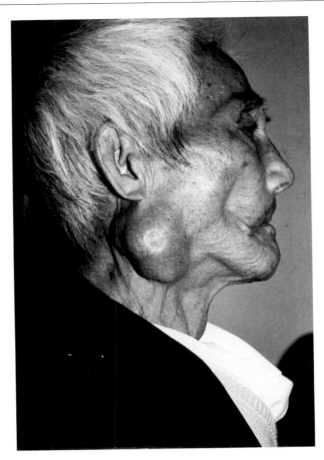

Fig. 2.35. Massive pleomorphic adenoma of the right parotid gland in a patient with thinning of the overlying skin but normal facial nerve function.

HISTOLOGIC FEATURES. Histologic examination demonstrates a varied pattern, consisting of epithelial and myoepithelial cells and a fibrocollagenous stroma that contains foci of myxoid, chondroid and/or bony areas (Fig. 2.36). The epithelial elements consist of flattened or cuboidal inner duct lining cells and outer myoepithelial cells (Fig. 2.37). The myoepithelial cells are usually prominent and appear as dark-staining, single or multiple layers of cells surrounding the ducts. The myoepithelial cells also are polygonal, fusiform or stellate and abut on the fibrocollagenous stroma of the tumor (Fig. 2.38). Hyaline-like, myxoid and cartilaginous areas are frequently seen in such tumors (Fig. 2.39). Trabecular, glandular, papillary, solid and cylindromatous patterns may be observed. Foci of squamous metaplasia, oncocytic change, mucus and sebaceous differentiation may be encountered (Fig. 2.40).

CYTOLOGIC FEATURES. The aspirate from a pleomorphic adenoma usually has a gel-like consistency. In most instances, the smears are appreciably cellular, although scanty material occasionally necessitates reaspiration. The smears are characteristic[38] and consist of a mixture of mesenchymal and epithelial elements (Fig. 2.41). These

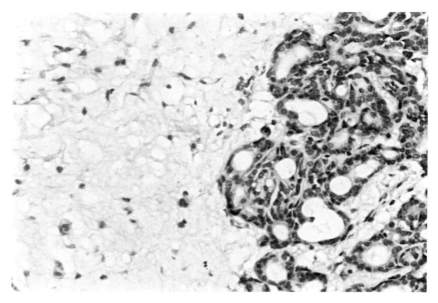

Fig. 2.36. Pleomorphic adenoma consists of a mixture of glandular and myxoid areas. Hematoxylin and eosin preparation. ×390.

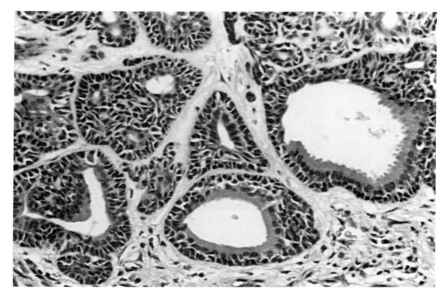

Fig. 2.37. Pleomorphic adenoma contains inner epithelial lining cells and outer myoepithelial cells. Hematoxylin and eosin preparation. ×390.

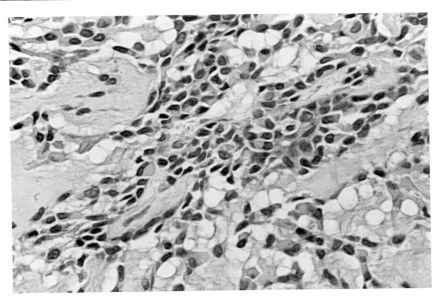

Fig. 2.38. Pleomorphic adenoma contains oval or elongated myoepithelial cells on a fibromyxoid stroma. Hematoxylin and eosin preparation. ×625.

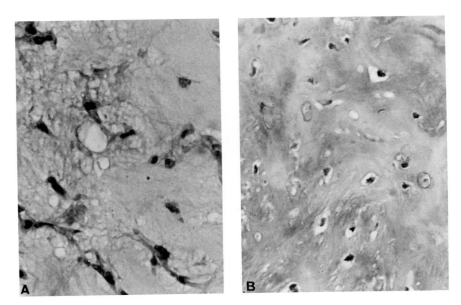

Fig. 2.39. Pleomorphic adenoma contains myxoid (a) and cartilage-like (b) areas. Hematoxylin and eosin preparation. ×390.

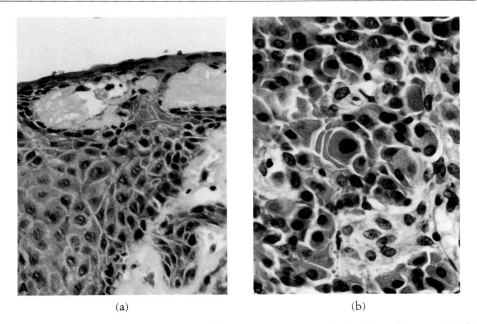

(a)   (b)

Fig. 2.40. Pleomorphic adenoma manifests squamous metaplastic (a) and oncocytic (b) changes. Hematoxylin and eosin preparation. ×390 and ×625.

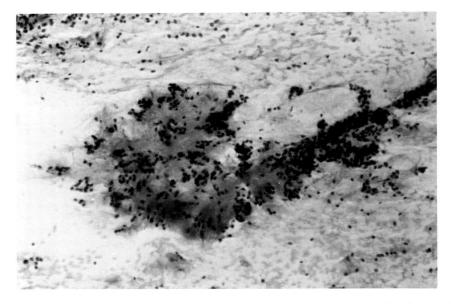

Fig. 2.41. Cytology specimen from a pleomorphic adenoma contains myxoid and epithelial elements. Papanicolaou preparation. ×150.

elements take the form of large fragments or clusters, although small groupings of cells and solitary cells are also seen. The epithelial component consists of small, uniform, cuboidal cells arranged in cohesive sheets, branching, trabecular or ductal formations or solid groupings (Figs. 2.42 and 2.43). The nuclei are round or oval and contain finely distributed chromatin and a small nucleolus (Fig. 2.43). The cytoplasm stains orangish brown with Papanicolaou's method and appears eosinophilic with hematoxylin and eosin stain. The cytoplasmic borders are ill-defined.

The myoepithelial cells appear as discrete, oval or cuboidal cells with abundant cytoplasm and round or oval nuclei (Fig. 2.44). The cytoplasm stains green with Papanicolaou's method and pink with hematoxylin and eosin. It has a dense, hyaline-like quality. The nucleus may be centrally or eccentrically located and has fine chromatin and a tiny nucleolus. Myoepithelial cells are also seen within the stromal elements and appear as oval to fusiform. Cystic change also occurs in pleomorphic adenomas and the aspirate in such instances consists of one or more milliliters of fluid that contains cellular debris and squamous cells, which usually line the cyst (Fig. 2.45). The squamous cells may be a source of misinterpretation, sometimes causing confusion with other squamous-lined cysts that occur in this area. Areas of oncocytic, squamous, sebaceous and mucous differentiation may occur in such tumors and may be reflected in the aspirate (Fig. 2.46). In one case that we studied, small, concentrically laminated bodies (Fig. 2.47), similar to corpora amylacea, were observed among the epithelial cell nests.[7] To our knowledge, this appearance has not been reported by other investigators, although psammoma bodies have been described in an acinic cell tumor.[39] Tyrosine crystals have also been reported in aspirates from pleomorphic adenoma,[40] although none was identified in our cases.

The epithelial elements usually merge gradually with the mesenchymal elements of the tumor. The mesenchymal or stromal elements consist of a loosely arranged, myxoid matrix or ground substance (Plate I.1) in which fine fibers can be seen (Fig. 2.48). The stromal cells, which are believed to be of myoepithelial origin, are in the ground substance. The stromal cells are round, oval or fusiform. Stellate cells with multiple cytoplasmic processes are also seen (Fig. 2.49). The mesenchymal elements are poorly stained by Papanicolaou's method, although in some preparations they stain gray or pale green. With hematoxylin and eosin, the matrix stains pink to purple. The chrondroid areas take up a greater concentration of stain and the stromal cells are enclosed in spaces, as seen in cartilaginous tissue (Fig. 2.50). The cytologic features of pleomorphic adenoma are summarized in Table 2.9.

A hyaline-cell variant of pleomorphic adenoma has recently been reported.[41] The cytoplasm of such cells has a glassy, hyaline quality. Electron microscopy reveals masses of intermediate filaments, which stain strongly for prekeratins with the immunoperoxidase method. Such lesions are best regarded as myoepitheliomas.

DIFFERENTIAL DIAGNOSIS. The cytologic diagnosis of pleomorphic adenoma is usually not difficult when needle aspiration biopsy is used.[3,7] Occasionally, a cellular, predominantly epithelial tumor may be mistaken for a monomorphic adenoma. Distinction between these two neoplasms, however, is not critical because their management is identical. Pleomorphism of epithelial cells sometimes poses a problem. Atypia of a few epithelial cells in a smear from an otherwise benign pleomorphic adenoma should not be regarded as evidence of a malignant process. Eneroth and Zajicek,[38] in a study of 316 pleomorphic adenomas, found 17 cases in

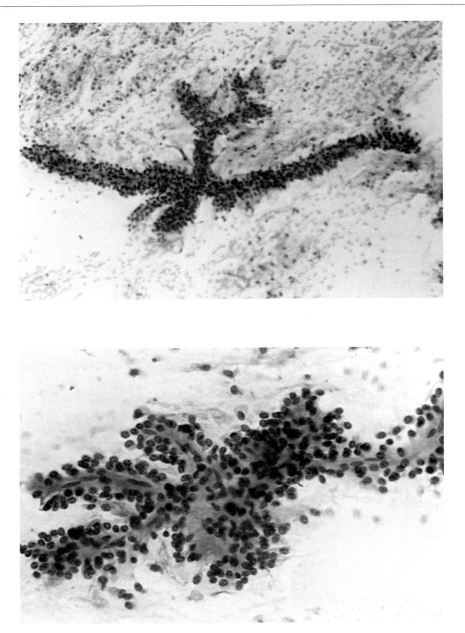

Figs. 2.42 and 2.43. Cytology specimen contains an epithelial component in the form of branching trabeculae of cells. Papanicolaou preparation. × 150 and × 390. (Figure 2.42 from Qizilbash et al: *Acta Cytol* 29:503–512, 1985, with permission.)

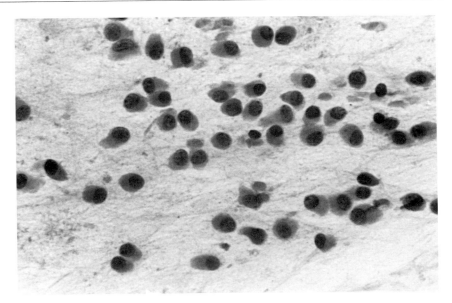

Fig. 2.44. Cytology specimen consists of oval cells that have dense cytoplasm and eccentric nuclei. These oval cells are myoepithelial cells. Papanicolaou preparation. ×625.

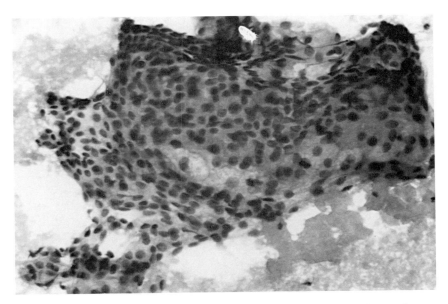

Fig. 2.45. Aspirate from pleomorphic adenoma with cystic degeneration and squamous metaplasia. Note sheets of benign squamous cells (same case as shown in Figure 2.40a). Papanicolaou preparation. ×390.

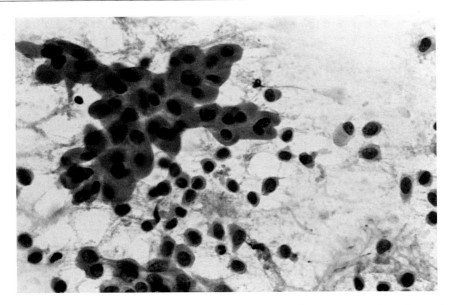

Fig. 2.46. Oncocytic cells in an aspirate of a pleomorphic adenoma. Note the polygonal cell outline with dense cytoplasm (same case as shown in Figure 2.40b). Papanicolaou preparation. ×625.

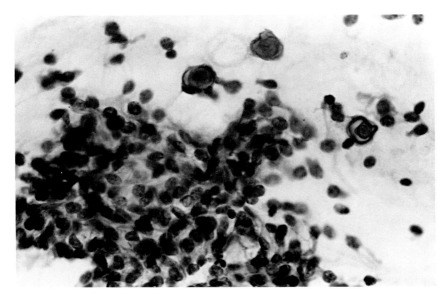

Fig. 2.47. Concentric, laminated bodies, similar to corpora amylacea, in an aspirate of a pleomorphic adenoma. Papanicolaou preparation. ×625.

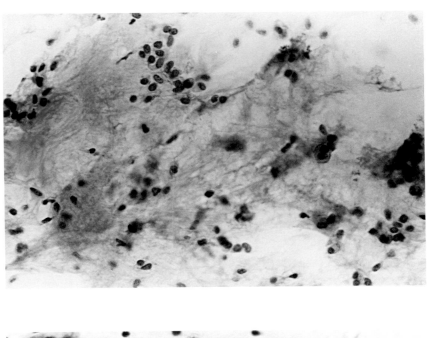

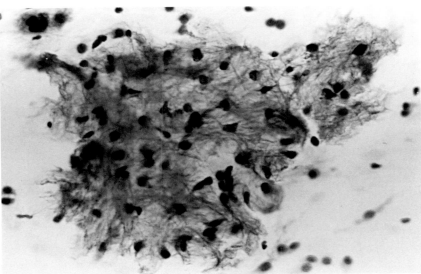

Figs. 2.48 and 2.49. Myxoid mesenchymal elements coexist with oval or stellate stromal cells of myoepithelial origin. Papanicolaou preparation. ×625.

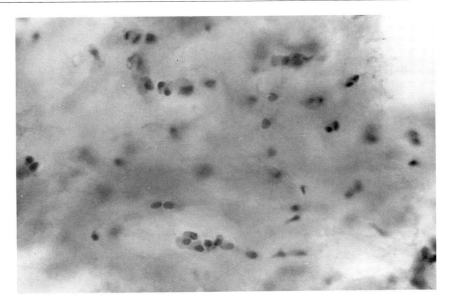

Fig. 2.50. Cytology specimen from a case of pleomorphic adenoma contains a cartilage-like area. Papanicolaou preparation. ×625.

which a cytologic diagnosis of malignancy was suspected on the basis of cellular atypia and polymorphous, carcinoma-like cells. On histologic study, these tumors were found to be benign. Because of the likelihood of overdiagnosis, these authors advise caution in the diagnosis of malignant mixed tumors on the basis of slight or moderate cellular atypia. On the other hand, when the smears contain numerous tumor cells that have cytologic features of malignant transformation, a diagnosis of cancer in a case of pleomorphic adenoma is justified; an infiltrative, destructive growth is usually documented on histologic examination in such cases.[38]

Monomorphic Adenoma

This benign neoplasm is composed of uniform-appearing epithelial cells and is devoid of the chondromyxoid stroma seen in pleomorphic adenomas. The World Health Organization[42] has classified monomorphic adenomas into three groups: papillary cystadenoma lymphomatosum (Warthin's tumor), oxyphilic adenoma (on-cocytoma) and other types, namely, basal cell adenoma, clear-cell adenoma, seba-ceous lymphadenoma and sebaceous adenoma.

TABLE 2.9. Pleomorphic Adenoma: Summary of Cytologic Features

Aspirates having a gel-like consistency
Cellular smears consisting of a mixture of mesenchymal and epithelial elements
Mesenchymal stroma, loosely arranged, myxoid to cartilagenous
Epithelial component, uniform cuboidal cells in branching, trabecular or solid forms

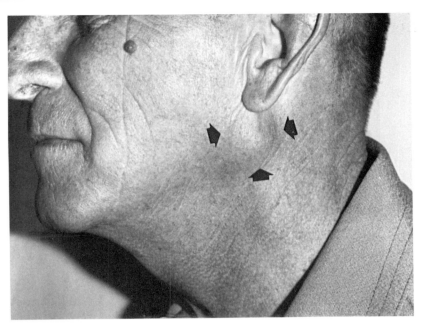

Fig. 2.51. Tumor of the left parotid gland (arrows) in a patient with a painless lump, the usual presentation. Facial nerve function was normal. The diagnosis on needle aspiration biopsy was Warthin's tumor.

Warthin's Tumor (papillary cystadenoma lymphomatosum)

This neoplasm is a variant of monomorphic adenoma in which the epithelial elements are regarded as neoplastic. A recent report suggested that the lymphoid elements within such tumors are a secondary immunologic response.[43] The mesenchymal areas so characteristic of pleomorphic adenomas are not seen in such tumors. Warthin's tumor almost always arises in the parotid gland on its inferior surface and comprises approximately 5 to 10 percent of all parotid tumors.[44] Rare cases have been reported in the minor salivary glands.[45] In approximately 5 to 10 percent of cases, the tumor is bilateral.[46] Multifocal involvement within a single parotid gland is not uncommon. This neoplasm is more common in men than in women and the average age at the time of diagnosis is 60 years (Fig. 2.51). Warthin's tumor is thought to arise from salivary gland inclusions within lymph nodes. Such inclusions are common in intraparotid or periparotid lymph nodes (Fig. 2.52), an observation that explains the almost exclusive localization of such tumors within or adjacent to parotid glands. Most patients with Warthin's tumor present with a painless mass in the parotid gland, commonly in the lower pole. The tumors are soft, often described as "doughy" or even cystic in consistency, and may fluctuate in size. They measure 1 to 10 centimeters in diameter. It is not unusual to confuse such lesions with enlarged lymph nodes.

Warthin's tumor presents as a soft, encapsulated mass with a smooth surface. Most

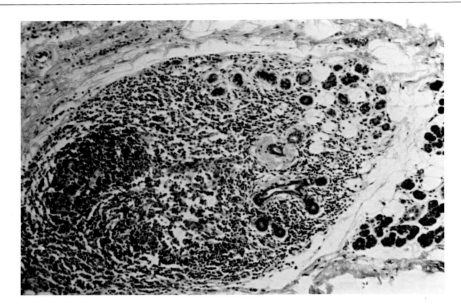

Fig. 2.52. Intraparotid lymph node contains salivary gland inclusions. Hematoxylin and eosin preparation. ×150.

such tumors are cystic, containing gray or brown, serous or mucoid, cloudy fluid. Solid portions of the tumor are gray to tan, resembling lymphoid tissue.

HISTOLOGIC FEATURES. The microscopic appearance is striking, with papillary processes lined by double-layered, oncocytic epithelium and supported by lymphoid stroma that contains follicles that have large reaction or germinal centers (Fig. 2.53). The inner lining cells are tall and columnar and contain oval nuclei arranged along their luminal ends. The cells of the outer, or basal, layer are cuboidal. The cytoplasm of both cell layers is eosinophilic and granular (Fig. 2.54). The granularity results from the large numbers of mitochondria in the cytoplasm of these so-called oncocytic cells. The contents of the cysts appear eosinophilic and stain with periodic acid-Schiff. Concentric, laminated bodies similar to corpora amylacea are occasionally found in the lumina of the cysts.[47]

CYTOLOGIC FEATURES. Aspiration of a Warthin's tumor usually yields a few drops of grayish, semisolid material or a few milliliters of turbid fluid. The background of the smear consists of amorphous and cellular debris mixed with lymphocytes and groupings of oxyphilic cells or oncocytes (Fig. 2.55). Macrophages and neutrophils may also be encountered. The lymphocytes are usually small and mature, although large cells normally seen in follicular centers may also be found. The epithelial cells occur in groupings and cohesive sheets (Fig. 2.56). Solitary cells also are observed. The cells are polyhedral and have an abundance of opaque to granular cytoplasm. The cytoplasmic cells borders are distinct. With hematoxylin and eosin stain, the cytoplasm appears eosinophilic, whereas with Papanicolaou's method, the cytoplasm stains green or brown. The nuclei are round or oval and usually only one is ob-

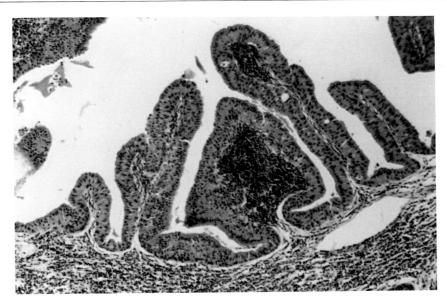

Fig. 2.53. Warthin's tumor. Note the double layer of oncocytic cells lining the papillary processes. Lymphoid tissue is an integral part of this tumor. Hematoxylin and eosin preparation. × 150.

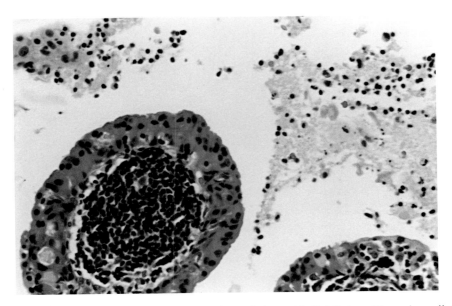

Fig. 2.54. Warthin's tumor. High-power view of the epithelial lining. Note the cellular debris in the lumen of the cystic portion of the tumor. Hematoxylin and eosin preparation. × 390.

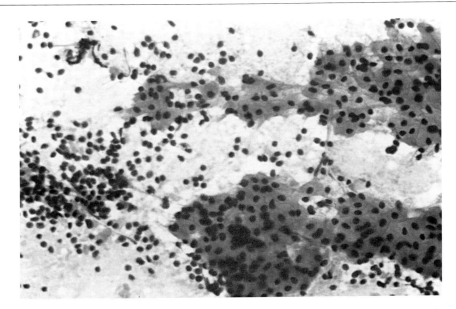

Fig. 2.55. Cytology specimen from a Warthin's tumor. Note the sheets of large, polygonal oncocytic cells coexisting with lymphoid cells. Papanicolaou preparation. ×390.

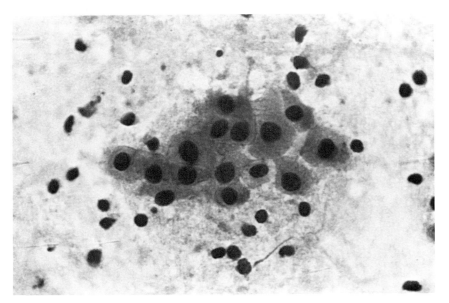

Fig. 2.56. A small grouping of oncocytic cells. Note the lymphocytes in the background. Papanicolaou preparation. ×625.

TABLE 2.10. Warthin's Tumor: Summary of Cytologic Features

Aspirates consisting of a few drops of mucoid material or a few milliliters of turbid
    fluid
Background containing amorphous, cellular debris
Mixture of lymphocytes and epithelial cells
Oncocytic cells in sheets and cohesive aggregates with dense, finely granular cytoplasm

served. The chromatin is finely granular and most nuclei possess a small nucleolus.
Occasionally, large papillary tissue fragments may be seen lying on edge in the
smear. In such instances, both cell layers seen on histologic examination can be
observed. Generally, one sees only sheets of large, oncocytic cells. Nuclear atypia is
not uncommon in oncocytes and cells with prominent nucleoli may be seen in the
aspirate. Care, therefore, should be exercised in not regarding these changes as
malignant. Occasionally, mucous and squamous cells may be seen in aspirates from
such tumors.

Mast cells may be encountered in smears from Warthin's tumor. In a recent study,
smears from 16 of 20 cases (80 percent) of Warthin's tumor contained mast cells.[48]
These cells were found in association with monolayer sheets of oncocytic cells. The
mast cells were identified with May-Grünwald-Giemsa stain and are not seen with
hematoxylin and eosin or Papanicolaou stain. The finding of mast cells should not be
regarded as diagnostic of Warthin's tumor because such cells also occur in 10 percent of mucoepidermoid tumors and in 5 percent of pleomorphic adenomas.[48] The
cytologic features of Warthin's tumor are summarized in Table 2.10.

A lesion similar to Warthin's tumor but without the lymphoid component is called
oncocytic papillary cystadenoma.[49]

DIFFERENTIAL DIAGNOSIS. Oncocytoma can be ruled out if lymphocytic cells are
observed. Moreover, in oncocytoma, the smears are highly cellular and rich in
groupings and sheets of oncocytic cells.

Differentiation from acinic cell neoplasms should generally pose no problem.
However, a rare acinic cell tumor with a heavy lymphocytic component may create a
diagnostic problem.[50] In such a case, epithelial cells and lymphocytes are found in
the smears and the correct diagnosis depends on the accurate identification of
epithelial cellular elements. In acinic cell neoplasms, the tumor cells tend to occur in
clusters and acini. The cytoplasm is more granular and foamy than that seen in
oncocytic tumors. Moreover, the smears lack the amorphous, cellular debris so
characteristic of Warthin's tumor.

Well-differentiated mucoepidermoid carcinoma may be cystic, but the aspirate
usually consists of goblet-like, mucus-containing cells and intermediate and squamous cells; in addition, mucous and inflammatory cells are usually observed in the
background. However, because squamous and mucous metaplasia may occur in
Warthin's tumor, the aspirate from such a lesion may contain squamous and glandular cells and the lesion may be mistaken for mucoepidermoid tumor. Nonetheless,
in addition to foci of squamous and glandular cells, such smears contain sheets of
characteristic oncocytic cells on a background of cellular debris and lymphocytes.
The latter appearance is a clue to the diagnosis of Warthin's tumor. The finding of

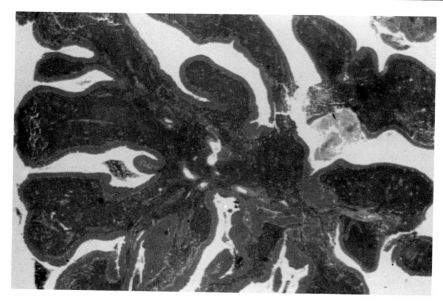

Fig. 2.57. Malignant lymphoma arising in a Warthin's tumor. Note the diffuse proliferation of lymphocytes in the papillary process of the lesion. Hematoxylin and eosin preparation. × 50.

atypical squamous cells may also lead to a false-positive diagnosis of squamous carcinoma.[8]

Branchial cleft cysts may occur in parotid glands and in the immediate vicinity. Smears from such lesions usually consist of benign squamous cells and lymphocytes in various proportions. Neutrophils and histiocytes may be seen if the cysts have become infected. However, oncocytes are not encountered. For further discussion, see Chapter 5.

Differentiation from benign lymphoepithelial lesion relies on the observation of oncocytic cells in Warthin's tumor and of cohesive clusters of ductal cells on a background of abundant mixed inflammatory cells in benign lymphoepithelial lesion. The development of malignant lymphoma in Warthin's tumor is a rare occurrence. Figures 2.57 and 2.58 are from a patient with Warthin's tumor and malignant lymphoma, small-cell type. The diagnosis of lymphoma in such a situation is difficult and depends on the identification of small or large, monomorphic lymphocytes in the smears.

Oncocytoma (oxyphilic adenoma)

Oncocytoma is a monomorphic adenoma composed of large, polyhedral cells that have granular, eosinophilic cytoplasm. These polyhedral cells are oxyphilic cells, or oncocytes. Such cells are rarely seen in the salivary glands of young persons, although they increase in number with age.[51] Oncocytes occur in the acini and ducts of normal salivary glands. The eosinophilic appearance of the cytoplasm is the result of mitochondrial hyperplasia.

Oncocytomas are rare tumors, comprising less than 1 percent of all salivary gland

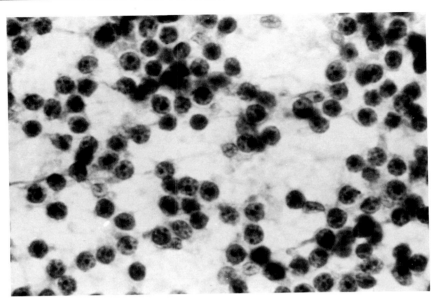

Fig. 2.58. Cytology specimen of the lesion shown in Figure 2.57. Note the monomorphic population of small lymphocytes. Small nucleoli are visible. Papanicolaou preparation. × 625.

neoplasms. They occur most commonly in the parotid gland, although they have been reported in the submandibular[52] and minor salivary glands.[53] Such tumors are slightly more common in women than in men and may be bilateral.[54] The average age at the time of diagnosis is 60 years. Although most oncocytomas are benign, a malignant variant has been described.[55] Patients usually present with a slow-growing, asymptomatic mass in the parotid gland and clinical differentiation from other benign tumors can be difficult. Such tumors are solid, firm and encapsulated and have a smooth, cream-colored to tan cut surface.

HISTOLOGIC FEATURES. The tumors are composed of cells which are uniform in appearance and polyhedral in shape (Fig. 2.59). The cytoplasm is finely granular and eosinophilic. The nucleus is centrally located and vesicular and contains a prominent nucleolus. The cells are arranged in columns or solid sheets with little supporting stroma of connective tissue. Acinar structures with central lumina may be seen in some such tumors. Unlike Warthin's tumor, oncocytomas have scanty supporting stroma and usually lack the lymphoid aggregates and germinal centers that are characteristically seen in Warthin's tumor. Lymphocytic infiltrates are occasionally seen in oncocytomas.

CYTOLOGIC FEATURES. The aspirate from an oncocytoma is cellular, consisting of numerous groupings of polygonal tumor cells that have an abundance of finely granular to dense-appearing, eosinophilic cytoplasm[56] (Fig. 2.60). The nuclei are eccentrically or centrally located and round and contain a prominent nucleolus. Occasional binucleated forms are observed (Fig. 2.61). Variation in nuclear size is not infrequently seen and care has to be exercised in not overdiagnosing such atypical features as malignant (Fig. 2.62). The background is usually clean, lacking

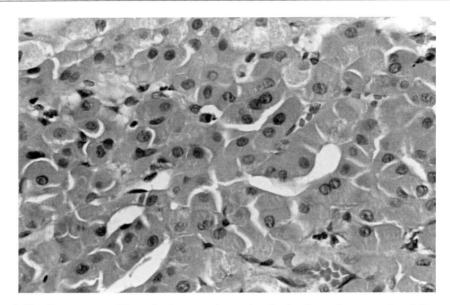

Fig. 2.59. Oncocytoma. Note the large, polygonal cells that have dense, eosinophilic cytoplasm. Hematoxylin and eosin preparation. ×625.

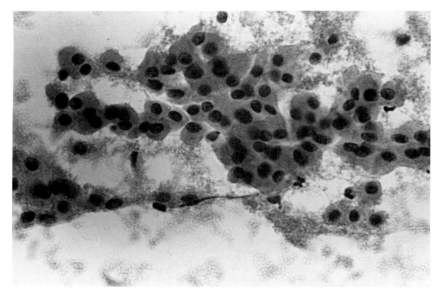

Fig. 2.60. Cytology specimen of the tumor shown in Figure 2.59. Note the similarity between the cells seen on cytologic study and those seen in paraffin sections. Hematoxylin and eosin preparation. ×625.

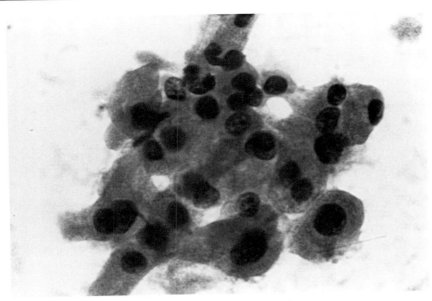

Fig. 2.61. Oncocytes that have nuclear atypia. Note the prominent nucleoli in some cells. A few binucleate forms are visible. Hematoxylin and eosin preparation. ×1000.

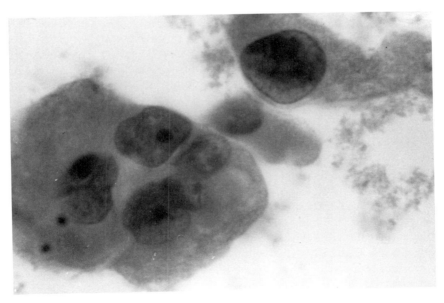

Fig. 2.62. Oncocytic cells from a patient with benign oncocytoma have nuclear changes that mimic those of a malignant process. Hematoxylin and eosin preparation. ×1500.

TABLE 2.11. Oxyphilic Adenoma: Summary of Cytologic Features

Cellular smears consisting of numerous groupings of large, polygonal cells with an abundance of finely granular to dense cytoplasm
Round or oval, centrally or eccentrically located nuclei containing prominent round nucleoli
Background clear, lacking the lymphocytes and debris of Warthin's tumor

the amorphous, cellular debris that is usually seen in Warthin's tumor.[56] The cytologic features of oncocytoma are summarized in Table 2.11.

DIFFERENTIAL DIAGNOSIS. The two lesions with which oncocytoma may be confused on cytologic examination are Warthin's tumor and acinic cell carcinoma.

Distinction between oncocytoma and Warthin's tumor usually is not difficult. First, the aspirate from Warthin's tumor consists of a few drops to a few milliliters of turbid fluid, unlike the aspirate from an oncocytoma, which consists of only a drop of semisolid material. Second, the background of such a smear is "dirty," consisting of amorphous, cellular debris, which is not seen in oncocytoma because it is a solid lesion. Third, the lymphocytic component that is characteristic of Warthin's tumor is lacking in oncocytoma. Finally, smears from an oncocytoma are rich in groupings and sheets of oncocytic cells, unlike smears from Warthin's tumor, which contain relatively few tumor cells.

Oncocytoma may on occasion be confused with acinic cell tumors. The cytoplasm of oncocytomas tends to be more dense than that of acinic cell neoplasms and may have a hyaline-like quality on hematoxylin and eosin stain. By contrast, the cytoplasm of acinic cell tumors is granular to foamy. Periodic acid-Schiff-positive, diastase-resistant granules can be identified in the cytoplasm of acinic cell tumors. In addition, smears from acinic cell tumors contain large numbers of bare nuclei in the background.

Basal Cell Adenoma

Basal cell adenoma of the salivary glands is an uncommon tumor, comprising less than 2 percent of all salivary gland neoplasms in most series.[57-59] This tumor was originally described by Kleinsasser and Klein[59] in 1967 in the European literature and by Batsakis[60] in 1972 in the North American literature. The mean age of patients is 60 years and the tumor has no predilection for either sex. Basal cell adenoma should not be confused with adenoid cystic carcinoma, which it closely resembles, because its biologic behavior differs. Adenoid cystic carcinoma is a slow-growing, relentless, malignant neoplasm and is often fatal, causing death within 15 years of diagnosis in 43 percent of cases.[61] By contrast, basal cell adenoma is a benign neoplasm that can be cured by simple surgical excision. However, rare malignant variants have been described. Such tumors usually present as a slowly enlarging, asymptomatic mass that involves the major salivary glands, commonly the parotid gland. They have also been reported in the minor salivary glands.[62]

Tumors that arise in the major salivary glands are solid, well-circumscribed lesions that have a grayish to pink cut surface. Some such tumors are encapsulated. Their size varies, although most such lesions measure 2 to 3 centimeters in diameter at the time of diagnosis.

HISTOLOGIC FEATURES. A number of different microscopic patterns have been described.[63] In the solid pattern, compact masses of uniform, basophilic cells are observed and the cells tend to palisade at the borders (Figs. 2.63 and 2.64). A few microcystic areas may be observed and there may be basosquamous whorling[64] (Fig. 2.63). The nuclei are round or oval and usually uniform. Mitoses are uncommon. The stroma is scanty and consists of loose connective tissue. Focal hyalinization may be seen, but the chondromyxoid stroma that is encountered in pleomorphic adenoma is lacking. In rare cases, extracellular hyaline material surrounds compact masses of basaloid cells and blood vessels. Because of its striking resemblance to skin appendage tumors, this variant has also been referred to as "dermal analogue tumor."[65,66]

In the canalicular, or tubular, type, anastomosing cords of cuboidal basaloid cells are seen enclosing microcystic spaces (Fig. 2.65), sometimes traversed by thin, mucoid strands and containing thin-walled capillaries and venules.[63] The cells contain round or oval, uniform nuclei. In the trabecular variant, the basaloid cells assume a ribbon-like configuration.

CYTOLOGIC FEATURES. The cytologic appearance of basal cell adenoma reflects the histologic architecture.[64] The smears are composed of small, uniform cells that have scanty, pale, basophilic cytoplasm and round or oval nuclei that contain finely granular chromatin (Fig. 2.66). The nuclei contain small chromocenters, although nucleoli are rarely seen. Aspirates from the basaloid variant of this tumor contain cells arranged in solid masses and irregular branching cords (Fig. 2.67). In addition, solitary cells are fairly numerous. An amorphous, eosinophilic, stromal substance may be adjacent to cell clusters (Fig. 2.66). However, the stromal material is never abundant and one has to search for them. The basisquamous whorling seen on histologic examination may also be demonstrated by cytologic studies (Fig. 2.68).

The canalicular variant is characterized by tight clusters of cells, with little stromal material surrounding empty microcystic spaces (Fig. 2.69). These spaces correspond to those observed on histologic examination and contain thin-walled capillaries and venules. The cytologic features of basal cell adenoma are summarized in Table 2.12.

DIFFERENTIAL DIAGNOSIS. One lesion with which basal cell adenoma is likely to be confused is adenoid cystic carcinoma. Cytologic examination demonstrates that both lesions are composed of similar basaloid cells; differences in the cellular pattern and the stromal substance are the only features that permit recognition of the tumor type.[64,67] Most adenoid cystic carcinomas that have been examined cytologically have globules or cylinders of hyaline material, making identification easy. However, when this feature is absent, as in the uncommon poorly differentiated solid variant of adenoid cystic carcinoma, differentiation from basal cell adenoma may be difficult. In poorly differentiated adenoid cystic carcinoma, the nuclei are generally large and contain coarse chromatin and prominent nucleoli, unlike the bland nuclei seen in basaloid adenomas. For further discussion, see pages 71–72, and 75.

Differentiation from pleomorphic adenoma should not be difficult because basal cell adenoma lacks the loose, chondromyxoid, mesenchymal elements encountered

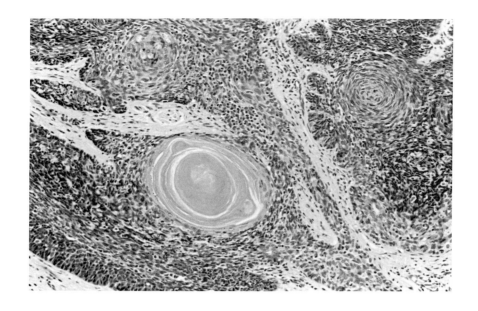

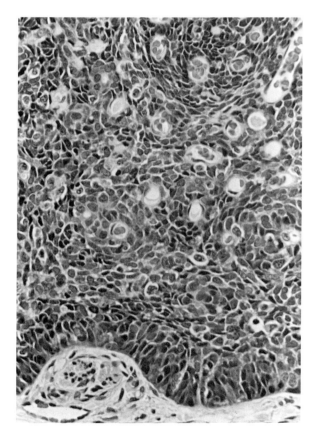

Figs. 2.63 and 2.64. Basal cell adenoma. Note the basosquamous whorling and the tendency of the cells to palisade at the borders. Hematoxylin and eosin preparations. ×150 and ×390. (From Hood et al: *Acta Cytol* 27:515–520, 1983, with permission.)

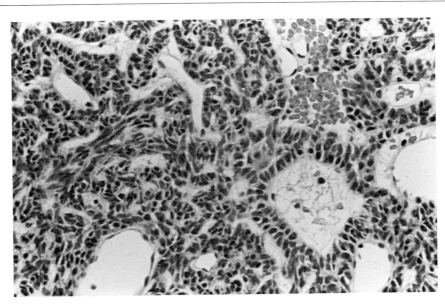

Fig. 2.65. Basal cell adenoma, canalicular type. Note the anastomosing cords of cuboidal, basaloid cells. Hematoxylin and eosin preparation. ×390. (From Hood et al: *Acta Cytol* 27:515–520, 1983, with permission.)

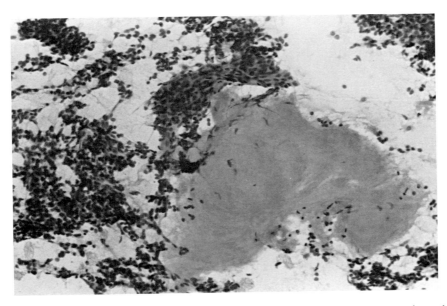

Fig. 2.66. Cytology specimen from a case of basal cell adenoma. Note the small, basophilic cells in sheets and clusters. Solitary cells are also visible. Dense, eosinophilic material is adjacent to the tumor cells. Hematoxylin and eosin preparation. ×390. (From Hood et al: *Acta Cytol* 27:515–520, 1983, with permission.)

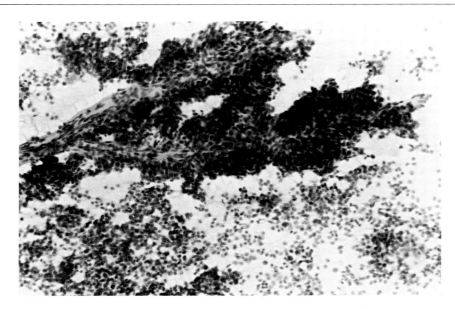

Fig. 2.67. Branching cords of basaloid tumor cells. Hematoxylin and eosin preparation. × 390. (From Qizilbash et al: *Acta Cytol* 29:503–512, 1985, with permission.)

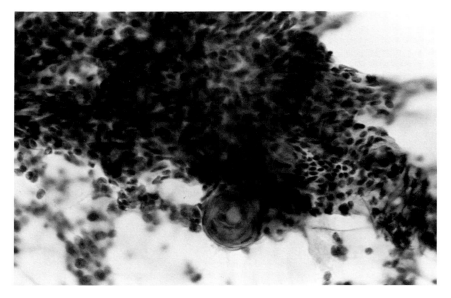

Fig. 2.68. High-power view of the tumor cells shown in Figure 2.67 reveals basosquamous whorling. Compare this appearance with that seen in Figure 2.63. Hematoxylin and eosin preparation. × 625. (From Hood et al: *Acta Cytol* 27:515–520, 1983, with permission.)

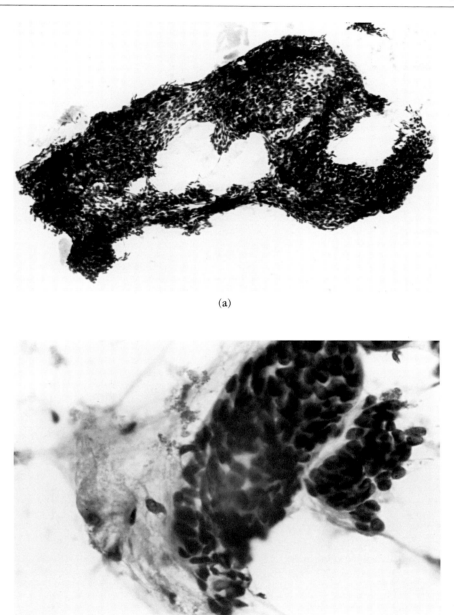

(a)

(b)

Fig. 2.69 (a and b). Two views of the canalicular variant of basal cell adenoma. Tight clusters of basaloid cells are seen. Empty spaces in (a), correspond to the stroma that contains vascular channels, as seen on histologic examination (a). Hematoxylin and eosin preparation. ×390. (b) ×625. (From Hood et al: *Acta Cytol* 27:515–520, 1983, with permission.)

TABLE 2.12. Basal Cell Adenoma: Summary of Cytologic Features

Aspirates in most cases cellular, consisting of small, uniform, basaloid cells in solid
masses or irregular branching cords; solitary cells in the background
Canalicular variant, arranged in tight clusters of cells surrounding empty microcystic
spaces
Round or oval, uniform nuclei lacking nucleoli
Loose, chondromyxoid stroma, similar to pleomorphic adenoma, not present

in pleomorphic adenoma. However, a predominantly cellular, pleomorphic adenoma is sometimes encountered and may be mistaken for basal cell adenoma. Distinction between these lesions is not clinically important because their management is similar.

Undifferentiated carcinomas occasionally are difficult to diagnose on cytologic examination. However, the cells of such tumors occur in small groupings and as solitary cells. Variation in nuclear size and shape is observed and the nuclear molding and nucleoli favor a diagnosis of undifferentiated carcinoma.

Clear-Cell Adenoma

This rare tumor has a propensity to arise in the parotid gland.[68] Like basal cell adenoma, it is a slow-growing tumor and is usually asymptomatic. Microscopy reveals that clear-cell adenomas are composed of an inner eosinophilic cell layer and outer layers of clear cells, which are rich in glycogen. In the differential diagnosis, acinic cell and mucoepidermoid tumors have to be considered. Batsakis uses the relatively nonspecific term clear-cell tumor to classify such neoplasms.[69] We have not seen a benign variant of this tumor on cytologic examination. A malignant variant is further discussed on page 99.

Sebaceous Adenoma and Lymphadenoma

Sebaceous tumors of the salivary glands are rare, although sebaceous differentiation is not infrequently seen in normal salivary glands. Benign and malignant primary sebaceous tumors have been reported.[70] In addition, focal sebaceous differentiation has been reported in pleomorphic adenoma, Warthin's tumor, mucoepidermoid carcinoma and, rarely, other salivary gland neoplasms.[70] Sebaceous adenoma and lymphadenoma will be discussed here and sebaceous carcinoma will be discussed along with other malignant lesions on pages 100 and 101.

Sebaceous lymphadenomas are slow-growing neoplasms that are composed of cysts lined by squamous and sebaceous cells and supported by a lymphoid-rich stroma.[70-72] When such a tumor lacks a lymphoid component, the term sebaceous adenoma is applied. Zajicek[73] has described two examples of this lesion that were composed of large, sebaceous cells with finely granular to vacuolated cytoplasm and a small, round or oval, uniform, eccentrically located nucleus. Lymphocytes are seen in the background in sebaceous lymphadenoma but are lacking in sebaceous adenoma.

MALIGNANT TUMORS

Adenoid Cystic Carcinoma

This slow-growing, malignant tumor was originally described in 1859 by Billroth as cylindroma.[74] Adenoid cystic carcinoma accounts for 2 to 5 percent of all tumors of the parotid gland.[75,76] In the submandibular and minor salivary glands, such tumors are more common, accounting for 15 and 30 percent of all tumors in these glands, respectively.[75,76] In addition to the salivary glands, sites of origin of adenoid cystic carcinoma include the lacrimal glands, ceruminous glands, bronchi, esophagus, breasts, skin, cervix and Bartholin's gland. Despite their initial slow growth, such tumors are associated with a poor long-term prognosis. Because of their infiltrative nature, perineural involvement is common (Fig. 2.70) and pain may be an early symptom. Lymph node metastases are uncommon, but numerous distant metastases develop late in the course of the disease and usually involve the lungs and bone. The five-year survival rate for patients with adenoid cystic carcinoma is approximately 70 percent; the survival rate decreases to about 40 percent at 15 years.[77] Such tumors develop in adult life and are most common between the ages of 40 and 70 years. Adenoid cystic carcinoma is slightly more common in women than in men.[76] Pain alone or in combination with swelling is the most common complaint in symptomatic patients.[76] However, almost half the patients present with an asymptomatic swelling.[76]

Such tumors are solid and appear to be well circumscribed, although they lack a definite capsule. Infiltration of the surrounding tissue is frequently observed.

HISTOLOGIC FEATURES. The cut surface is firm and gray to pink. Adenoid cystic carcinomas have been divided into three grades on the basis of histologic criteria.[78] Grade 1 tumors have a cribriform or cylindromatous pattern (Fig. 2.71), grade 2 tumors consist of an equal mixture of cribriform and solid patterns, and grade 3 tumors are composed predominantly of solid, basaloid cells or anaplastic cells (Fig. 2.72).

The tumor cells are relatively uniform, have small, round or oval nuclei and scanty cytoplasm and are arranged in anastomosing cords; there are cystic spaces surrounded by ductal lining cells or myoepithelial cells. Both cell types are observed. Myoepithelial cells are said to produce mucoid or hyaline-like material that surrounds small strands of tumor cells. The hyaline-like, acellular substance has been shown by electron microscopy to consist of layers of basal lamina.[79] In grade 3, or anaplastic, tumors, the cells are arranged in solid, basaloid masses. Cystic spaces are not encountered and cellular pleomorphism is more marked in such tumors than in well-differentiated tumors.

CYTOLOGIC FEATURES. Despite its name, adenoid cystic carcinoma is a solid tumor and aspirates usually consist of one or two drops of semisolid, cellular material. The typical branching, cylindromatous pattern seen on histologic examination is also seen in most aspirates from adenoid cystic carcinoma.[80,81] In smears, this branching pattern is found to be composed of round or branching multilayer clusters of uniform epithelial cells (Figs. 2.73, 2.74 and 2.75) arranged around cores of homoge-

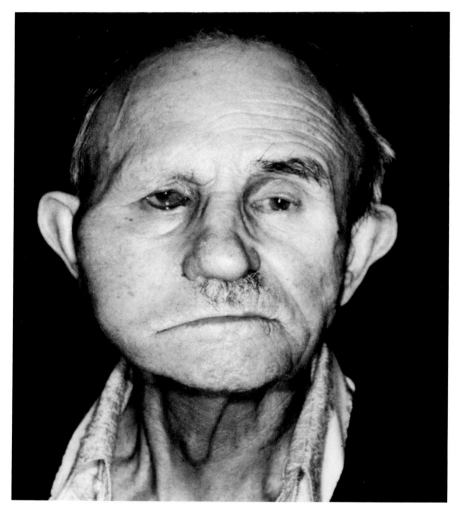

Fig. 2.70. Adenoid cystic carcinoma of the right parotid gland. The tumor has invaded the facial nerve, causing total facial paralysis.

neous, acellular material that stains pink with hematoxylin and eosin and translucent with Papanicolaou's method (Plate I.3). Eneroth and Zajicek[80] refer to these translucent "cylinders" as mucoid globules. As was noted earlier, these cylinders consist of layers of basal lamina.[79] Recent ultrastructural studies on a needle aspirate specimen from adenoid cystic carcinoma showed similar findings.[82] Because these clusters are thick and three-dimensional, it may be necessary to adjust the focus of the microscope to appreciate the cores of acellular material. When the cells appear in large, solid masses or sheets, they form a relatively regular mosaic arrangement, with the peripheral cells having their long axis directed along the borders of the cell clusters[81] (Fig. 2.74). In some tumors, there is an abundance of homogeneous, acellular material that is observable in the aspirates. In such cases, globules of hyaline substance are seen in the smears and basaloid, epithelial tumor cells arranged along the bor-

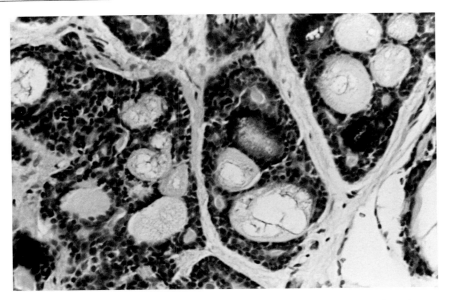

Fig. 2.71. Adenoid cystic carcinoma, cylindromatous type. Hematoxylin and eosin preparation. ×390.

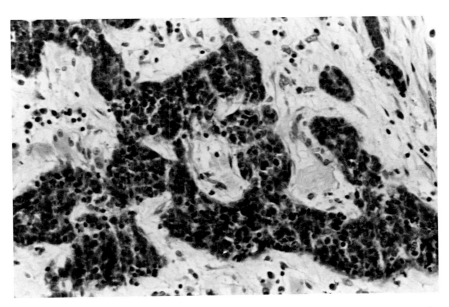

Fig. 2.72. Adenoid cystic carcinoma, solid, poorly differentiated type. Hematoxylin and eosin preparation. ×390.

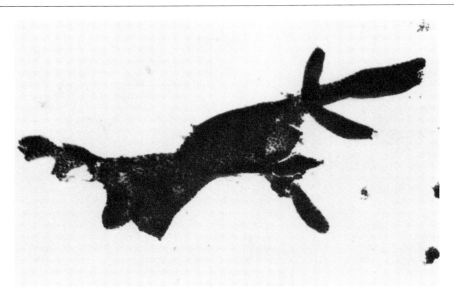

Fig. 2.73. Cytology specimen from a case of adenoid cystic carcinoma contains a branching, multilayered fragment of tumor cells. Papanicolaou preparation. × 150.

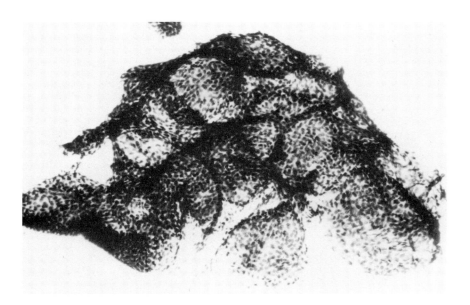

Fig. 2.74. Three-dimensional tissue fragment from an adenoid cystic carcinoma. Note the pale "mucous cylinders" outlined by a peripherally arranged row of cells, giving a mosaic-like appearance. Papanicolaou preparation. × 150. (From Hood et al: *Acta Cytol* 27:515–520, 1983, with permission.)

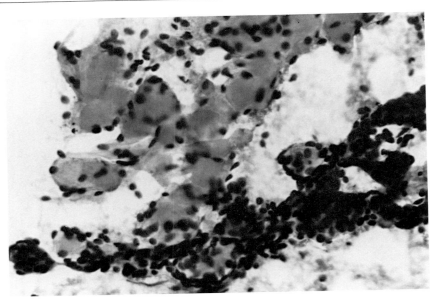

Fig. 2.75. Aspirate of an adenoid cystic carcinoma contains hyaline globules. Papanicolaou preparation. ×390. (From Hood et al: *Acta Cytol* 27:515–520, 1983, with permission.)

ders of the acellular material (Fig. 2.75). Cells in small, loose groupings or dispersed cells are observed in most cases of adenoid cystic carcinoma. Careful inspection reveals small nucleoli. In some cases, the nucleoli are large and prominent (Figs. 2.76 and 2.77). Occasionally, the mucoid globules do not stain with Papanicolaou's method and empty spaces are surrounded by basaloid tumor cells.

In poorly differentiated tumors, the aspirates usually contain small groupings of cells or solitary cells (Fig. 2.78). Mucoid globules are not seen and the tumor cells also have more atypia than do those of well-differentiated tumors.[80,81] The cells of such tumors have more pleomorphism with nuclear changes that are definitely of a malignant nature. Prominent nucleoli are observed in such cases (Fig. 2.79). The cytologic features of adenoid cystic carcinoma are summarized in Table 2.13.

DIFFERENTIAL DIAGNOSIS. Differentiation of pleomorphic adenoma from adenoid cystic carcinoma is no longer as difficult as it was during the pioneering years of clinical aspiration cytology at the Radiumhemmet.[80] The two lesions with which adenoid cystic carcinoma may be confused are basal cell adenoma and undifferentiated carcinoma.

Basal cell adenoma may mimic adenoid cystic carcinoma and distinction between the two lesions may be difficult. Both lesions are composed of basaloid cells and only differences in the cellular pattern and stroma permit recognition of the tumor type.[81,83] As was noted previously, the vast majority of adenoid cystic carcinomas consist of basophilic tumor cells arranged around cores of a homogeneous, acellular, basal lamina material. This pattern is diagnostic of adenoid cystic carcinoma and is not seen in any other salivary gland neoplasm. However, in the absence of a basal lamina material, confusion with basal cell adenoma may occur. In such instances,

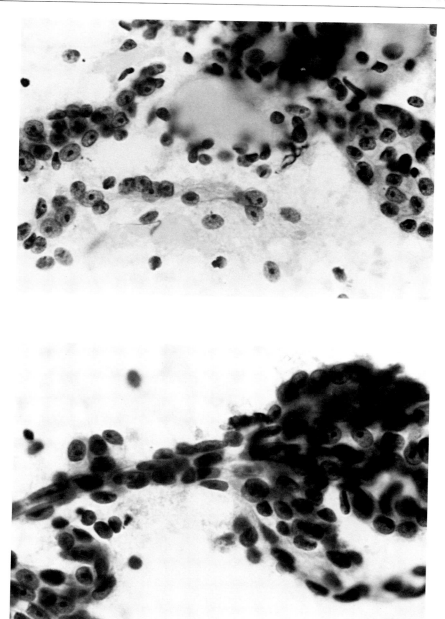

Figs. 2.76 and 2.77. High-power view shows basaloid cells that have indistinct cytoplasm. Note the prominent nucleoli. Papanicolaou preparation. ×625.

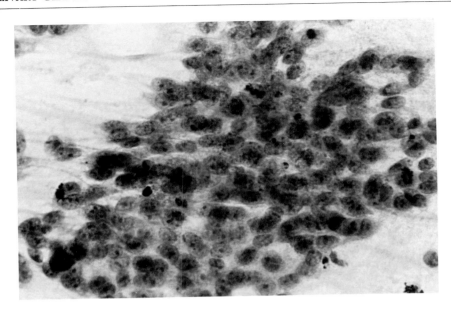

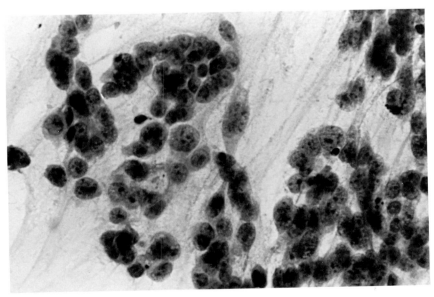

Figs. 2.78 and 2.79. Aspirate of the poorly differentiated adenoid cystic carcinoma shown in Figure 2.72. The malignant nature of the cells is obvious, although a diagnosis of adenoid cystic carcinoma may be difficult to make on the basis of the cytologic appearance alone. Papanicolaou preparation. ×625.

TABLE 2.13. Adenoid Cystic Carcinoma: Summary of Cytologic Features

Well Differentiated	Poorly Differentiated
Aspirates consisting of one or two drops of semisolid material	Aspirates consisting of one or two drops of semisolid material
Round, ball-like or branching, multilayered groupings of basophilic cells surrounding homogeneous, acellular material	Cells in loose groupings or solitary cells; acellular material lacking
Small, uniform nuclei, some containing small nucleoli	Increased nuclear atypia and prominent nucleoli
Appearance diagnostic	Differential diagnosis includes basal cell adenoma and undifferentiated carcinoma

attention to nuclear detail is necessary to arrive at the correct diagnosis. The nuclei of basal cell adenomas are regular and contain bland chromatin and no nucleolus. Poorly differentiated adenoid cystic carcinoma, however, has more marked cellular atypia, with variation in nuclear size and nucleoli.

Undifferentiated carcinoma occurs in the salivary glands and distinction from a solid variant of poorly differentiated adenoid cystic carcinoma may pose a problem. Smears from undifferentiated carcinoma usually contain cells that have a high nuclear to cytoplasmic ratio, decreased cohesiveness and nuclear changes of a malignant nature. However, differentiation between these entities is occasionally difficult. Figures 2.98 and 2.99 are from a case of undifferentiated carcinoma of the parotid gland that mimicked a solid variant of poorly differentiated adenoid cystic carcinoma.

The real challenge lies in the diagnosis of metastatic adenoid cystic carcinoma and differentiation from other small-cell neoplasms. Lymph node metastases in adenoid cystic carcinoma are uncommon and in one study the cervical lymph nodes were involved in only 15 percent of cases.[76] Visceral metastases commonly occur in the lungs and bones and needle aspiration is a simple method for documenting metastases and distinguishing between secondary deposits of adenoid cystic carcinoma and other cytologically similar tumors.

Figure 2.80 is from a patient with adenoid cystic carcinoma of the parotid gland metastatic to the bone. A bone marrow aspirate stained with the Wright-Giemsa method contains the characteristic reddish mucoid globules surrounded by densely packed, round tumor cells. If homogeneous, acellular material is observed, the diagnosis is relatively easy. If such material is lacking however, the diagnosis may be difficult.

In metastatic adenoid cystic carcinoma, the site of the lesion aspirated must also be considered in arriving at the correct diagnosis. In a lymph node, differentiation from poorly differentiated adenocarcinoma, undifferentiated carcinoma, neuroendocrine carcinoma and even lymphoma may be difficult. In the bone, such small-cell tumors as Ewing's sarcoma, neuroblastoma and lymphoma also have to be considered. In the lungs, poorly differentiated adenocarcinoma, small-cell undifferentiated carcinoma and carcinoid enter into the differential diagnosis.[84]

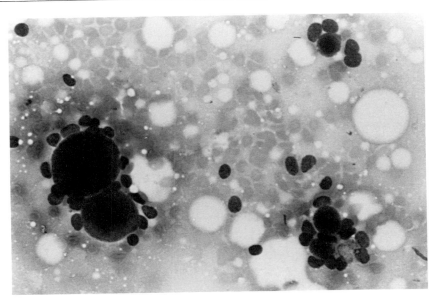

Fig. 2.80. Adenoid cystic carcinoma metastatic to bone. A bone marrow aspirate contains magenta globules surrounded by a rim of small, round cells. Wright-Giemsa preparation. ×625.

Mucoepidermoid Carcinoma

Mucoepidermoid tumors were originally described by Stewart and associates,[85] who classified them as benign or malignant. Most investigators now regard such tumors as malignant and classify them as low-grade or high-grade cancers.[86,87] Such tumors comprise approximately 5 to 10 percent of all major salivary gland neoplasms and most mucoepidermoid carcinomas occur in the parotid gland. These tumors occur in all age groups. They are the most common malignant salivary gland neoplasms in children.[88] In adults, they occur commonly in the third to fifth decades. They have no predilection for either sex. Most such tumors present as painless masses, although high-grade lesions may be fixed to adjacent tissues and thus are not as readily movable as low-grade ones (Fig. 2.81). Low-grade mucoepidermoid carcinoma may develop slowly over a period of years, whereas high-grade lesions usually grow rapidly. Low-grade tumors recur locally, especially if surgical excision is incomplete. Distant metastases are rare. The five-year survival rate for patients with low-grade tumors is 90 percent.[87,89] High-grade tumors recur locally and metastasize to regional lymph nodes, lungs and bone. The five-year survival rate for patients with high-grade mucoepidermoid carcinomas is approximately 40 percent.[89,90]

Low-grade tumors are well circumscribed but characteristically lack a capsule. Some tumors are cystic, containing mucus or bloody fluid. High-grade tumors are infiltrative and tend to be solid. They have a firm, gray cut surface with areas of necrosis.

HISTOLOGIC FEATURES. Low-grade tumors are composed predominantly of mucus-secreting, columnar cells with variable numbers of intermediate and squamous cells

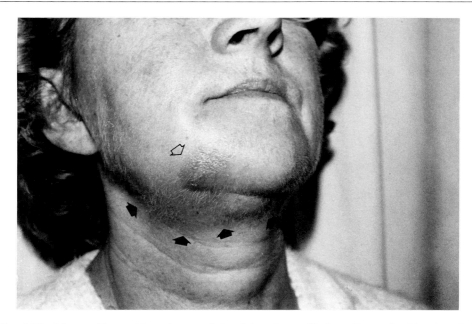

Fig. 2.81. Mucoepidermoid carcinoma of the right submandibular salivary gland has invaded the overlying skin. The tumor outline is indicated by black arrows and the skin involvement by an open arrow.

(Fig. 2.82). Mucus-filled cysts are common and lined by tall, columnar cells. Distended, goblet-like cells are also encountered. The glandular cells take up mucin stains. The cells are uniform and nuclear atypia is not observed. Mitoses are extremely uncommon. High-grade tumors are composed predominantly of squamous and poorly differentiated cells with scanty glandular elements (Fig. 2.83). Cytologic atypia is seen and mitoses are easily found. Clear-cell areas may be observed.

CYTOLOGIC FEATURES. Aspirates from low-grade tumors usually consist of a few drops of mucoid material. If a cyst is needled, one or more milliliters of clear or blood-tinged fluid may be recovered.[91] After the cyst fluid is evacuated, it is advisable to reneedle the mass. The mass should always be reneedled if it fails to disappear, recurs or is abnormal cytologically. In low-grade tumors (Fig. 2.84), the smears consist of a mixture of intermediate and mucus-secreting cells[91] (Plate I.2). Squamous cells may also be seen. The cells are arranged in sheets or irregular tissue fragments. The glandular component consists of columnar or large, oval cells that have foamy, pale-staining cytoplasm and small, uniform, centrally or eccentrically located nuclei that vary only slightly in size (Fig. 2.85). The chromatin is fine to moderately coarse and small nucleoli can be identified. The intermediate cells appear smaller than the glandular cells and have a scant amount of eosinophilic cytoplasm and small, round, uniform nuclei (Fig. 2.86). A variable number of cells have features of immature metaplastic squamous cells with prominent cell borders. Such cells have more cytoplasm than do the intermediate cells; the nuclei of the former cells appear slightly larger than those of the intermediate cells that have a similar

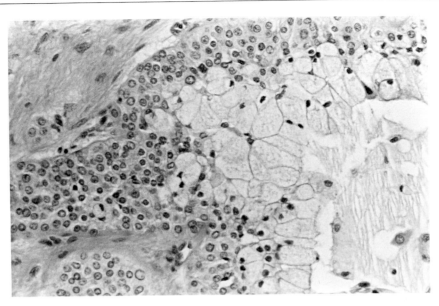

Fig. 2.82. Mucoepidermoid carcinoma, low grade. Mucus-secreting, columnar cells coexist with squamous cells. Hematoxylin and eosin preparation. ×390.

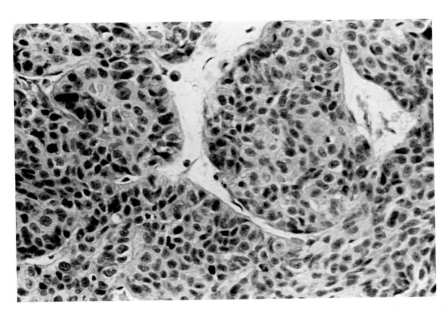

Fig. 2.83. Mucoepidermoid carcinoma, high grade, poorly differentiated. The glandular component may be evident only after staining with mucicarmine. Hematoxylin and eosin preparation. ×390.

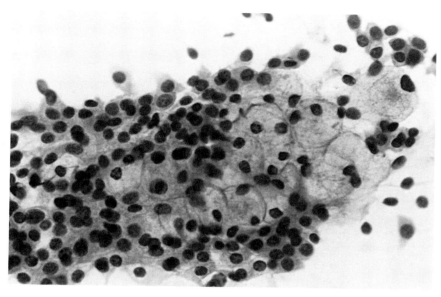

Fig. 2.84. Cytology specimen from a low-grade mucoepidermoid carcinoma. Note the mixture of cell types. Papanicolaou preparation. ×625. (From Qizilbash et al: *Acta Cytol* 29:503–512, 1985, with permission.)

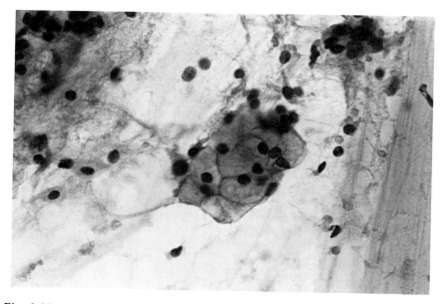

Fig. 2.85. A grouping of mucus-secreting cells. Papanicolaou preparation. ×625.

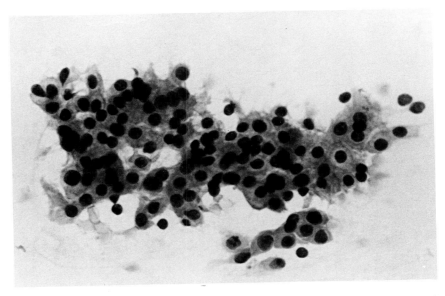

Fig. 2.86. A monolayer sheet of intermediate cells. Papanicolaou preparation. ×625.

chromatin pattern. Keratinization is rarely seen and intercellular bridges are difficult to demonstrate. The background of smears varies, depending on the amount of mucus and cellular debris. With Papanicolaou's method, the mucus stains almost translucent to pale pink. Red blood cells, neutrophils, lymphocytes and a few histiocytes may also be seen mixed with mucus in the background.

Aspirates from high-grade tumors usually consist of one or two drops of semisolid material. Smears are usually cellular, consisting of cell clusters and sheets of poorly differentiated malignant squamous cells (Figs. 2.87 and 2.88). Occasionally, pearl formations are observed (Fig. 2.87). Glandular cells are not common and at times cannot be found. A definitive diagnosis of mucoepidermoid carcinoma cannot be made if such cells are not detected.[91] However, if there is no known primary tumor, the finding, of poorly differentiated squamous tumor cells in a smear should arouse suspicion of high-grade mucoepidermoid carcinoma. Table 2.14 summarizes the cytologic features of low-grade and high-grade mucoepidermoid carcinomas seen in needle aspirates.

DIFFERENTIAL DIAGNOSIS. Low-grade mucoepidermoid carcinoma must be distinguished from chronic sialadenitis with prominent squamous and mucous metaplasia. Smears from such lesions are relatively acellular, consisting of occasional small clusters of squamous and glandular cells. In addition, the background contains inflammatory cells and elongated or spindle-shaped fibroblasts. Normal salivary gland components, such as acini and ductal elements, may also be encountered.

Necrotizing sialometaplasia is a benign, self-healing lesion that mainly involves the minor salivary glands.[92] This lesion most likely is a response to ischemic injury of the glands and results in squamous epithelial hyperplasia, squamous metaplasia of the ducts and acini and an inflammatory reaction to extravasated mucus. Smears

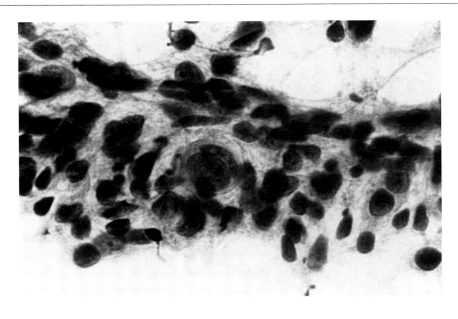

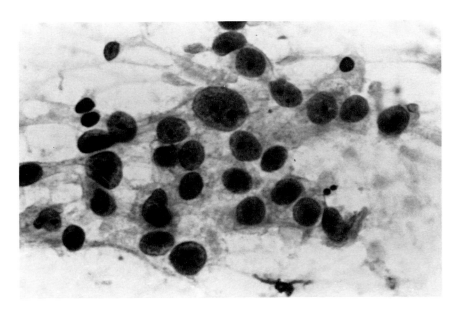

Figs. 2.87 and 2.88. Cytology specimen from a high-grade mucoepidermoid carcinoma. Note the poorly differentiated appearance of the cells. A "pearl" formation is evident in Figure 2.87. Papanicolaou preparation. × 1000.

TABLE 2.14. Mucoepidermoid Carcinoma: Summary of Cytologic Features

Low Grade	High Grade
Aspirates consisting of a few drops to a few milliliters of mucoid material	Aspirates consisting of one or two drops of semisolid material
Mixture of mucus-secreting, columnar or goblet-like cells, intermediate and squamous cells	Poorly differentiated and squamous cells; glandular cells difficult to identify
Small, round or oval, uniform nuclei	Nuclear atypia more marked with frankly malignant features
May be confused with Warthin's tumor and other benign lesions	Usually confused with squamous, poorly differentiated or undifferentiated carcinoma

from such lesions consist of squamous and glandular cells and their appearance may mimic that of mucoepidermoid carcinoma. Another rare lesion that may cause confusion with mucoepidermoid carcinoma on cytologic examination is adenomatoid hyperplasia of the mucous salivary glands.[93] In this lesion, the surface squamous epithelium also is hyperplastic and smears consist of a mixture of squamous and mucous cells. Both these lesions involve the minor salivary glands and the history along with the clinical findings may be of help in arriving at the diagnosis. Because one-third of mucoepidermoid carcinomas involve the minor salivary glands,[94] the examiner should keep this possibility in mind to avoid misdiagnosis.

Mucous cysts and mucoceles also must be considered in the differential diagnosis of well-differentiated mucoepidermoid tumors. Smears from such lesions consist of mucus, inflammatory cells, histiocytes, which occasionally mimic glandular cells, and few epithelial cells. After aspiration, such cysts usually disappear. However, if they persist or recur after evacuation, they should be reneedled or excised for histologic study.

Another lesion that should be considered in the differential diagnosis of well-differentiated mucoepidermoid carcinoma is Warthin's tumor, which was discussed previously.

With increased awareness, misdiagnosis of well-differentiated mucoepidermoid carcinoma is no longer as common as it was during the 1950s and early 1960s, as noted by Zajicek and coworkers.[91] Cytologic criteria for the diagnosis of salivary gland neoplasms have been devised largely by Zajicek and colleagues and use of these criteria permits a correct diagnosis in virtually all cases.

Poorly differentiated mucoepidermoid carcinomas may mimic other poorly differentiated tumors, notably squamous cell carcinoma and undifferentiated carcinoma. A definitive diagnosis of poorly differentiated mucoepidermoid carcinoma relies on the identification of squamous and glandular elements. Because mucous glandular cells are sparse and difficult to find in needle aspirates from such tumors, it is not always possible to make a definitive diagnosis on the basis of cytologic findings alone; surgical excision and histologic study are required in many cases. Mucin stains, however, should be performed on the smears in such cases. Smears from a carcinoma that arises in a pleomorphic adenoma likewise may consist of squamous, poorly differentiated or undifferentiated malignant cells and differentiation from poorly differentiated mucoepidermoid carcinoma may be difficult.

Metastatic squamous cell carcinoma commonly involves the lymph nodes in the head and neck and is also a common source of metastases to the parotid and submandibular glands. For this reason, an attempt should be made to rule out an occult primary tumor in the oral cavity or upper respiratory tract in cases in which poorly differentiated squamous cells are found in the aspirate. Distinction between primary and metastatic carcinoma is important because the management of these entities differs. High-grade mucoepidermoid carcinoma is usually managed by radial excision of the gland and neck nodes, whereas metastatic squamous cell carcinoma is often managed by radiotherapy. Two of our cases of high-grade mucoepidermoid carcinoma were diagnosed as poorly differentiated squamous cell carcinoma on the basis of cytologic study. No primary lesion was found in either case and only surgical excision and histologic examination allowed us to arrive at a diagnosis of mucoepidermoid carcinoma.

Acinic Cell Carcinoma

Acinic cell carcinoma is an uncommon tumor, accounting for approximately 3 percent of all salivary gland tumors. Such carcinomas are commonly found in the parotid gland, although rare examples have been described in the other major salivary glands.[95] Approximately 3 percent of such tumors are bilateral.[96] They are more common in women than in men and occur at all ages, although there is a peak incidence in the fifth decade. Acinic cell carcinoma is the second most common malignant salivary gland tumor in children, surpassed in frequency only by mucoepidermoid carcinoma.[96] Such tumors arise from stem cells of the intercalated ducts and differentiate in a manner characteristic of acinar cells. Like most salivary gland tumors, acinic cell carcinomas grow slowly. Most patients present with an asymptomatic mass. Occasionally, the tumor is painful. Local recurrence is not uncommon and depends on the surgical method used to remove the primary tumor. Local excision of the primary tumor is associated with a recurrence rate of 67 percent, whereas total parotidectomy is associated with a recurrence rate of 10 percent.[97] Metastasis to lymph nodes occurs in 10 percent of cases and distant metastasis to the lungs and bones occurs in approximately 15 percent of cases.[98] The five-year survival rate for patients with acinic cell carcinoma is 90 percent and falls to 56 percent at 20 years, according to one report.[97]

Most tumors of this kind measure less than 5 centimeters in diameter at the time of diagnosis. They are round or lobulated, soft masses and usually are well circumscribed but not completely encapsulated. The cut surface is grayish yellow. Hemorrhage and necrosis are common. A rare cystic variant has also been reported[99] and is shown in Figures 2.89 and 2.90.

HISTOLOGIC FEATURES. Acinic cell carcinomas have a solid, microcystic, papillary cystic or follicular growth pattern. The tumor cells are cuboidal or polyhedral and have basophilic cytoplasm that contains granules of variable size (Fig. 2.91). The granules are similar to the zymogen granules seen in normal serous acinar cells. They stain with periodic acid-Schiff, are resistant to diastase and do not take up mucin stains. Their nuclei appear uniform and occasional mitoses are observed. Papillary areas are prominent in some tumors and foci of clear cells are seen in others. The stroma is scanty, although in some tumors, wide, dense bands of hy-

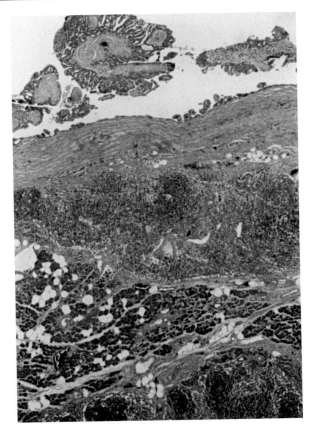

Fig. 2.89. Cystic acinic cell carcinoma of a parotid gland. The tumor is largely necrotic and cystic; however, attached to the wall are foci of small, papillary folds lined by acinic cells. Hematoxylin and eosin preparation. ×50.

alinized tissue are observed. In the follicular variant, a dense, lymphoid infiltrate is observed with germinal centers.

CYTOLOGIC FEATURES. Aspirates usually consist of one or two drops of semisolid material mixed with blood. In rare instances, the tumor is cystic and must be reneedled after the fluid has been evacuated.[3] The smears are usually extremely cellular, consisting of sheets and solid groupings of cells, some of which resemble glandular configurations (Fig. 2.92). The tumor cells are large and have an abundance of orange to pink, foamy cytoplasm and distinct cell borders (Fig. 2.93). The nuclei appear uniform in size, although the chromatin may be moderately coarse and prominent nucleoli may be identified. Periodic acid-Schiff-positive, diastase-resistant granules can be demonstrated within the cytoplasm of the tumor cells.[7] A striking feature of a typical smear is the large number of naked tumor cell nuclei. The naked nuclei most likely are an artifact, resulting from trauma at the time of aspiration and preparation of the smears. Care should be exercised in not confusing bare tumor nuclei with lymphocytes. However, in the rare follicular variant of acinic

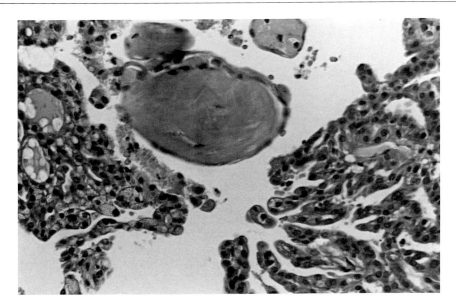

Fig. 2.90. High-power view of the tumor shown in Figure 2.89. Hematoxylin and eosin preparation. ×390.

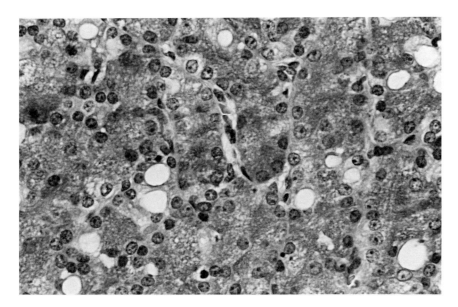

Fig. 2.91. Acinic cell carcinoma. A solid variant composed of trabeculae of granular cells. Hematoxylin and eosin preparation. ×625.

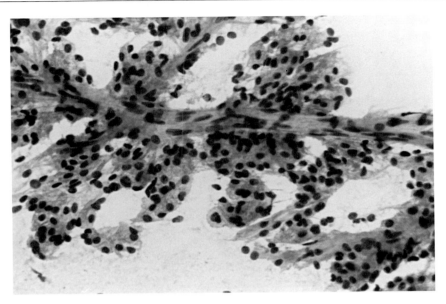

Fig. 2.92. Cytology specimen from an acinic cell carcinoma. Note the capillary lined by endothelial cells. Attached to the sides of the capillary are loose aggregates of acinic tumor cells. Hematoxylin and eosin preparation. ×390.

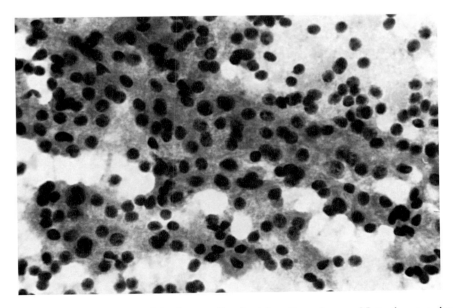

Fig. 2.93. High-power view of the large cells of acinic cell carcinoma. Note the granular or finely foamy nature of the cytoplasm. Bare nuclei are in the background. Hematoxylin and eosin preparation. ×625.

TABLE 2.15. Acinic Cell Carcinoma: Summary of Cytologic Features

Aspirates usually consisting of one or two drops of semisolid, cellular material; tumors
  cystic in rare cases
Cellular smears consisting of sheets and solid groupings of tumor cells, some in an
  acinus-like configuration
Large tumor cells with an abundance of foamy or coarsely granular cytoplasm
Periodic acid-Schiff-positive diastase-resistant granules in cytoplasm of tumor cells
Uniform nuclei with moderately coarse chromatin and small or prominent nucleoli
Lymphocyte-sized, bare nuclei in background
Absence of fat or ductal lining cells
Lymphocytes usually absent in smears, except in the follicular variant

cell carcinoma, the stroma is rich in lymphoid cells that have germinal centers and
aspirates from such tumors yield lymphoreticular elements as well as epithelial
tumor cells.[100] The background of the smears usually consists of an amorphous, pale
pink material.

In well-differentiated tumors, nuclear pleomorphism is minimal, although the
cells are larger than the acinar cells of normal parotid glands. The tumor cells are not
mixed with fat or ductal cells, a feature commonly seen in nonneoplastic aspirates.[3]
However, in poorly differentiated tumors, cellular atypia and nuclear pleomorphism
are more evident and the prominent nucleoli that are encountered make a cytologic
diagnosis of a malignant process less difficult. If the characteristic foamy cytoplasm is
not observed, it may be impossible to further categorize such a tumor.[3] In the
papillary-cystic variant, laminated, calcific structures that resemble psammoma
bodies are sometimes discovered on cytologic examination.[101] Figures 2.94 and 2.95
are from the cystic variant shown in Figure 2.89. In that case, an abundance of
necrotic material in combination with a few small groupings of degenerated tumor
cells made the diagnosis difficult. The cytologic features of acinic cell carcinoma are
summarized in Table 2.15.

DIFFERENTIAL DIAGNOSIS. Well-differentiated acinic cell carcinoma should not be
confused with nonneoplastic salivary gland tissue. Aspirates from acinic cell carcinomas are rich in tumor cells and bare epithelial nuclei are plentiful in the background. Fat cells and ductal epithelium are not encountered.[3,7] Aspirates from
nonneoplastic lesions, on the other hand, consist of small fragments of salivary gland
tissue in which intact acinar elements, fat and ductal cells can be recognized. Free
acinar cells, as seen in tumors, are usually not found in aspirates from normal or
nonneoplastic salivary glands. Moreover, in aspirates from acinic cell carcinoma, the
tumor cells are larger and have more pleomorphism than do serous cells from
normal salivary glands.

Differentiation from Warthin's tumor may pose a problem, as was originally
reported by Zajicek.[3] However, attention to the cytoplasmic detail and background
material leads the examiner to the correct diagnosis in most cases. Generally, the
cytoplasm of acinic tumor cells appears granular to foamy, whereas the cytoplasm of
oncocytes is more dense, especially when hematoxylin and eosin stain is used.
Moreover, tumor cells from acinic neoplasms assume a small, glandlike configuration, a finding that is extremely rare in Warthin's tumor. Solitary dissociated cells are

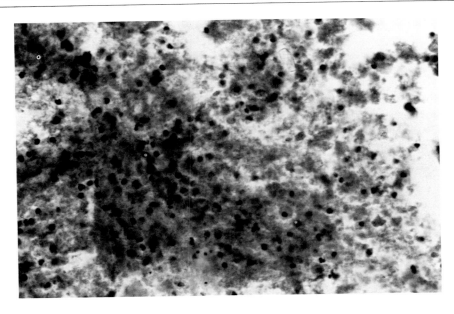

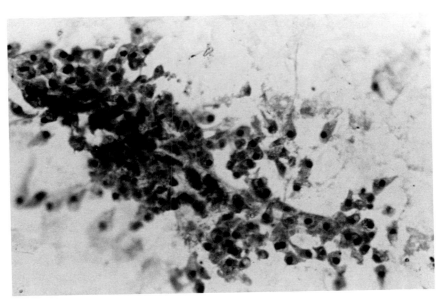

Figs. 2.94 and 2.95. Cystic acinic cell carcinoma (same case as shown in Figure 2.89). The aspirate contains necrotic, cellular debris and focal aggregates of tumor cells that show degenerative changes. Papanicolaou preparation. ×390.

common in acinic cell tumors, whereas oncocytes occur in sheets and groupings in Warthin's tumor. Periodic acid-Schiff reagent can be used if the diagnosis is in doubt. Periodic acid-Schiff-positive, diastase-resistant granules can be identified in many well-differentiated acinic cell carcinomas. The background material in Warthin's tumor contains lymphocytes and amorphous, cellular debris, an appearance that differs from the bare tumor nuclei seen in acinic cell neoplasms. Acinic cell carcinomas occasionally have a lymphoid-rich stroma, in which case differentiation from Warthin's tumor is based on the arrangement and the cytologic features of the tumor cells rather than on the type of background.[3,100] The finding of lymphocytes in combination with acinar tumor cells may also suggest metastatic carcinoma in a lymph node.[3,100] In such instances, the examiner must be certain that a lymph node was needled before making the diagnosis. However, it may not be possible to ascertain that a lymph node was needled because lymph nodes normally occur adjacent to and within parotid glands and the needle could inadvertently enter a lymph node. In such instances, lymphoid tissue and tumor cells may be aspirated together.

Carcinoma ex Pleomorphic Adenoma

Such tumors contain elements of benign pleomorphic adenoma and carcinoma. Metastases consist only of a carcinomatous element. Such tumors account for less than 5 percent of all pleomorphic adenomas.[102] They involve the major and minor salivary glands but occur most commonly in the parotid gland. Such tumors are more common in women than in men and develop most often in the sixth decade. The typical presentation is that of a long-standing, slowly enlarging tumor that has recently had a rapid increase in size. However, such tumors sometimes develop rapidly in patients with no history of a pleomorphic adenoma. Pain, facial nerve palsy or fixation to surrounding tissues is encountered in up to 50 percent of patients. Metastases are not uncommon and usually involve the lymph nodes, bone and lungs.[102] The five-year survival rate of patients is approximately 50 percent.[103]

HISTOLOGIC FEATURES. The tumors are usually solitary and well circumscribed and have a smooth or bosselated surface. Infiltration into adjacent tissues may be noted. Areas of hemorrhage and necrosis are common. Benign and malignant elements must be identified to make the diagnosis. The benign portion may be reduced to a microscopic focus or may occupy most of the lesion. Transformation into adenocarcinoma is frequent. Less commonly, undifferentiated, squamous cell, mucoepidermoid or adenoid cystic carcinoma are encountered. Features that suggest malignant change include infiltration into surrounding tissues, foci of necrosis and hemorrhage and vascular and perineural invasion. Cellularity and nuclear atypia are insufficient evidence of a malignant process.

CYTOLOGIC FEATURES. The cytologic diagnosis of carcinoma in a pleomorphic adenoma by means of needle aspiration biopsy has rarely been reported. The literature contains only a handful of cases.[104-107] Aspirates usually contain the major components of such tumors. However, benign and malignant elements may be encountered in the same smear.[104] Depending on the dominant pattern, the smears may consist of frankly malignant cells that are undifferentiated or that have a glandu-

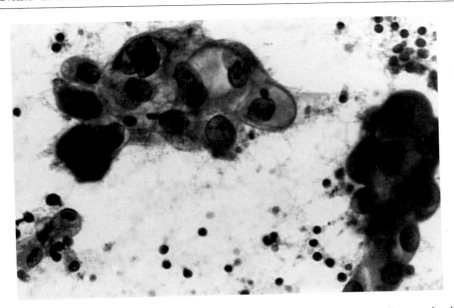

Fig. 2.96. Adenocarcinoma ex pleomorphic adenoma. The smear contains malignant glandular cells. Papanicolaou preparation. × 1000.

lar, squamous or adenoid cystic pattern, reflecting the histologic appearance of the tumor. Benign stromal elements of pleomorphic adenoma may be found adjacent to malignant cells, an observation that has been well illustrated by Linsk and colleagues.[107] A recent report has documented the cytologic diagnosis of adenoid cystic carcinoma in a pleomorphic adenoma by means of needle aspiration biopsy.[106] Figure 2.96 is from a case of poorly differentiated adenocarcinoma arising in a pleomorphic adenoma of the parotid gland that had metastasized to a regional lymph node. Smears from the tumor and the involved lymph node contained only malignant glandular cells. The history of a recent increase in size of a long-standing tumor in the parotid gland with regional lymph node enlargement suggested the diagnosis. Table 2.16 summarizes the cytologic features of carcinoma ex pleomorphic adenoma seen in needle aspirates.

DIFFERENTIAL DIAGNOSIS. The diagnosis of carcinoma ex pleomorphic adenoma is not difficult if the cellular aspirate contains unequivocal malignant cells and benign fragments of pleomorphic adenoma. Such cases are, however, rare and in a series of 316 histologically benign pleomorphic adenomas, cytologically malignant cells in

TABLE 2.16. Carcinoma ex pleomorphic adenoma: Summary of Cytologic Features

Diagnosis of needle aspirates difficult
Diagnosis relies on benign mesenchymal stroma and malignant epithelial elements
Malignant elements, usually squamous, glandular or undifferentiated
Slight or moderate cellular atypia, not sufficient for diagnosis of a malignant lesion

addition to benign elements of pleomorphic adenoma were encountered in only five cases.[104] If the aspirate contains only a malignant element, cytologic examination can lead only to a diagnosis of a malignant tumor; depending on the pattern of differentiation, such a lesion can be classified as adenocarcinoma, squamous carcinoma or undifferentiated carcinoma. Distinction between primary malignant tumors of the salivary glands and carcinoma ex pleomorphic adenoma is not possible in such cases. There is no problem clinically, however, because the management of most primary malignant tumors of the salivary glands involves surgical intervention, the exception being advanced anaplastic tumors, for which radiotherapy is the treatment of choice. A history of a long-standing mass with recent rapid increase in growth and fixation in conjunction with the cytologic findings suggest the diagnosis. It should be stressed that mild to moderate atypia of a few cells in an otherwise benign pleomorphic adenoma is insufficient evidence of malignant change. Eneroth and Zajicek,[104] in a study of 316 pleomorphic adenomas, found 17 cases in which the cytologic diagnosis of a malignant process was suspected because of cellular atypia and polymorphous, carcinoma-like cells. On histologic examination, however, all 17 tumors were found to be benign. Because of the likelihood of overdiagnosis, these authors advise caution in the diagnosis of carcinoma ex pleomorphic adenoma on the basis of slight or moderate cellular atypia alone. On the other hand, when the aspirates contain many tumor cells with definite cytologic features of malignant transformation, a diagnosis of carcinoma ex pleomorphic adenoma is justified.

Malignant Mixed Tumor

In this uncommon tumor, the stromal and epithelial elements appear malignant.[108,109] Chen has described a variant of this tumor in which both elements appear benign histologically, yet the tumor has metastasized.[110] Needle aspiration biopsy of such tumors has rarely been reported; to our knowledge, only two reports of malignant mixed tumor aspirates have been published.[111,112]

Primary Squamous Cell Carcinoma

This rare tumor occurs in the major and minor salivary glands. It accounts for 1 percent of all parotid gland tumors.[113,114] Such tumors are more common in men than in women and the peak incidence is in the fifth and sixth decades. They most likely arise from foci of squamous metaplasia in the epithelial lining of the ducts of the salivary glands. It is often impossible to be certain that such a lesion is not a metastasis from a primary head or neck tumor (e.g., in the skin, oropharynx or nasopharynx). A search for a primary tumor outside the salivary glands is mandatory. Patients usually have a history of a rapidly enlarging tumor, with fixation to overlying skin and adjacent tissues (Fig. 2.97). Local infiltration and lymph node metastases are common, although distant visceral metastases are rare. The five-year survival rate of patients with such tumors is approximately 30 percent.[115]

HISTOLOGIC FEATURES. Such tumors are solid and have ill-defined edges with infiltration into adjacent tissues. The cut surface is gray and there are areas of necrosis and hemorrhage. The usual spectrum of well-differentiated to poorly differentiated tumors is encountered. Keratinization is seen in most cases.

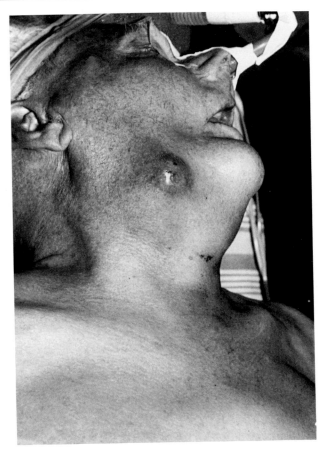

Fig. 2.97. Squamous cell carcinoma of the right submandibular gland has invaded the overlying skin.

CYTOLOGIC FEATURES. The aspirates usually contain numerous tumor cells. Depending on the degree of differentiation of the tumor, the cells may be solitary or occur in loose groupings or in sheets and clusters. A mixture of these patterns is usually seen. Elongated, keratinized cells with crisp, eosinophilic cytoplasm and cells that have pearl formations are seen when the tumor is well-differentiated. Fragments of keratinized cytoplasm, the so-called ghost cells, may also be seen. In nonkeratining tumors, the cells occur in sheets and branching trabeculae. The cells have a high nuclear to cytoplasmic ratio, with overlapping of nuclei. The chromatin is fine to coarse and nucleoli are observed. Primary squamous cell carcinomas appear identical to metastatic tumors on cytologic examination of needle aspirates. Illustrations of such lesions are depicted in Chapter 3.

DIFFERENTIAL DIAGNOSIS. Lesions that must be ruled out in the differential diagnosis include metastatic squamous cell carcinoma, high-grade mucoepidermoid carcinoma and squamous cell carcinoma ex pleomorphic adenoma.

Primary squamous cell carcinoma cannot be diagnosed unless thorough investigation has ruled out an occult primary tumor. Cytologic study merely allows the demonstration of malignant squamous cells. Whether the tumor is primary or metastatic can be determined only from the history, physical findings and other investigations.

High-grade mucoepidermoid carcinomas masquerade as squamous cell carcinomas because of their paucity of glandular elements. Periodic acid-Schiff and mucicarmine stains may be helpful, although a definitive diagnosis sometimes depends on histologic examination of a surgical specimen.

Squamous cell carcinoma arising in a pleomorphic adenoma poses a similar dilemma. If benign stromal and malignant squamous elements coexist, then a diagnosis of squamous cell carcinoma arising in a pleomorphic adenoma can be made with confidence.

Undifferentiated Carcinoma

This primary tumor of the salivary glands accounts for less than 3 percent of all major tumors of the salivary glands.[116] Undifferentiated carcinoma occurs in both sexes equally, and although this tumor involves all age groups, it is most common in the seventh and eighth decades.[116] Most patients present with a rapidly enlarging, painful mass. Facial paralysis may be observed. Such tumors may be primary, arising from the ductal epithelium, or may originate from a pleomorphic adenoma. In the latter situation, a history of a long-standing, previously painless mass is characteristic. This rapidly growing tumor infiltrates surrounding tissues and secondarily involves regional lymph nodes. Distant metastases are common and occur in the lungs, bone and liver. The five-year survival rate of patients with such tumors is approximately 20 percent.

HISTOLOGIC FEATURES. Like squamous cell carcinoma, undifferentiated carcinomas have poorly defined margins with infiltration into surrounding tissues. They are firm lesions and the cut surface is gray. Areas of hemorrhage and necrosis are common. Such tumors have a variable appearance, being composed of masses or trabeculae of large, round or polygonal cells. Spindle cell variants also occur. Areas of necrosis are common and mitoses are plentiful. A small-cell variant, similar to oat cell carcinoma of the bronchus, has recently been described[117,118] and is illustrated in Figure 2.98.

CYTOLOGIC FEATURES. Aspirates from such tumors are cellular, consisting of solitary cells and small, loose groupings of large, pleomorphic tumor cells that have a high nuclear to cytoplasmic ratio. The nuclei are round or oval and contain coarse chromatin and prominent nucleoli. Spindle-shaped cells may be seen.

We recently examined an aspirate from a patient with undifferentiated carcinoma (Fig. 2.99) composed of small, uniform cells that had round or oval nuclei. Small nucleoli were observed, but the nuclei lacked the pleomorphism typically seen in undifferentiated carcinomas. Histologic examination (Fig. 2.98) revealed that the tumor was not a basaloid or solid variant of poorly differentiated adenoid cystic carcinoma. Grimelius stain demonstrated fine, black granules in the tumor cells, suggesting neuroendocrine differentiation. Unfortunately, electron microscopy was

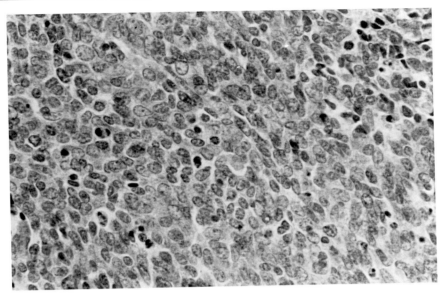

Fig. 2.98. Histologic appearance of small-cell undifferentiated carcinoma. Hematoxylin and eosin preparation. ×390.

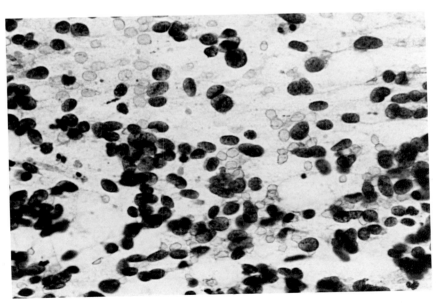

Fig. 2.99. Small-cell undifferentiated carcinoma of parotid gland is composed of cells that have small, round or oval nuclei and small nucleoli. Papanicolaou preparation. ×625.

not done. Similar cases have been reported previously.[117,118] In one case, electron microscopy did not demonstrate neurosecretory granules.[118]

DIFFERENTIAL DIAGNOSIS. Small-cell undifferentiated tumor may be confused with malignant lymphoma and the basaloid variant of poorly differentiated adenoid cystic carcinoma. This diagnostic problem was discussed previously.

Tumors composed of large, polygonal cells must be differentiated from poorly differentiated squamous cell carcinoma and adenocarcinoma. Cells from all three lesions may appear similar. Foci of squamous differentiation may be evident in poorly differentiated tumors, facilitating the diagnosis of squamous carcinoma. If no such foci are encountered, distinction among these entities may be difficult. In poorly differentiated adenocarcinoma, the tumor cells are cuboidal or polygonal and have a high nuclear to cytoplasmic ratio and large, hyperchromatic nuclei. Nucleoli are prominent. The cytoplasm of some tumor cells is vacuolated, suggesting glandular differentiation. If vacuolation is not observed, differentiation of poorly differentiated adenocarcinoma from undifferentiated carcinoma and poorly differentiated squamous carcinoma may be difficult.

Adenocarcinoma

The salivary glands are the site of origin of a variety of adenocarcinomas, including papillary adenocarcinoma,[119] papillary-cystic carcinoma,[120] mucus-producing adenopapillary carcinoma[121] and salivary duct carcinoma.[122] The first three terms probably refer to the same entity. These rare neoplasms occur in the major and minor salivary glands, although they are more common in the latter glands. They usually grow slowly and are asymptomatic.

HISTOLOGIC FEATURES. On gross inspection, papillary tumors are firm and rubbery. Histologic examination shows that they are composed of papillary processes that may project into cystic spaces lined by cuboidal epithelium. Solid areas are also encountered. Adenocarcinomas of the salivary glands are regarded as low-grade malignant tumors, as judged by local invasion and metastasis to regional lymph nodes. The prognosis of patients with such tumors is excellent.

Carcinoma of the salivary duct is a rare variant of adenocarcinoma of the salivary glands that resembles ductal carcinoma of the breasts on histologic examination. Such tumors arise in the major and minor salivary glands. Twelve cases have been reported and most have arisen from Stensen's duct.[122] Patients present with painful, rapidly enlarging masses and facial nerve involvement.

Gross inspection demonstrates that carcinomas of the salivary duct are grayish white and firm. Necrosis is observed. Microscopy reveals that such tumors mimic comedocarcinoma of the breasts, having papillary and cribriform patterns. The tumor cells are large and have pleomorphic nuclei and eosinophilic cytoplasm. This tumor is extremely aggressive, being capable of metastasizing to regional lymph nodes and distant sites.

CYTOLOGIC FEATURES. Aspirates from papillary adenocarcinomas consist of solitary, mucus-containing cells and small groupings of such cells. The tumor cells are cuboidal or polygonal and have large nuclei. Signet-ring forms are also observed.[3]

We have not seen a case of carcinoma of the salivary duct diagnosed by needle aspiration biopsy, although a recent report described demonstration of such a tumor by this technique.[123] The neoplastic cells in the aspirate consisted largely of naked, round or oval nuclei. There was variation in nuclear size and coarse, unevenly distributed chromatin and one or two small nucleoli. The cytoplasm in some cells appeared vacuolated due to degeneration. No papillary structures were seen.

DIFFERENTIAL DIAGNOSIS. Aspirates from well-differentiated mucoepidermoid carcinoma may mimic those from papillary adenocarcinoma. However, in mucoepidermoid tumors, there usually are two cell populations, goblet-like glandular cells coexisting with intermediate and squamous cells. The goblet-like cells have foamy cytoplasm, unlike the vacuolated cytoplasm seen in papillary adenocarcinoma, which gives the cells a signet-ring appearance.

Adenocarcinoma ex pleomorphic adenoma may have similar appearance to adenocarcinoma of salivary glands and the two lesions may thus be difficult to distinguish on cytologic examination. This point was mentioned previously.

Clear-Cell Carcinoma

This rare tumor has been given a variety of names in the literature. Terms commonly used to describe such tumors include clear-cell adenoma,[124] clear-cell carcinoma,[125] glycogen-rich clear-cell tumor[126,127] and clear-cell myoepithelioma.[128] Most such lesions arise in the parotid gland, although some involve the submandibular and minor salivary glands. The mean age of patients at diagnosis is 60 years and the tumor is more common in women than in men. Tumors that appear encapsulated on gross inspection and are found to be composed of uniform cells on histologic examination are classified as adenomas[126,129] and those that have infiltrative tendencies, with nuclear atypia and necrosis, are regarded as malignant.[127] The clinical features of such lesions are similar to those of other carcinomas of the salivary glands. They may present as a painless mass or may be associated with facial nerve involvement and pain. Recurrence is not uncommon and regional lymph node metastasis has been documented.[127]

HISTOLOGIC FEATURES. Clear-cell carcinomas are composed of large cells with clear cytoplasm that contains glycogen. Solid variants have no discernible ductlike structures, whereas other types have glands lined by an inner, dark-staining layer of cells surrounded by clear-cell areas.

CYTOLOGIC FEATURES. Such tumors consist of round or polygonal cells that have clear cytoplasm. The nuclei may be uniform and round or slightly pleomorphic. Areas of necrosis may be identified. We have seen only one example of this lesion. The aspirate contained extensive areas of necrosis and only outlines of ghost cells were visible. A definitive diagnosis could not be made by examination of the smear alone. Histologic study revealed a glycogen-rich, clear-cell carcinoma that had extensive areas of necrosis. Metastases were found in the regional lymph nodes.

DIFFERENTIAL DIAGNOSIS. Acinic cell tumors, mucoepidermoid carcinoma with clear-cell areas, metastatic follicular carcinoma of the thyroid and renal cell carci-

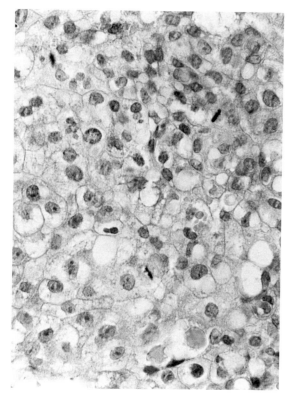

Fig. 2.100. Sebaceous carcinoma metastatic to parotid gland. Note the polygonal tumor cells that have foamy cytoplasm filled with vacuoles. Hematoxylin and eosin preparation. ×625.

noma must be considered in the differential diagnosis. It may be difficult to differentiate among these entities by cytologic study of needle aspirates.

Sebaceous Carcinoma

This invasive tumor is composed of sebaceous cells that have a variable degree of differentiation. Only 19 cases have been reported.[130] Such tumors occur in a wide age range, but the incidence peaks in the third and eighth decades. The tumor has no predilection for either sex. Patients usually present with a painful mass over the parotid gland and skin involvement.

HISTOLOGIC FEATURES. Sebaceous carcinomas are circumscribed, having pushing or infiltrative margins. They are firm and the cut surface is grayish white to grayish yellow. Such tumors are composed of lobules of variable size separated by fibrous septa. The lobules consist of sheets of sebaceous cells that have a variable degree of cytoplasmic vacuolation (Fig. 2.100). The nuclei are pleomorphic and have coarse chromatin and prominent nucleoli. Mitoses are a common finding. The vacuoles do not stain with mucicarmine but do stain with oil-red-O.

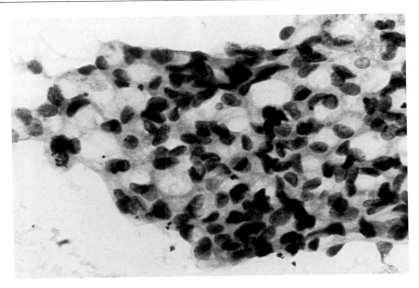

Fig. 2.101. Aspirate of a sebaceous carcinoma contains a sheet of poorly differentiated tumor cells. The cytoplasm, however, appears vacuolated. Papanicolaou preparation. ×625.

CYTOLOGIC FEATURES. We have not seen a primary sebaceous carcinoma of the salivary glands on needle aspiration biopsy cytology. However, we have seen two metastatic sebaceous carcinomas, one from the eyelid that involved the parotid region and one from the skin of the face that involved the submandibular area. Because the histologic features of primary carcinoma of the sebaceous glands of the parotid are similar to those of primary carcinoma of the sebaceous glands in the skin or of the meibomian glands of the eyelids, we will describe the cytologic features of these two cases.[131]

The aspirates were cellular, consisting of large aggregates of tumor cells, similar to the lobules seen on histologic examination. One smear contained small clusters and groupings of malignant tumor cells. The cells were large and had a moderate amount of cytoplasm and indistinct cell borders. The cytoplasm was finely reticulated and had a variable degree of vacuolation (Fig. 2.101). In the cell clusters, the nuclei of the tumor cells overlapped and contained coarse chromatin and prominent nucleoli. Tumor diastasis was seen in the background and necrosis and pyknosis of some cells was observed. Oil-red-O stain demonstrated intracellular globules of lipid material in the tumor cells.

DIFFERENTIAL DIAGNOSIS. Sebaceous carcinoma must be differentiated from poorly differentiated squamous cell carcinoma. Careful attention to nuclear detail helps make the diagnosis of a malignant process. In the cells of poorly differentiated squamous cell carcinoma, the cytoplasm is not as abundant as it is in the cells of sebaceous carcinoma. Moreover, the finely reticular to vacuolated nature of the cytoplasm in the cells of the latter tumor is a clue to the diagnosis. Distinction between primary sebaceous carcinoma of the parotid gland and metastatic sebaceous

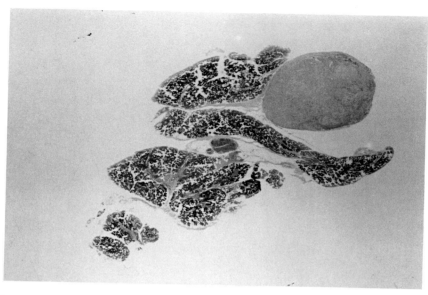

Fig. 2.102. Whole-mount section from a case of sebaceous carcinoma metastatic to an intraparotid lymph node. Hematoxylin and eosin preparation. ×4.

carcinoma is not possible on the basis of cytologic examination alone. The history and clinical findings should always be taken into account in such cases. In our patient who had parotid involvement, histologic examination of the resected parotid gland revealed metastasis confined to an intraparotid lymph node. This is illustrated in Figure 2.102.

Malignant Lymphoma

Involvement of the salivary glands by lymphoma may be primary[132] or secondary.[133] Primary lymphoma usually is associated with benign lymphoepithelial lesion[134,135] or Sjögren's syndrome.[136] Sjögren's syndrome is also associated with lymphoma that involves extrasalivary sites.[137] Lymphomas that occur in association with benign lymphoepithelial lesion and Sjögren's syndrome usually are B-cell lymphomas.[136] Lymphomas are occasionally associated with Warthin's tumor; this topic was discussed previously (page 60, Figs. 2.57 and 2.58). Non-Hodgkin's and Hodgkin's lymphomas may also develop primarily within intraparotid lymph nodes and later involve other lymphoid sites.[7,136] Such lesions may present as a parotid mass and distinction from primary tumors of the salivary glands depends on further investigations. Needle aspiration biopsy in this situation usually provides information that the clinician can use in planning management. Two of our salivary gland tumors presented in this fashion.[7]

Secondary involvement of the salivary glands by lymphoma and leukemia can occur during the course of generalized disease.[133] The diagnosis in most such cases can be confirmed by needle aspiration biopsy. Involvement of the salivary glands by lymphoma is a common occurrence in Africa. Wright[138] found such involvement in eight of 50 cases of Burkitt's lymphoma at autopsy. Involvement of the salivary glands is uncommon in North America, however. The reader is referred to Chapter 3 for the diagnosis and discussion of lymphomas.

Mesenchymal Tumors

Benign and malignant soft-tissue tumors have been reported in the salivary glands. The cytologic diagnosis of such neoplasms has rarely been reported. Mavec and associates[139] reported seven cases of benign mesenchymal tumors in a total of 274 histologically proven salivary gland tumors. Of these seven tumors, the aspirates were unsatisfactory in two cases; four cases were neurofibromas and one was a lipoma. Of the 91 primary malignant neoplasms, five were examples of malignant mesenchymal tumors. Of these five tumors, two were lymphomas and three were neurofibrosarcomas. The lymphomas were diagnosed correctly on cytologic examination and the neurofibrosarcomas were classified only as mesenchymal tumors.

Of the benign tumors, lipomas usually are not difficult to diagnose by aspiration biopsy cytology. In most cases, the aspirate consists of one or two transparent drops of fat that contain small clusters of fat cells with prominent cell borders and small, uniform, round or oval, eccentrically located nuclei. The cytologic features of other mesenchymal tumors are similar to those of tumors in other sites; this topic is discussed in greater detail in Chapter 4.

Metastatic Neoplasms

Carcinoma metastatic to the parotid gland is not uncommon, although involvement of the submandibular gland is an unusual occurrence. Involvement of the parotid gland usually results from metastases to the intraparotid lymph nodes.[140] Figure 2.102 shows a whole-mount section of a parotid gland with metastatic carcinoma in an intraparotid lymph node. Hematogenous metastases are rarely encountered. There are no lymph nodes in the submandibular and sublingual glands. The lymph nodes in and around the parotid glands drain lymph from the scalp, face, external ears, maxilla, nasopharynx, palate and tonsils. Enlarged lymph nodes in and around the parotid glands are difficult to differentiate clinically from primary tumors of these glands (Fig. 2.3). Aspiration biopsy cytology is an easy and reliable method for making the diagnosis. The two malignant lesions that most commonly metastasize to the parotid region are squamous cell carcinoma and malignant melanoma.[7] Metastases in the salivary glands less frequently are from carcinoma of the kidneys, stomach, breasts, lungs or pancreas[133,141,142] or from carcinoma of the sebaceous glands.[7]

Malignant Melanoma

Melanoma of the head or neck frequently metastasizes to the parotid lymph nodes.[7] Needle aspiration biopsy smears from such cases consist of numerous solitary, round or oval tumor cells (Fig. 2.103). The cells have a high nuclear to cytoplasmic ratio and round, centrally or eccentrically located nuclei. Binucleate forms may also be encountered. Nucleoli are usually prominent and a few cells have round, pale, cytoplasmic inclusions within the nuclei. Careful inspection may reveal golden

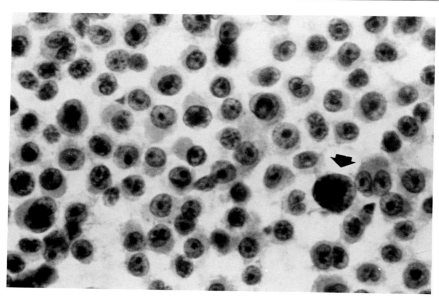

Fig. 2.103. Melanoma metastatic to an intraparotid lymph node. The aspirate consists of solitary tumor cells. Binucleate cells are also present. One cell (arrow) contains melanin. Hematoxylin and eosin preparation. ×625.

brown pigment within the cytoplasm. Occasionally, such tumors are heavily pigmented, many tumor cells containing melanin. Spindle cell, anaplastic giant-cell and small-cell undifferentiated patterns are also seen in aspirates from patients with malignant melanoma; this topic is discussed in greater detail in Chapter 3.

In one of our cases, metastatic melanoma was diagnosed even though the primary lesion had not been found.[7] Needle aspiration biopsy smears contained typical melanoma cells. Biopsy was followed by total parotidectomy and resection of adjacent lymph nodes. Histologic study revealed a large intraparotid lymph node completely replaced by metastatic melanoma. The primary lesion was never discovered and the patient died of widespread metastatic disease 42 months after diagnosis.

Squamous Cell Carcinoma

This lesion is the most common tumor that metastasizes in or near the salivary glands.[7,140] Most metastases in this region are from squamous cell carcinoma of the oral cavity, laryngopharyngeal area, nasopharynx or skin. Needle aspiration biopsy smears consist of numerous solitary and small collections of malignant squamous cells. The degree of differentiation is usually evident in the smears. The cytologic features of such tumors are similar to those of the primary tumors described on pages 94 to 96 and are illustrated in Chapter 3.

Other Tumors

The salivary glands may also be involved in cases of carcinoma of the sebaceous glands,[7] kidneys, stomach, breasts and lungs.[133,141,142] Needle aspiration biopsy smears from such cases reflect the histologic pattern of the primary tumor. The reader is referred to Chapter 3 for further discussion of this topic. When the salivary glands become involved by direct spread of a malignant tumor, the primary lesion is most likely a sarcoma.[143] Direct spread, however, is a rare occurrence.

DIAGNOSTIC PITFALLS

The examiner should be aware of the pitfalls of needle aspiration biopsy cytology of the salivary glands because many of the pitfalls can be avoided. A cytologic diagnosis should not be attempted on an inadequate aspirate. Experience in obtaining and preparing smears helps minimize the frequency of unsatisfactory specimens. Admixture with blood, poorly fixed and dried specimens and scanty material all may give rise to problems in interpretation. Sampling errors can occur and are more common in inexperienced hands. However, if there is a suspicious mass but needle aspiration biopsy cytology results in a nondiagnostic report, the lesion is reaspirated. In most cases, the second aspirate is usually diagnostic. If the second aspirate is not diagnostic and a malignant process is suspected on clinical grounds, surgical excision of the mass is mandatory. As was already emphasized, interpretative skills are gained only from experience with a large volume of material and from thorough knowledge of the normal and pathologic morphologic appearances of the salivary glands. The pitfalls that deserve special mention will now be briefly discussed.

Neoplasms That Simulate Cysts

A number of neoplasms in the salivary glands may be cystic and care has to be taken not to regard such lesions as simple retention cysts. Aspirates from cystic lesions should be sent to the cytology laboratory for interpretation. If any mass remains after aspiration or if the mass recurs, it should be reaspirated and the material sent for cytologic study. Table 2.3 lists the neoplasms of the salivary glands that can mimic cysts.

Cellular Atypia in Cytology Preparations

Mild to moderate atypia in the nuclei of a few cells in an otherwise benign aspirate compatible with pleomorphic adenoma should not be mistaken as evidence of a malignant process. Pleomorphism of epithelial cells is seen in about 5 percent of cases of pleomorphic adenoma and care should be exercised in not overdiagnosing such lesions as malignant. In cases of carcinoma ex pleomorphic adenoma, the smear contains not only frankly malignant cells but also necrotic debris in the background, evidence of an infiltrative, destructive lesion.

Oncocytic cells may have mild to moderate nuclear atypia and yet not be malignant. Such cells are usually found in Warthin's tumor and in oncocytic adenoma. They are occasionally seen in pleomorphic adenoma. In Warthin's tumor, the amorphous, cellular debris seen in the background along with lymphocytes points to the diagnosis. Malignant change is rarely encountered in cases of oncocytoma and the chance of detecting such a change on needle aspiration biopsy cytology is extremely small. Distinction between benign and malignant oncocytes by needle aspiration biopsy is difficult.

In the follow-up of surgically resected lesions or after radiotherapy, localized thickening occasionally develops in the scar tissue or deeper down. In such cases, the examiner must be careful not to mistake fibroblasts that have atypical and bizarre nuclear changes for malignant cells. Moreover, radiotherapy also results in atypical changes in the epithelial lining cells of the salivary ducts and such changes may mimic a malignant lesion.

Basaloid Tumors

Differentiation among basal cell adenoma, adenoid cystic carcinoma and undifferentiated carcinoma is sometimes difficult. The finding of acellular, hyaline material or mucoid globules is diagnostic of adenoid cystic carcinoma. However, as was noted previously, in poorly differentiated tumors, one has to rely on nuclear abnormalities to arrive at the diagnosis. Similarly, small-cell undifferentiated tumors may be difficult to diagnose.

Mucoepidermoid Tumors

Differentiation of low-grade tumors from Warthin's tumor, mucocele, necrotizing sialometaplasia and adenomatoid hyperplasia of the salivary glands has already been discussed. A recent report that described adenomatoid hyperplasia of the minor salivary glands of the palate, which was initially diagnosed as low-grade mucoepidermoid carcinoma, emphasizes the importance of a correct diagnosis because of its therapeutic and prognostic implications.[146] In the major salivary glands this should not pose any difficulty because adenomatoid hyperplasia occurs in the mucus-secreting minor salivary glands. High-grade mucoepidermoid carcinoma masquerades as undifferentiated or poorly differentiated squamous cell carcinoma because glandular cells are difficult to identify in such lesions without the use of mucin stains. If poorly differentiated tumor cells are seen in aspirates from the salivary glands and no primary tumor can be found, the slide should be decolorized and restained with mucicarmine or alcian blue stain to look for mucin in the tumor cells.

Lymphocytes in Smears

A large number of lymphocytes in the smears can pose a diagnostic problem. Table 2.7 lists the lesions in which lymphocytes are encountered. In chronic sialadenitis, lymphocytes usually are not numerous and a mixture of cell types is present. Lymphoepithelial lesions may mimic lymphoma and if there are no epithelial cells, differentiation relies on the characteristics of the lymphoreticular cells. In lymphoepithelial lesions, there usually is a mixture of cell types and small aggregates of elongated, epithelioid histiocytes may be encountered. Warthin's tumor usually consists of sheets of oncocytic cells with a mixture of lymphocytes and cellular debris in the background. Reactive follicular hyperplasia of the lymph nodes usually is not difficult to diagnose because in most cases, a polymorphous infiltrate is seen along with tingible-body histiocytes. Aspirates from granulomatous lesions contain the characteristic elongated, epithelioid cells in loose clusters and multinucleated cells may also be observed. In lymphoma, there is a monomorphic pattern, whereas the diagnosis of Hodgkin's disease requires the identification of Reed-Sternberg cells. This topic is discussed in greater detail in Chapter 3.

COMPLICATIONS OF ASPIRATION BIOPSY CYTOLOGY

Needle aspiration biopsy cytology is a safe technique that is associated with no major complication. Severe patient discomfort or formation of salivary fistulas or hematomas has not occurred in any of our cases.[7] No complication occurred in the series reported by Frable,[5] but Mavec and colleagues[139] reported a few small hematomas in their series of 652 aspirations. The danger of seeding of tumor cells in the needle tract or in the puncture site in the skin was investigated by Engzell and associates.[145] These authors found no recurrence involving the skin or the site of the needle puncture in 157 patients with pleomorphic adenoma who were treated surgically and followed up for 10 years. In another report involving seven pleomorphic adenomas, histologic examination of the area surrounding the surgical excision, including serial sections of the needle tract after needle aspiration biopsy, also failed to demonstrate tumor seeding.[38] If there is concern that tumor cells may be implanted along the needle tract, the puncture site can be tatooed and excised at the time of operation. Tatooing and excision were performed in most of our cases of parotid tumors; subsequent histologic examination of the excised needle tract and puncture site failed to show evidence of tumor implantation. We are not aware of any reports of local tumor implantation caused by fine-needle aspiration biopsy of the salivary glands, although the use of large-bore needles has led to this complication in other sites.

Dissemination of tumor cells through vascular channels is a potential danger of needle aspiration biopsy. However, experiments in rabbits suggest that needling does not result in release of cancer cells into lymph nodes and the bloodstream[145] and certainly the risk of dissemination of tumor cells via the bloodstream or by implantation is much less with needle aspiration biopsy than with open biopsy, which is the approach still used by some surgeons.

RESULTS OF ASPIRATION BIOPSY CYTOLOGY

We previously reported our experience with needle aspiration biopsy cytology of the salivary glands.[9] In our hands, the overall diagnostic accuracy of this technique was 97.9 percent. There was no false-positive diagnosis, making the technique's specificity 100 percent. The diagnostic accuracy for malignant neoplasms was 87.5 percent. There were three false-negative diagnoses: a metastatic squamous cell carcinoma, a non-Hodgkin's lymphoma and a Hodgkin's lymphoma that involved the intraparotid lymph nodes. Tables 2.17, 2.18 and 2.19 summarize our updated expe-

TABLE 2.17. Fine-Needle Aspiration Biopsy Cytology: Benign Neoplasms of the Salivary Glands

Pathologic Diagnosis	Number of Cases	ABC Diagnosis		
		Diagnostic	Benign	Malignant
Pleomorphic adenoma	79	73	4	2
Monomorphic adenoma	5	4	1	—
Warthin's tumor	17	15	2	—
Total	101	92	7	2

TABLE 2.18. Fine-Needle Aspiration Biopsy Cytology: Primary Malignant Neoplasms of the Salivary Glands

Pathologic Diagnosis	Number of Cases	ABC Diagnosis		
		Diagnostic	Benign	Malignant
Adenoid cystic carcinoma	7	7	—	—
Acinar cell carcinoma	7	5	1	1
Mucoepidermoid carcinoma	6	3	1	2
Squamous carcinoma	2	2	—	—
Adenocarcinoma	3	2	—	1
Undifferentiated carcinoma	1	1	—	—
Carcinoma ex pleomorphic adenoma	1	—	—	1
Non-Hodgkin's lymphoma arising in Warthin's tumor	1	1	—	—
Total	28	21	2	5

TABLE 2.19. Fine-Needle Aspiration Biopsy Cytology: Neoplasms Metastatic to the Salivary Glands and Intraparotid Lymph Nodes

Pathologic Diagnosis	Number of Cases	ABC Diagnosis		
		Diagnostic	Benign	Malignant
Squamous cell carcinoma	14	13	1	—
Malignant melanoma	4	4	—	—
Sebaceous carcinoma	2	2	—	—
Merkel cell carcinoma	1	1	—	—
Poorly differentiated carcinoma	2	2	—	—
Waldenström's macro-globulinemia	1	1	—	—
Malignant lymphoma	1	—	1	—
Hodgkin's disease	1	—	1	—
Total	26	23	3	—

TABLE 2.20. Fine-Needle Aspiration Biopsy Cytology: Benign Tumors of the Salivary Glands—Diagnostic Accuracy of Selected Reports

Authors	Type of Lesion	Number of Cases	Diagnostic Accuracy* of ABC (percent)
Eneroth and Zajicek	Benign mixed tumor	316	92.4
Persson et al.	Benign tumor of salivary glands	150	97.4
Webb	Benign tumor of salivary glands	24	95.8
Sismanis et al.	Benign tumor of salivary glands	18	72.2
Frable	Benign tumor of salivary glands	49	98.0
Layfield et al.	Benign tumor of salivary glands	71	82.0

*Specific Histologic Diagnosis.

rience with benign and malignant tumors of the salivary glands. The current results are similar to those published previously. The diagnostic accuracy for benign neoplasms is about 98 percent. For primary malignant tumors, it is 93 percent, and for metastatic tumors, it is 88 percent. Table 2.20 summarizes the results of needle aspiration biopsy in the cytologic diagnosis of benign tumors and Table 2.21 the results for malignant tumors from selected reports.[2,4-6,8,38] The difficulties encountered in the diagnosis of malignant neoplasms of the salivary glands have been

TABLE 2.21. Fine-Needle Aspiration Biopsy Cytology: Malignant Tumors of the Salivary Glands—Diagnostic Accuracy of Selected Reports

Authors	Type of Lesion	Number of Cases	Diagnostic Accuracy* of ABC (percent)
Persson et al.	Malignant tumor of salivary glands	33	69.7
Webb	Primary and metastatic tumors of salivary glands	13	92.3
Sismanis et al.	Malignant tumor of salivary glands	17	64.7
Frable	Malignant tumor of salivary glands	32	84.3
Layfield et al.	Malignant tumor of salivary glands	51	74.0

*Specific Histologic Diagnosis.

reviewed by Zajicek.[3] Before 1963, the diagnostic accuracy for malignant tumors was low (31 percent). However, with increasing experience, the diagnostic accuracy has improved, so that from 1963 to 1967, 82 percent of the malignant tumors were diagnosed as malignant and 63 percent were identified by type on histologic examination. Since 1967, the diagnostic accuracy has increased still further, so that virtually all carcinomas of the salivary glands are now correctly diagnosed at the Radiumhemmet.[3] Zajicek has emphasized that experience is essential because a wide variety of tumors occur in the salivary glands. Once the necessary experience and skill have been acquired, the diagnostic accuracy of needle aspiration biopsy cytology approaches that of surgical pathology.

REFERENCES

1. Eneroth CM, Franzen S, Zajicek J: Cytologic diagnosis on aspirates from 1000 salivary gland tumours. *Acta Oto-Laryngol Suppl* 224:168–172, 1967.

2. Persson PS, Zettergren L: Cytologic diagnosis of salivary gland tumours by aspiration biopsy. *Acta Cytol* 17:351–354, 1973.

3. Zajicek J: Aspiration biopsy cytology. Part I. Cytology of supradiaphragmatic organs. *Monogr Clin Cytol* 4:30–65, 1974.

4. Webb AJ: Cytologic diagnosis of salivary gland lesions in adult and pediatric surgical patients. *Acta Cytol* 17:51–58, 1973.

5. Frable WJ: *Thin Needle Aspiration Biopsy.* Philadelphia, Saunders, 1983, pp 119–151.

6. Sismanis A, Merriam JM, Kline TS, et al: Diagnosis of salivary gland tumours by fine needle aspiration biopsy. *Head Neck Surg* 3:482–489, 1981.

7. O'Dwyer P, Farrar WB, James AG, et al: Needle aspiration biopsy of major salivary gland tumours. *Cancer (Philadelphia)* 57:554–557, 1986.

8. Layfield LJ, Tan P, Glasgow BJ: Fine needle aspiration of salivary gland lesions. *Arch Pathol Lab Med* 111:346–353, 1987.

9. Qizilbash AH, Sianos J, Young JEM, et al: Fine needle aspiration biopsy cytology of major salivary glands. *Acta Cytol* 29:503–512, 1985.

10. Sisson GA, Sommers GW: Branchiogenic cysts within the parotid gland. *Arch Otolaryngol* 96:165–167, 1972.

11. Batsakis JG: *Tumours of Head and Neck.* Baltimore, Williams & Wilkins, 1979, pp 55–67.

12. Donohue WB, Bolden TE: Tuberculosis of the salivary glands: A collective review. *Oral Surg* 14:576–588, 1961.

13. Hammer JE, Scofield HH: Cervical lymphadenopathy and parotid gland swelling in sarcoidosis: A study of 31 cases. *J Amer Dent Assoc* 74:1224–1230, 1967.

14. Miglets AW, Viall JH, Kataria YP: Sarcoidosis of the head and neck. *Laryngoscope* 87:2038–2048, 1977.

15. Tarpley TM Jr, Anderson L, Lightbody P, et al: Minor salivary gland involvement in sarcoidosis. *Oral Surg* 33:755–762, 1972.

16. Qizilbash AH, Elavathil LJ, Chen V, et al: Aspiration biopsy cytology of lymph nodes in malignant lymphoma. *Diagn Cytopathol* 1:18–22, 1985.

17. Godwin JT: Benign lymphoepithelial lesion of the parotid gland. *Cancer (Philadelphia)* 5:1089–1103, 1952.

18. Mikulicz J: Uber eine eigenartige symmetrische erkrarkung der thranen-und mund-speich eldrusen, in *Bertrage zur Chururgie-Festschrift Gewidmet Theodor Billroth.* Stuttgart, Enke, 1982, pp 610–630.

19. Font RL, Yanoff M, Zimmerman LE: Benign lymphoepithelial lesion of the lacrimal gland and its relationship to Sjögren's syndrome. *Amer J Clin Pathol* 48:365–376, 1967.

20. Waldron CA: The histopathology of Sjögren's syndrome in labial salivary gland biopsies. *Oral Surg* 37:217–229, 1974.

21. Azzopardi JG, Evans TJ: Malignant lymphoma of parotid associated with Mikulicz's disease (benign lymphoepithelial lesion). *J Clin Pathol* 24:744–752, 1971.

22. Batsakis JG, Bernacki EG, Rice DH, et al: Malignancy and the benign lymphoepithelial lesion. *Laryngoscope* 85:389–399, 1975

23. Schmid U, Helborn D, Lennert K: Development of malignant lymphoma in myoepithelial sialadenitis (Sjögren's syndrome). *Virchows Arch A* 395:11–43, 1982.

24. Arthaud JB: Anaplastic parotid carcinoma ("malignant lymphoepithelial lesion") in seven Alaskan natives. *Amer J Clin Pathol* 57:275–286, 1972.

25. Wallace AC, MacDougall JT, Hildes JA, et al: Salivary gland tumours in Canadian Eskimos. *Cancer (Philadelphia)* 16:1338–1353, 1963.

26. Leegaard J, Lindman H: Salivary gland tumours: Clinical picture and treatment. *Acta Oto-Laryngol* 263:155–159, 1970.

27. Davies JNP, Dodge OG, Burkitt DP: Salivary gland tumors in Uganda. *Cancer (Philadelphia)* 17:1310–1322, 1964.

28. Thackray AC: Salivary gland tumours. *Proc R Soc Med* 61:1089–1090, 1968.

29. Batsakis JG, Regezi JA: The pathology of head and neck tumours: Salivary glands. Part I. *Head Neck Surg* 1:59–68, 1978.

30. Eversole LR: Histogenetic classification of salivary tumours. *Arch Pathol* 92:433–443, 1970.

31. Evans RW, Cruickshank AH: *Epithelial Tumours of the Salivary Glands.* Philadelphia, Saunders, 1970, pp. 11–26.

32. Deppisch LM, Toker C: Mixed tumors of the parotid gland. An ultrastructural study. *Cancer (Philadelphia)* 24:174–184, 1969.

33. Kondo T, Muragishi H, Imaizumi M: A cell line from a human salivary gland mixed tumor. *Cancer (Philadelphia)* 27:403–410, 1971.

34. Hubner G, Klein HJ, Kleinsasser O, et al: Role of myoepithelial cells in the development of salivary gland tumors. *Cancer (Philadelphia)* 27:1255–1261, 1971.

35. Mylius EA: The identification and the role of the myoepithelial cell in salivary gland tumors. *Acta Pathol Microbiol Scand* 50 (Suppl 139):1–81, 1960.

36. David R, Buchner A: Elastosis in benign and malignant salivary gland tumors. A histochemical and ultrastructural study. *Cancer (Philadelphia)* 45:2301–2310, 1980.

37. Dardick I, van Nostrand AWP, Jeans MTD, et al: Pleomorphic adenoma. I. Ultrastructural organization of "epithelial" regions. *Hum Pathol* 14:780–797, 1983.

38. Eneroth CM, Zajicek J: Aspiration biopsy of salivary gland tumours. III. Morphologic studies on smears and histologic sections from 368 mixed tumors. *Acta Cytol* 10:440–454, 1966.

39. Bottles K, Lowhagen T: Psammoma bodies in the aspiration cytology smears of an acinic cell tumour. *Acta Cytol* 27:191–192, 1985.

40. Bottles K, Ferrell LD, Miller TR: Tyrosine crystals in fine needle aspirates of a pleomorphic adenoma of the parotid gland. *Acta Cytol* 28:490–492, 1984.

41. Schultenover SJ, MacDonald EC, Ramsay I: Hyaline cell pleomorphic adenoma. Diagnosis by fine needle aspiration biopsy. *Acta Cytol* 28:593–597, 1984.

42. Thackray AC, Sobin LH: *Histologic Typing of Salivary Gland Tumours*. Geneva, World Health Organization, 1972, pp 20–22.

43. Allegra SR: Warthin's tumour: A hypersensitivity disease? *Hum Pathol* 2:403–420, 1971.

44. Chaudhry AP, Gorlin RJ: Papillary cystadenoma lymphomatosum (adenolymphoma). *Amer J Surg* 95:923–931, 1958.

45. Veronesi U, Corbetta L: Adenolymphoma of the lower lip. *Acta Oto-Laryngol* 52:1–6, 1960.

46. Kavka SJ: Bilateral simultaneous Warthin's tumors. *Arch Otolaryngol* 91:302, 1970.

47. David R, Buckner A: Corpora amylacea in adenolymphoma (Warthin's tumor). *Amer J Clin Pathol* 69:173–175, 1978.

48. Bottles K, Lowhagen T, Miller TR: Mast cells in the aspiration cytology differential diagnosis of adenolymphoma. *Acta Cytol* 29:513–515, 1985.

49. Kuhn AJ: Cystadenoma of the parotid gland and larynx. *Arch Otolaryngol* 73:404–406, 1961.

50. Palma O, Torri AM, deCristofaro JA, et al: Fine needle aspiration cytology in two cases of well differentiated acinic cell carcinoma of the parotid glands. Discussion of diagnostic criteria. *Acta Cytol* 29:516–521, 1985.

51. Meza-Chavez L: Oxyphilic granular cell adenoma of the parotid gland (oncocytoma). Report of 5 cases and study of oxyphilic granular cells (oncocytes in normal parotid gland). *Amer J Pathol* 25:523–538, 1949.

52. Beltaos E, Maurer WJ: Oncocytoma of the submaxillary salivary gland. *Arch Otolaryngol* 84:193–197, 1966.

53. Cohen MA, Batsakis JG: Oncocytic tumours (oncocytomas) of minor salivary glands. *Arch Otolaryngol* 88:97–99, 1968.

54. Blanck C, Eneroth CM, Jacobsson PA: Oncocytoma of the parotid gland: Neoplasm or nodular hyperplasia? *Cancer (Philadelphia)* 25:919–925, 1970.

55. Gray SR, Cornog JL, Seo IS: Oncocytic neoplasms of salivary glands. Report of 15 cases including two malignant oncocytomas. *Cancer (Philadelphia)* 38:1306–1317, 1976.

56. Eneroth CM, Zajicek J: Aspiration biopsy of salivary gland tumours. II. Morphologic studies on smears and histologic sections from oncocytic tumours (45 cases of papillary cystadenoma lymphomatosum and 4 cases of oncocytoma). *Acta Cytol* 9:355–361, 1965.

57. Evans RW, Cruickshank AH: *Epithelial Tumours of the Salivary Glands*. Philadelphia, Saunders, 1970, pp 58–76.

58. Headington JT, Batsakis JG, Beals, FF, et al: Membranous basal cell adenoma of parotid gland, dermal cylindromas and trichoepitheliomas: Comparative histochemistry and ultrastructure. *Cancer (Philadelphia)* 39:2640–2649, 1977.

59. Kleinsasser O, Klein HJ: Basalze iladenone der speicheldrusen. *Arch Klin Exp Ohren Nasen Kehlkopfheilkd* 189:301–316, 1967.

60. Batsakis JG: Basal cell adenoma of the parotid gland. *Cancer (Philadelphia)* 29:226–230, 1972.

61. Conley J, Dingman DL: Adenoid cystic carcinoma in the head and neck (cylindroma). *Arch Otolaryngol* 100:81–90, 1974.

62. Fantasia JE, Neville BW: Basal cell adenomas of the minor salivary glands. *Oral Surg* 50:433–440, 1980.

63. Crumpler C, Scharfenberg JC, Reid RJ: Monomorphic adenomas of salivary glands: Trabecular-tubular, canalicular and basaloid variants. *Cancer (Philadelphia)* 38:198–200, 1976.

64. Hood IC, Qizilbash AH, Salama SS, et al: Basal cell adenoma of parotid. Difficulty of differentiation from adenoid cystic carcinoma on aspiration biopsy. *Acta Cytol* 27:515–520, 1983.

65. Batsakis JG, Brannon RB: Dermal analogue tumours of major salivary glands. *J Laryngol Otol* 95:155–164, 1981.

66. Reingold IM, Keasbey LE, Graham JH: Multicentric dermal-type cylindromas of the parotid gland in a patient with florid turbid tumour. *Cancer (Philadelphia)* 40:1702–1710, 1977.

67. Zajicek J: Aspiration biopsy cytology. Part I. Cytology of supradiaphragmatic organs. *Monogr Clin Cytol* 4:37–39, 1974.

68. Corridan M: Glycogen-rich clear cell adenoma of the parotid gland. *J Pathol Bacteriol* 72:623–627, 1956.

69. Batsakis JG: Clear cell tumours of salivary glands. *Ann Otol Rhinol Laryngol* 89:196–197, 1980.

70. Gnepp DR: Sebaceous neoplasms of salivary gland origin. A review. *Pathol Annu* 18:71–102, 1983.

71. Wassan SM: Sebaceous lymphadenoma of parotid gland. *Cancer (Philadelphia)* 28:1019–1022, 1971.

72. Rawson AJ, Horn RC: Sebaceous glands and sebaceous gland-containing tumours of the parotid salivary gland. *Surgery* 27:93–101, 1950.

73. Zajicek J: Aspiration biopsy cytology. Part I. Cytology of supradiaphragmatic organs. *Monogr Clin Cytol* 4:40–42, 1974.

74. Billroth T: Beobachtungen uber geschwulste der speichisdersen. *Virchows Arch A* 17:357–375, 1859.

75. Batsakis JG, Regezi JA: The pathology of head and neck tumours: Salivary glands part 4. *Head Neck Surg* 1:340–349, 1979.

76. Spiro RH, Huvos AG, Strong EW: Adenoid cystic carcinoma of salivary origin. A clinicopathologic study of 242 cases. *Amer J Surg* 128:512–520, 1974.

77. Conley J, Dingman DL: Adenoid cystic carcinoma in the head and neck (cylindroma). *Arch Otolaryngol* 100:81–90, 1974.

78. Eby LS, Johnson DS, Baker HW: Adenoid cystic carcinoma of the head and neck. *Cancer (Philadelphia)* 29:1160–1168, 1972.

79. Tandler B: Ultrastructure of adenoid cystic carcinoma. *Lab Invest* 24:504–512, 1971.

80. Eneroth CM, Zajicek J: Aspiration biopsy of salivary gland tumours. IV. Morphologic studies on smears and histologic sections from 45 cases of adenoid cystic carcinoma. *Acta Cytol* 13:59–63, 1969.

81. Hood IC, Qizilbash AH, Salama SSS, et al: Basal cell adenoma of parotid. Difficulty of differentiation from adenoid cystic carcinoma on aspiration biopsy. *Acta Cytol* 27:515–520, 1983.

82. Geisinger KR, Reynolds GD, Vance RP, et al: Adenoid cystic carcinoma arising in a pleomorphic adenoma of the parotid gland. An aspiration cytology and ultrastructural study. *Acta Cytol* 29:522–526, 1985.

83. Zajicek J: Aspiration biopsy cytology. Part I. Cytology of supradiaphragmatic organs. *Monogr Clin Cytol* 4:37–39, 1974.

84. Anderson RJ, Johnston WW, Szpak CA: Fine needle aspiration of adenoid cystic carcinoma metastatic to the lung. Cytologic features and differential diagnosis. *Acta Cytol* 29:528–532, 1985.

85. Stewart FW, Foote FW, Becker WF: Mucoepidermoid tumours of the salivary gland. *Ann Surg* 122:820–844, 1945.

86. Eneroth CM, Hjertman L, Soderberg G: Mucoepidermoid carcinomas of the salivary gland. *Acta Oto-Laryngol* 73:68–74, 1972.

87. Healey WV, Perzin KH, Smith L: Mucoepidermoid carcinoma of salivary gland origin. *Cancer (Philadelphia)* 26:368–388, 1970.

88. Krolls SO, Trodahl JN, Boyers RC: Salivary gland lesions in children. *Cancer (Philadelphia)* 30:459–469, 1972.

89. Thorvaldsson SE, Beahrs OH, Woolner LP, et al: Mucoepidermoid tumours of the major salivary glands. *Amer J Surg* 120:432–438, 1970.

90. Spiro RH, Huvos AG, Strong EW: Cancer of the parotid gland. A clinicopathological study of 288 primary cases. *Amer J Surg* 130:452–459, 1975.

91. Zajicek J, Eneroth CM, Jakobsson P: Aspiration biopsy of salivary gland tumours. VI. Morphologic studies on smears and histologic sections from mucoepidermoid carcinoma. *Acta Cytol* 20:35–41, 1976.

92. Spark RP, Duncan BG: Necrotizing sialometaplasia. *Ann Otol Rhinol Laryngol* 87:409–411, 1978.

93. Arafat A, Brannon RB, Ellis GL: Adenomatoid hyperplasia of mucus salivary glands. *Oral Surg* 52:51–55, 1981.

94. Cornog JL, Gray SR: Surgical and clinical pathology of salivary gland tumours, in Rankow RM, Polayes IM (eds): *Diseases of the Salivary Glands*. Philadelphia, Saunders, 1976, pp 99–142.

95. Abrams AM, Cornyn J, Scofield HH, et al: Acinic cell adenocarcinoma of the major salivary glands. *Cancer (Philadelphia)* 18:1145–1162, 1965.

96. Batsakis JG, Chinn E, Weimert TA, et al: Acinic cell carcinoma. A clinicopathologic study of 35 cases. *J Laryngol Otol* 93:325–340, 1979.

97. Chong GC, Beahrs OH, Woolner LB: Surgical treatment of acinic cell carcinoma of the parotid glands. *Surg Gynecol Obstet* 138:65–68, 1974.

98. Batsakis JG, Chinn E, Regezi JA, et al: The pathology of head and neck tumours: Salivary glands part II. *Head Neck Surg* 1:167–180, 1978.

99. Hanson TA: Acinic cell carcinoma of the parotid gland presenting as a cyst. *Cancer (Philadelphia)* 36:570–575, 1975.

100. Palma O, Torri AM, deCristofaro JA, et al: Fine needle aspiration cytology in two cases of well differentiated acinic cell carcinoma of the parotid glands. Discussion of diagnostic criteria. *Acta Cytol* 29:516–521, 1985.

101. Bottles K, Lowhagen T: Psammoma bodies in the aspiration cytology smears of an acinic cell tumour. *Acta Cytol* 29:191–192, 1985.

102. LiVolsi VA, Perzin KH: Malignant mixed tumours arising in salivary glands. 1. Carcinomas arising in benign mixed tumours. A clinicopathologic study. *Cancer (Philadelphia)* 39:2209–2239, 1977.

103. Gerughty RM, Scofield HH, Brown FM, et al: Malignant mixed tumours of salivary gland origin. *Cancer (Philadelphia)* 24:471–486, 1969.

104. Eneroth CM, Zajicek J: Aspiration biopsy of salivary gland tumours. III. Morphologic studies of smears and histologic sections from 368 mixed tumours. *Acta Cytol* 10:440–454, 1966.

105. Frable WJ: *Thin Needle Aspiration Biopsy.* Philadelphia, Saunders, 1983, pp 133–135.

106. Geisinger KR, Reynolds GD, Vance RP, et al: Adenoid cystic carcinoma arising in a pleomorphic adenoma of the parotid gland. An aspiration cytology and ultrastructural study. *Acta Cytol* 29:522–526, 1985.

107. Linsk JA, Franzen S, Terrone-Donnorso R: Aspiration biopsy cytology of the salivary glands, in Linsk JA, Franzen S (eds): *Clinical Aspiration Cytology.* Philadelphia, Lippincott, 1983, pp 85–104.

108. Batsakis JG: *Tumours of Head and Neck.* Baltimore, Williams & Wilkins, 1979, pp 26–30.

109. LiVolski VA, Perzin KH: Malignant mixed tumors arising in salivary glands. l. Carcinomas arising in benign mixed tumours. A clinicopathologic study. *Cancer (Philadelphia)* 39:2209–2239, 1977.

110. Chen KTK: Metastasizing pleomorphic adenoma of the salivary gland. *Cancer (Philadelphia)* 42:2407–2411, 1978.

111. Koss LG, Woyke S, Olszewski W: *Aspiration Biopsy. Cytologic Interpretation and Histologic Bases.* Tokyo, Igaku-Shoin, 1984, pp 214–220.

112. Linsk JA, Franzen S, Terrone-Donnorso R: Aspiration biopsy cytology of the salivary glands, in Linsk JA, Franzen S (eds): *Clinical Aspiration Cytology.* Philadelphia, Lippincott, 1983, pp 85–104.

113. Batsakis JG, McCaltchey KD, Johns M, et al: Primary squamous cell carcinoma of the parotid gland. *Arch Otolaryngol* 102:355–357, 1976.

114. Evans RW, Cruickshank AH: *Epithelial Tumours of Salivary Glands.* Philadelphia, Saunders, 1970, pp 253–254.

115. Spiro RH, Huvos AG, Strong EW: Cancer of the parotid gland. A clinicopathological study of 288 primary cases. *Amer J Surg* 130:452–459, 1975.

116. Evans RW, Cruickshank AH: *Epithelial Tumors of Salivary Glands.* Philadelphia, Saunders, 1970, pp 242–244.

117. Koss LG, Spiro RH, Hajdu S: Small cell (oat cell) carcinoma of minor salivary gland origin. *Cancer (Philadelphia)* 30:737–741, 1972.

118. Wirman JA, Battifora HA: Small cell undifferentiated carcinoma of salivary gland origin. *Cancer (Philadelphia)* 37:1840–1848, 1976.

119. Edwards EG: Tumours of minor salivary glands. *Amer J Clin Pathol* 34:455–463, 1960.

120. Spiro RH, Koss LG, Hajdu S, et al: Tumours of minor salivary gland origin. A clinicopathologic study of 492 cases. *Cancer (Philadelphia)* 31:117–129, 1973.

121. Eneroth CM: Histologic and clinical aspects of parotid tumours. *Acta Oto-Laryngol Suppl* 191:5–99, 1964.

122. Chen KTK, Hafez GR: Infiltrating salivary duct carcinoma. A clinicopathologic study of five cases. *Arch Otolaryngol* 107:37–39, 1981.

123. Rivka G, Strauss M, Zohar Y, et al: Salivary duct carcinoma of the parotid gland. Cytologic and histopathologic study. *Acta Cytol* 29:454–456, 1985.

124. Perzin KH: Systemic approach to the pathologic diagnosis of salivary gland tumours. *Progr Surg Pathol* 4:137–179, 1982.

125. Echevarria RA: Ultrastructure of acinic cell carcinoma and clear cell carcinoma of the parotid gland. *Cancer (Philadelphia)* 20:563–571, 1967.

126. Corridan M: Glycogen-rich clear cell adenoma of the parotid. *J Pathol Bacteriol* 72:623–627, 1956.

127. Mohamed AH: Ultrastructure of glycogen-rich clear cell carcinoma of the palate. *J Oral Pathol* 5:103–121, 1976.

128. Batsakis JG: Clear cell tumours of salivary glands. *Ann Otol Rhinol Laryngol* 89:196–197, 1980.

129. Goldman RL, Klein HZ: Glycogen-rich adenoma of the parotid gland. An uncommon benign clear cell tumour resembling certain clear cell carcinomas of salivary origin. *Cancer (Philadelphia)* 30:749–754, 1972.

130. Gnepp DR: Sebaceous neoplasms of salivary gland origin. A review. *Pathol Annu* 18:71–102, 1983.

131. Hood IC, Qizilbash AH, Salama SSS, et al: Needle aspiration cytology of sebaceous carcinoma. *Acta Cytol* 28:305–312, 1984.

132. Schmid U, Helbron D, Lennert K: Primary malignant lymphoma localized in salivary glands. *Histopathology* 6:673–687, 1982.

133. Patey DH, Thackray AC, Keeling DH: Malignant disease of the parotid. *Brit J Cancer* 19:712–737, 1965.

134. Azzopardi JG, Evans DJ: Malignant lymphoma of parotid associated with Mikulicz's disease (benign lymphoepithelial lesion). *J Clin Pathol* 24:744–752, 1971.

135. Batsakis JG, Bernacki EG, Rice DH, et al: Malignancy and the benign lymphoepithelial lesion. *Laryngoscope* 85:389–399, 1975.

136. Schmid U, Helbron D, Lennert K: Development of malignant lymphoma in myo-epithelial sialadenitis (Sjogren's syndrome). *Virchows Arch A* 395:11–43, 1982.

137. Pinkus GS, Dekker A: Benign lymphoepithelial lesion of parotid glands associated with reticulum cell carcinoma. *Cancer (Philadelphia)* 25:121–127, 1970.

138. Wright DH: Burkitt's tumour. A post-mortem study of 50 cases. *Brit J Surg* 51:245–251, 1964.

139. Mavec P, Eneroth CM, Franzen S, et al: Aspiration biopsy of salivary gland tumours. I. Correlation of cytologic reports from 652 aspirations with clinical and histologic findings. *Acta Oto-Laryngol* 58:472–484, 1964.

140. Conley J, Arena S: Parotid gland as a focus of metastasis. *Arch Surg* 87:757–764, 1963.

141. Januska JR, Leban HS: Pulmonary metastasis to the submandibular gland. *J Oral Surg* 36:50–51, 1978.

142. Yarington CT Jr: Metastatic malignant disease to the parotid gland. *Laryngoscope* 91:517–519, 1981.

143. Evans RW, Cruickshank AH: *Epithelial Tumours of the Salivary Glands.* Philadelphia, Saunders, 1970, 276.

144. Aufdemorte TB, Ramsay I, Holt GR, et al: Focal adenomatoid hyperplasia of salivary glands. A differential diagnostic problem in fine-needle aspiration biopsy. *Acta Cytol* 29:23–28, 1985.

145. Engzell U, Esposti PL, Rubio C, et al: Investigation on tumour spread in connection with aspiration biopsy. *Acta Radiol* 10:385–398, 1971.

3

Lymph Nodes

INTRODUCTION

One of the earliest reports of lymph node aspiration was by Greig and Gray[1] in 1904 for the identification of trypanosomes in a patient with clinical suspicion of sleeping sickness. Subsequently, Guthrie[2] used lymph node puncture in the diagnosis of various diseases, including lymphoma, leukemia and metastatic carcinoma. Despite its introduction in the 1930s at the Memorial Hospital, New York,[3,4] the technique of aspiration biopsy did not gain widespread popularity in North America until recently. Today, aspiration biopsy has an important role in the investigation of patients with lymphadenopathy at any site. Its primary purpose is to confirm the existence of a malignant process, either primary[5-13] or metastatic,[4,5,13-19] although it also has an important role in the diagnosis of various inflammatory disorders.[5,6,8,16,20,21]

INDICATIONS FOR NEEDLE ASPIRATION BIOPSY

Persistence of clinically abnormal lymph node enlargement from any suspected cause is an indication for aspiration biopsy. In the head and neck, lymph node enlargement most often presents as an undiagnosed "lump in the neck." The lymph nodes of the neck are superficial and easily accessible to aspiration biopsy. Nodes of the neck are the largest nodal group investigated by aspiration biopsy.[6] It is important to note that the etiologic basis of a "lump in the neck" may not be ascertained until aspiration biopsy has established whether the lump is a lymph node involved in a benign or malignant process or, alternatively, a soft-tissue or other tumor (e.g., lipoma, rhabdomyosarcoma, carotid body tumor or salivary neoplasm), cyst (e.g., branchial cleft cyst, thyroglossal cyst or salivary cyst), abscess, hematoma or some other lesion. Aspiration biopsy is more helpful in this situation than in any other. It allows a definitive diagnosis of "unknown" masses in the neck in almost every case.

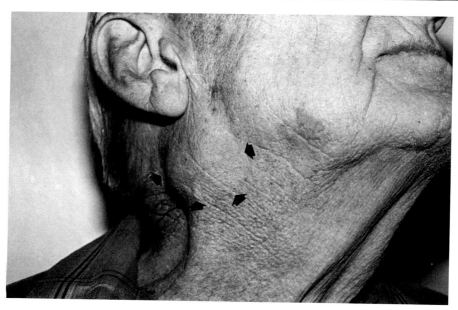

Fig. 3.1. Metastatic carcinoma involving the lymph node of the upper posterior triangle (arrows). Needle aspiration biopsy allowed a cytologic diagnosis of metastatic squamous cell carcinoma. The primary tumor was a small carcinoma of the posterior portion of the tongue.

Its usefulness has been well demonstrated in the following areas:

1. *Diagnosis of Metastatic Cancer:* The lymph nodes of the head and neck are common sites for metastases (Fig. 3.1) from primary tumors in the head and neck and from below the clavicle. Aspiration biopsy is an easy and practical technique for making the diagnosis immediately and without costly investigations.[15]

2. *Diagnosis of Primary Malignant Lymphoma:* Lymphoma can be diagnosed with a high degree of accuracy by use of aspiration biopsy[12] (Fig. 3.2), although excisional biopsy is usually required subsequently. Aspiration biopsy allows the selection of patients with lymphoma for further investigation and makes it possible to avoid unnecessary surgical intervention in patients with lymphadenopathy due to hyperplasia or infection.

3. *Staging of Lymphoma:* In the work-up of patients who are known to have lymphoma or in whom the diagnosis of recurrent disease is suspected, aspiration biopsy can be invaluable[7] and can make it possible to avoid unnecessary surgical intervention.

4. *Diagnosis of Specific and Nonspecific Chronic Inflammatory Diseases:* Aspiration biopsy can be particularly helpful in the diagnosis of inflammatory lesions, including granulomatous disorders[20] (Fig. 3.3).

5. *Special Studies:* Aspiration biopsy provides easy access to tumor tissue for electron microscopy[22,23] and to immunologic markers[24] and makes possible the performance of other special studies.[25,26] When used in conjunction with routine cytology methods, these additional studies are helpful in making the diagnosis.

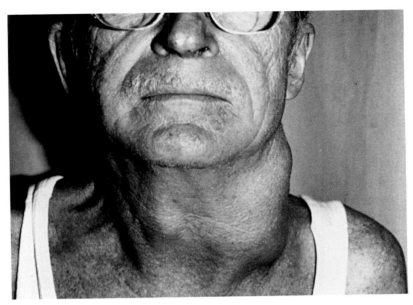

Fig. 3.2. Non-Hodgkin's lymphoma of the lymph nodes. Several nodes were involved and the involvement was confluent. The diagnosis was made by needle aspiration biopsy followed by surgical biopsy.

NORMAL LYMPH NODES

ANATOMIC STRUCTURES. Lymph nodes are encapsulated, oval or bean-shaped structures of lymphoid tissue distributed along the course of lymphatic vessels. They vary from 0.2 to 2.0 centimeters in greatest diameter. Each node receives lymph via afferent lymphatic vessels that enter the convex surface of the node. Lymph is then filtered in the node and exits via the efferent lymphatic vessels at the hilum. The major functions of lymph nodes are lymphopoiesis, filtration of lymph and processing of antigens. Lymph nodes are widely distributed in the body and large numbers of nodes are found in the head and neck, thorax, abdomen, axillae, groin, limbs and in association with most major body organs. The locations of the major nodal groups in the head and neck are shown in Figure 3.4.

HISTOLOGIC FEATURES. The overall structure of a lymph node is depicted in Figure 3.5. Within a lymph node, the lymphoid tissue is conveniently divided into an outer part, referred to as the cortex, and an inner part next to the hilum, referred to as the medulla. The intervening area is called the paracortex. A node is surrounded by a connective tissue capsule from which thin, fibrous trabeculae extend inward into the substance of the node. These septa provide structural support and carry blood vessels. Beneath the capsule is a subcapsular sinus into which the afferent lymphatic vessels open. This sinus sends branches into the cortical lymphoid tissue, through which it communicates with the sinuses in the medulla. The medullary sinuses deliver lymph to the lymphatic vessels that leave the node. The sinuses are lined by

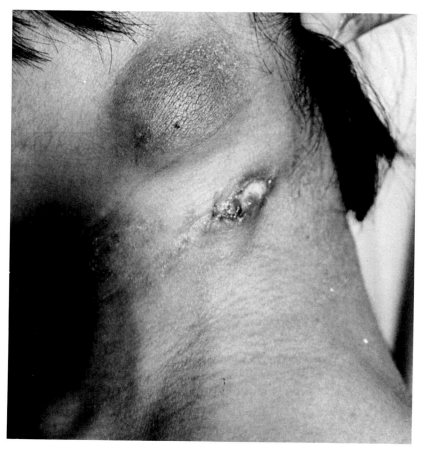

Fig. 3.3. Tuberculous lymphadenitis. Needle aspiration yielded necrotic material that contained histiocytes and multinucleated giant cells.

flattened endothelial cells and contain macrophages as well as lymphocytes, immunoblasts, plasma cells and neutrophils.

The cortical area includes the lymphoid follicles with their germinal centers and represents the bursa-dependent, or B-cell, area of the lymph node. The B lymphocytes secrete immunoglobulins and confer humoral immunity. The lymphoid follicles are round nodules, consisting of a peripheral area of small, dark-staining lymphocytes and the central, pale germinal centers. The germinal centers contain lymphocytes in different stages of maturation, histiocytes (tingible-body macrophages) and dendritic reticular cells. The small, or so-called mature, lymphocytes are the resting cells, which are approximately 6 to 8 micrometers in diameter. The dense nucleus of a small lymphocyte is almost structureless and is surrounded by a narrow rim of cytoplasm. The intermediate lymphocytes are larger than the mature lymphocytes and represent the transitional form between the small lymphocytes and the large lymphocytes. The nucleus of an intermediate lymphocyte is round or clefted and appears paler than that of a resting lymphocyte. Small nucleoli are

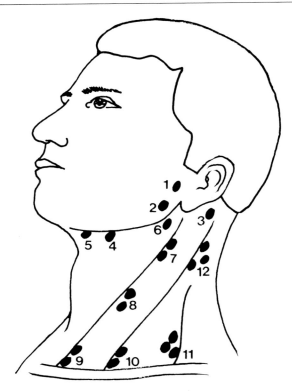

Fig. 3.4. Anatomic locations of the lymph nodes of the neck. 1, Preauricular; 2, parotid; 3, postauricular; 4, submandibular; 5, submental; 6, digastric-omohyoid; 7, upper jugular; 8, middle jugular; 9, lower jugular; 10, supraclavicular; 11, postcervical, lower; 12, postcervical, upper.

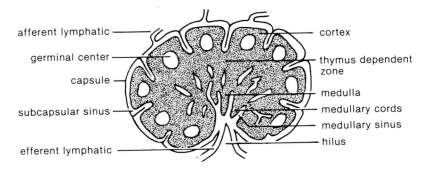

Fig. 3.5. Diagrammatic structure of a lymph node.

usually present. The large lymphocytes have a greater amount of cytoplasm than do the other lymphocytes. The nucleus of a large lymphocyte is round or indented. The chromatin is fine, giving the nucleus a vesicular appearance. One or more prominent nucleoli are present. The germinal centers vary in size, becoming larger under conditions of antigenic stimulation. As a result of antigenic stimulation, small resting lymphocytes within the germinal centers undergo blast cell transformation. The transformed cells are large, have abundant cytoplasm and contain round, pale-staining nuclei that are about four times the size of a mature lymphocyte. They contain several nucleoli, which are often adjacent to the nuclear membrane. These lymphocytes are the so-called centroblasts of Lennert[27] and the large, noncleaved lymphocytes of Lukes and Collins.[28] These noncleaved lymphoid cells are the dividing forms of the follicular center cells.[28] The large, noncleaved cells may divide further or be transformed into immunoblasts, which outside the germinal centers become plasma cells.

The paracortex, which consists of the area between the lymphoid follicles and the medullary cords, represents the thymus-dependent area of the node. The T lymphocytes may be small or large. The nuclei are predominantly noncleaved. Similar to B lymphocytes, T lymphocytes also change into immunoblasts and may undergo active proliferation or enter the pool of circulating lymphocytes. T lymphocytes play an important part in cell-mediated immunity.

The medulla is composed of cords of lymphocytes and plasma cells separated by medullary sinuses. This area is the major site of plasma cell proliferation and production of antibodies.

CYTOLOGIC FEATURES. The cellular elements from a normal lymph node can be identified on cytologic examination of lymph node aspirates obtained for staging patients with known malignant disease elsewhere or of lymph node aspirates obtained during surgical intervention. Cells in such aspirates are similar to those seen on histologic examination[8] and contain a mixed population of lymphocytes, histiocytes and other cells.

Lymphocytes

The lymphocytes seen may be divided into small, intermediate and large.

Small Lymphocytes

Resting, or small, lymphocytes are the predominant cell type and are similar to those seen in peripheral blood smears. They measure approximately 6 to 8 micrometers in diameter. The nucleus of a small lymphocyte appears dense as a result of clumping of chromatin and a nucleolus is not identifiable. A scant rim of cytoplasm may be visible around the nucleus.

Intermediate Lymphocytes

These cells are also referred to as prolymphocytes and are approximately 8 to 11 micrometers in diameter. The nucleus of an intermediate lymphocyte may be round or, less frequently, cleaved. The chromatin is less clumped than that of a small lymphocyte and appears coarse. A small nucleolus may be identifiable in these cells. A scant rim of basophilic cytoplasm may be visible around the nucleus.

Large Lymphocytes

These cells are normally seen in the center of the follicle and hence are also referred to as follicular center cells. Other terms used to describe these cells include lymphoblasts, poorly differentiated lymphocytes, transformed lymphocytes and reticulum cells. They are larger than intermediate lymphocytes and have a vesicular, round or cleaved nucleus that contains fine chromatin. One or more large nucleoli are usually present. The nucleus may be round or cleaved.

Immunoblasts also are large cells that have a large, round nucleus and a prominent, usually centrally located nucleolus. The cytoplasm is abundant and stains red with methyl-green pyronine. In properly prepared smears, immunoblasts can be differentiated from large lymphocytes. These cells become prominent and are relatively easy to identify in reactive hyperplasia.

Histiocytes

These cells are also referred to as phagocytes, macrophages or tingible-body macrophages. They are large and have an abundance of granular to foamy cytoplasm. The cell margins may be ill-defined. The small nucleus is round or oval and contains one or more small nucleoli. Phagocytosed cellular debris and pigment may occur within the cytoplasm of such cells. Histiocytes are characteristically seen in follicular hyperplasia.

Other Cell Types

A few plasma cells, neutrophils, eosinophils and mast cells are also present in normal lymph node aspirates and may be identifiable on microscopic examination. Giant cells are rarely encountered in so-called normal smears but are seen in various granulomatous disorders, reactive conditions, including infectious mononucleosis, Hodgkin's lymphoma and, occasionally, in acute lymphadenitis. Lymphoglandular bodies are small, spherical, pale bluish structures that are usually seen in lymph node aspirates stained by the Romanowsky method but are not seen in Papanicolaou-stained material. They represent cytoplasmic fragments and their presence in large numbers is characteristic of lymphoid tissue.[8,29]

BENIGN ENLARGEMENT OF LYMPH NODES

Reactive Lymphoid Hyperplasia

Enlargement of a lymph node may be the result of hyperplasia of some or all of its cellular constituents caused by the stimulation of lymphoid cells by a variety of antigens. In most cases, no specific agent is found, whereas in others, the hyperplasia is determined to be a response to viral, bacterial or fungal agents. Most cases of

TABLE 3.1. Reactive Lymphoid Hyperplasia

Follicular hyperplasia
Sinus histiocytosis
Diffuse hyperplasia
Mixed hyperplasia

hyperplasia resolve spontaneously within weeks. However, at times, an enlarged lymph node fails to decrease in size after several weeks of observation; in such instances, lymphoma may be suspected on clinical grounds. In such cases, needle aspiration is justified, particularly if other investigations have failed to reveal the cause of the enlargement.

HISTOLOGIC FEATURES. Reactive lymphoid hyperplasia has been divided into four morphologic subtypes on the basis of histologic criteria[30,31] (Table 3.1).

Most cases of hyperplasia are of the "follicular" type. This pattern is seen in rheumatoid arthritis and angiofollicular hyperplasia, although in most cases no cause is apparent. The follicles are greatly enlarged and vary in size and shape (Fig. 3.6). The germinal centers are prominent and contain a mixture of small and large lymphocytes that have round or cleaved nuclei (Fig. 3.7). Mitoses are frequent. A large number of tingible-body macrophages are encountered.

In the "sinus histiocytosis" type, the sinuses are greatly enlarged and there is compression of the nodal parenchyma. The sinuses are filled with proliferated histiocytic cells that have an abundance of foamy, eosinophilic cytoplasm. Ingested red blood cells and leukocytes are visible in the cytoplasm of the histiocytic cells. The

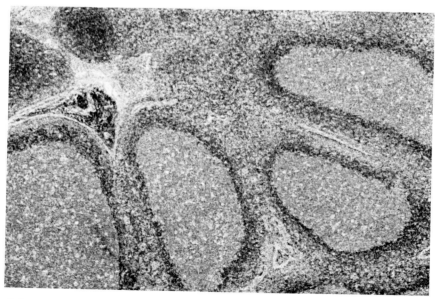

Fig. 3.6. Follicular hyperplasia. Enlarged follicles composed of pale germinal centers. Hematoxylin and eosin preparation. × 50.

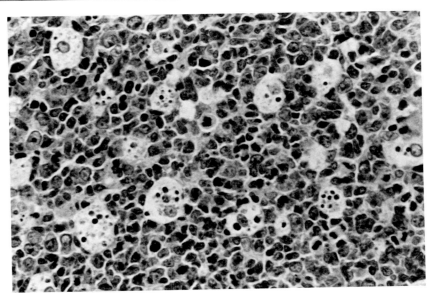

Fig. 3.7. Follicular hyperplasia. High-power view of a germinal center composed of a mixture of small and large lymphocytes. Numerous tingible-body macrophages are visible. Hematoxylin and eosin preparation. ×625.

medullary cords contain large numbers of blood vessels and lymphocytes. This pattern is usually seen in uninvolved lymph nodes that drain malignant neoplasms and in sinus histiocytosis with massive lymphadenopathy, as described by Rosai and Dorfman.[32]

The "diffuse" type is characterized by lymphoid hyperplasia with effacement of lymph node architecture. The follicles are small or absent. Within the parenchyma one sees lymphocytes, plasma cells, immunoblasts and macrophages. This type is usually seen in some viral infections, following vaccination and in dermatopathic lymphadenitis. It also is seen in immunoblastic lymphadenopathy,[33] where in addition to immunoblasts and plasma cells there is proliferation of arborizing small vessels.

In the "mixed" variant, combinations of various hyperplastic subtypes are noted with large follicles, distended sinuses and proliferation of intrafollicular lymphocytes and immunoblasts (Fig. 3.8). Such a pattern is seen in infectious mononucleosis and in toxoplasma lymphadenitis.

CYTOLOGIC FEATURES. The needle aspirate from a reactive lymph node usually consists of a semisolid drop of grayish lymphoid material. The smears are cellular, consisting of a mixed population of lymphoid cells. The smears are dispersed, although in the thick portions of the smear, some clumping of cells may be observed. The hallmark of a reactive smear is a polymorphous cell pattern. It may not be possible to distinguish the various histologic subtypes on cytologic examination. Most smears are of the follicular pattern and consist of a mixed cell population, with small lymphocytes being the dominant cell type (Fig. 3.9). These cells are admixed

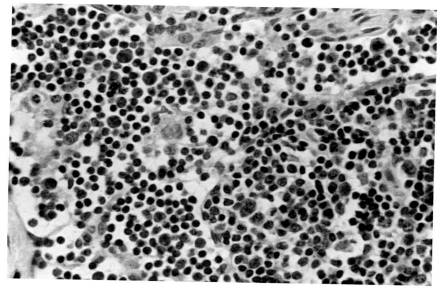

Fig. 3.8. Infectious mononucleosis. Distended sinuses contain a mixture of lymphocytes and immunoblasts. Hematoxylin and eosin preparation. ×390.

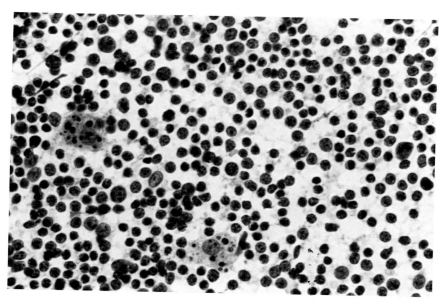

Fig. 3.9. Follicular hyperplasia. Cytology specimen contains a mixture of small and large lymphocytes and tingible-body macrophages. Papanicolaou preparation. ×390.

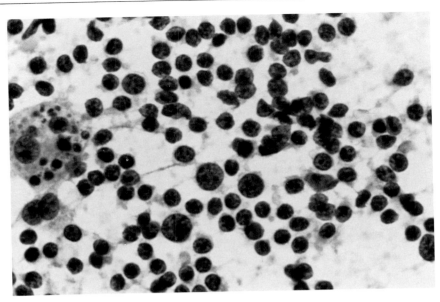

Fig. 3.10. High-power view of the lesion shown in Figure 3.9. Papanicolaou preparation. ×625.

with intermediate and large, immature-looking lymphocytes that have, round cleaved or noncleaved nuclei and contain nucleoli (Fig. 3.10). Immunoblasts that have an abundance of basophilic cytoplasm, a large, circular, noncleaved nucleus and one or more prominent nucleoli are also seen in such smears. Mitoses may be seen in the large, noncleaved, follicular center cells. In addition to lymphocytes, the smears contain macrophages, plasma cells, neutrophils and eosinophils. Fibroblasts and endothelial cells may also be found. A cell that is characteristically noted in aspirates from follicular hyperplasia is the tingible-body macrophage (Figs. 3.9 and 3.10). These cells are histiocytic cells that have abundant cytoplasm and contain phagocytosed cellular debris. The nucleus of a tingible-body macrophage is round or oval and contains a small nucleolus. Although all the features described in the preceding text are characteristic of follicular hyperplasia, some of them may be seen in the other subtypes. The common denominator is the mixed cell pattern.

In the sinus histiocytosis type, one sees, in addition to lymphocytes and plasma cells, a large number of histiocytes that have granular, eosinophilic cytoplasm. Multinucleated histiocytes may also be found. The nuclei are round or oval and contain small or medium-sized nucleoli. Small loose groupings of histiocytes that have delicate, elongated cytoplasmic processes may also be encountered. In the diffuse variety, a mixed cell population is the rule, with plasma cells and immunoblasts being numerous. In infectious mononucleosis, a mixed cellular pattern is seen, with numerous transformed lymphocytes and immunoblasts (Fig. 3.11). Multinucleated cells that resemble Reed-Sternberg cells are occasionally seen (Fig. 3.11, *inset*). The cytologic features of lymphoid hyperplasia are summarized in Table 3.2.

DIFFERENTIAL DIAGNOSIS. Reactive lymphoid hyperplasia must be differentiated from Hodgkin's and non-Hodgkin's lymphoma. In the usual case of follicular or the

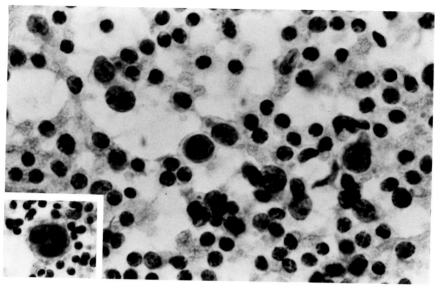

Fig. 3.11. Infectious mononucleosis. Cytology specimen contains large transformed lympho-cytes coexisting with small lymphocytes and plasma cells. A Reed-Sternberg-like cell is also visible (*inset*). Papanicolaou preparation. ×625.

mixed variant of hyperplasia, differentiation from lymphoma is not difficult. The finding of a mixed cell population and tingible-body macrophages suggest the diagnosis. Occasionally, diffuse hyperplasia mimics lymphocytic small-cell lymphoma. Careful attention to cell types is important because diffuse hyperplasia also involves other cell types. In non-Hodgkin's lymphoma, a monomorphic population of cells is usually encountered. Differentiation from Burkitt's lymphoma is discussed on page 156. Hodgkin's lymphoma, especially the lymphocytic predominant and mixed-cellularity types, may mimic the diffuse and mixed types of reactive lymphoid hyper-plasia. The diagnosis relies on the finding of typical Reed-Sternberg cells in the proper cellular environment. In reactive conditions, such as angioimmunoblastic lymphadenopathy or infectious mononucleosis, atypical histiocytic cells that resem-ble Reed-Sternberg cells may be seen. However, careful attention to the other cells usually helps in the differentiation of Hodgkin's lymphoma from these disorders. In infectious mononucleosis and other reactive states, large, transformed lymphocytes or immunoblasts occur in large numbers and are a clue to the diagnosis. The sinus histiocytosis variant of hyperplasia must be differentiated from histiocytosis X. This

TABLE 3.2. Reactive Lymphadenopathy: Summary of Cytologic Features

Cellular smears, cells dispersed
Mixed cell population, with small, intermediate and large transformed lymphocytes; im-munoblasts, eosinophils, neutrophils, plasma cells and histiocytes also present
Tingible-body macrophages
Mitotic figures frequent

TABLE 3.3. Common Causes and Patterns of Granulomatous Lymphadenopathy

Classical Epithelioid Granulomas
    Tuberculosis
    Histoplasmosis
    Sarcoidosis
    Tuberculoid leprosy
    Lymph nodes draining malignant tumors
    Hodgkin's disease
    Chronic granulomatous disease of childhood
Granulomas with Central Abscesses
    Cat-scratch fever
    Lymphogranuloma venereum
    Yersinia*
Scattered Aggregates of Epithelioid Histiocytes
    Toxoplasmosis
    Syphilis
    Lepromatous leprosy
    Hodgkin's disease
    Lennert's lymphoma

*Granulomas confined to mesenteric lymph nodes.

distinction is sometimes extremely difficult. The finding of eosinophils admixed with histiocytes suggests histiocytosis X. Plasma cells are more commonly seen along with histiocytes in the reactive sinus histiocytosis variant of hyperplasia.

Granulomatous Lymphadenopathy

Granulomas occur in lymph nodes in a wide variety of infective and noninfective diseases (Table 3.3). Such lesions may be solitary or multiple and small or large and may involve one or more groups of lymph nodes. Lymph nodes in the head and neck are common sites for granulomatous inflammation[34-38] (Fig. 3.12).

HISTOLOGIC FEATURES. Granulomas are composed of oval or fusiform epithelioid histiocytes, lymphocytes and plasma cells. Multinucleated giant cells are admixed with the epithelioid histiocytes. Fibroblasts and neutrophils may also be seen. In tuberculosis, the center of the granuloma characteristically undergoes a coagulative type of necrosis, leaving no cellular debris, and is referred to as caseous necrosis (Fig. 3.13). The histologic diagnosis is made by identifying the beaded, rod-shaped, acid-fast tubercle bacillus by Ziehl-Neelsen or other special stains. In sarcoidosis, one sees a number of well-demarcated, noncaseating granulomas unlike the caseating ones seen in tuberculosis (Fig. 3.14). Although sarcoidosis more commonly involves the hilar lymph nodes, involvement of the nodes of the neck or salivary glands is a well-recognized feature of the disease.[6] Small, noncaseating granulomas can also be found in lymph nodes that drain malignant neoplasms and occur in Hodgkin's lymphoma.

In cat-scratch fever and lymphogranuloma venereum, the granulomas have central abscesses that are often stellate.[36,39,40] This appearance is characteristic. In cat-

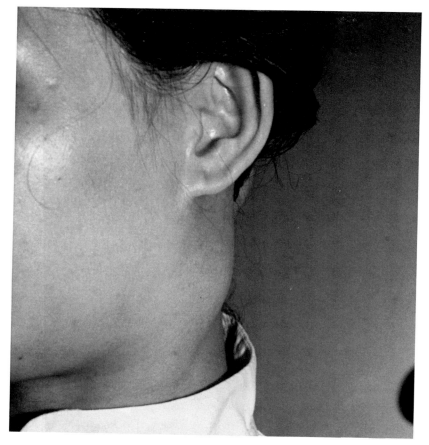

Fig. 3.12. Large, nonmalignant, inflammatory nodes in a young asymptomatic woman. Aspiration biopsy cytology revealed granulomatous inflammation. (Tuberculosis.)

scratch fever, although the axillary lymph nodes are most often involved, cervical lymphadenopathy also occurs. The disease commonly afflicts children with a history of cat-scratch.[36] In lymphogranuloma venereum, involvement of the inguinal, perianal and pelvic lymph nodes is most commonly encountered, although other nodal groups may be involved.

Toxoplasmosis results in asymptomatic enlargement of the lymph nodes in otherwise healthy adults, although in immunodeficient persons and newborn fetuses, several organs may be involved. The posterior cervical lymph nodes are most commonly involved, although other nodes of the head and neck may be affected.[34] A mixed type of reactive lymphoid hyperplasia occurs in the lymph nodes along with small, granuloma-like aggregates of histiocytes in the cortex and paracortical areas. Classical granulomas are not seen. Toxoplasma organisms are rarely observed in lymph nodes. Geimsa stain may show groups of trophozoites within macrophages or as solitary cysts.[34]

In lepromatous leprosy, aggregates of histiocytes are found in the sinuses that

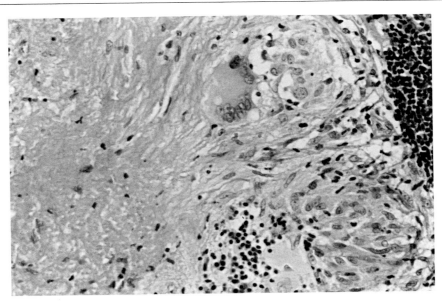

Fig. 3.13. Tuberculous lymphadenitis. Caseous necrosis is seen on the left with epithelioid histiocytes and multinucleated giant cells to the right. Hematoxylin and eosin preparation. ×390.

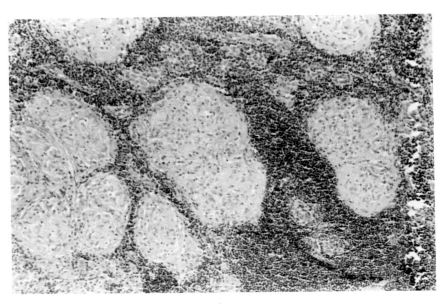

Fig. 3.14. Noncaseating granulomas. Hematoxylin and eosin preparation. ×150.

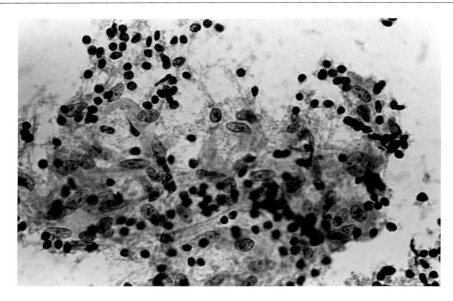

Fig. 3.15. A small grouping of epithelioid histiocytes. Cytology specimen shows oval or elongated nuclei and ill-defined cytoplasmic processes. Papanicolaou preparation. ×625.

contain acid-fast organisms, whereas in the tuberculoid variant, noncaseating granulomas occur.[41]

Granulomas occasionally occur in syphilis, although one more commonly sees follicular hyperplasia. Isolated histiocytes and multinucleated giant cells are found in the lymph node parenchyma.[42]

Classical epithelioid granulomas with or without necrosis may also occur in patients with Hodgkin's lymphoma.

CYTOLOGIC FEATURES. The cytologic findings in aspirates from patients with granulomatous lymphadenitis are characteristic, consisting of a background of lymphoid cells on which exist small loose groupings of epithelioid histiocytes. The epithelioid cells have poorly defined, slender cytoplasmic processes and an elongated nucleus that contains finely granular chromatin and small nucleoli (Fig. 3.15). Multinucleated giant cells may be found as solitary cells or in association with epithelioid histiocytes (Fig. 3.16). Giant cells are not always encountered and a careful search may be required to find such cells. In some cases, the entire granuloma is aspirated and can be seen in the smear. When there is caseation or necrosis, degenerating cells are seen on a background of granular, necrotic debris (Fig. 3.17).

By themselves, the collections of epithelioid cells and occasional giant cells are not diagnostic of a specific disease. However, granular, necrotic debris in the background is suggestive of necrotizing granulomatous inflammation and such a pattern mandates consideration of tuberculosis. In a recent report on 39 cases of tuberculosis in which needle aspiration was performed, Bailey and colleagues[20] found granulomatous inflammation in only 18 cases. In the other 21 cases, large amounts of necrotic debris were seen in the absence of epithelioid cells. Samples from 15 cases with and 19 cases without granulomas were submitted for culture and fluores-

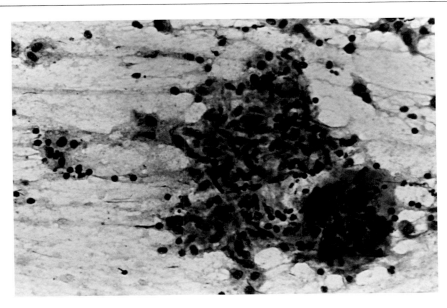

Fig. 3.16. Multinucleated giant histiocytes. Papanicolaou preparation. ×390.

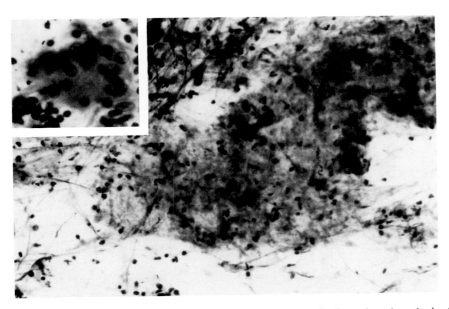

Fig. 3.17. Necrotizing granulomatous inflammation in a case of tuberculous lymphadenitis. The inset shows a multinucleated giant histiocyte. Papanicolaou preparation. ×390. (*Inset*, ×625.)

cence studies. Auramine-rhodamine staining of smears was positive in four of the 15 cases (27 percent of those with granulomas) and in nine of 19 (47 percent of those without granulomas). *Mycobacterium tuberculosis* organisms were isolated in 12 of the 15 (80 percent) cases with granulomas and in 16 of the 19 (84 percent) cases without granulomas. In only two smears, however, were multinucleated giant cells found. It is advisable, therefore, that when granulomatous inflammation is noted in an aspirate, especially if it is associated with necrosis, or when necrotic debris is seen, tuberculosis should be suspected and if no material was initially submitted for bacteriologic studies, aspiration should be repeated so that fluorescence and culture studies can be performed. Rajwanshi and associates[37] have reviewed their experience in a report on 160 aspirates from patients with tuberculosis. Acid-fast bacilli were demonstrated in 40 percent of their cases.

Silverman[39] recently described the cytologic features of cat-scratch fever, as diagnosed by needle aspiration biopsy. Characteristic granulomas with peripherally located, epithelioid, histiocytic cells and centrally located neutrophils were noted.

A recent report[43] has documented the efficacy of aspiration biopsy cytology for the diagnosis of sarcoidosis of the head and neck. All six cases in that report were diagnosed by this technique. Epithelioid and multinucleated giant cells were found in the smears and small, complete granulomas were observed in some cases.

Aspiration biopsy cytology has also recently been used for the diagnosis of toxoplasmosis and leprosy.[44,45]

Acute or Chronic Lymphadenitis

Needle aspiration biopsy is rarely performed in cases of acute lymphadenitis because the diagnosis is usually apparent on the basis of clinical findings. However, this technique can have an important role in the diagnosis of selected inflammatory disorders. Viral inclusions or other diagnostic organisms may be detected. In this situation, organisms of tuberculosis, actinomycosis, various fungi, cat-scratch fever, toxoplasmosis and leprosy may be identifiable.[5,20,21,46] Needle aspiration biopsy is also an ideal technique for obtaining material for culture.

Generalized Persistent Lymphadenopathy and Acquired Immune Deficiency Syndrome

Generalized persistent lymphadenopathy is common in homosexual men and is regarded as a prodrome of acquired immune deficiency syndrome. Bottles and coworkers[47] have recently reported the cytologic findings obtained by needle aspiration biopsy in homosexual patients with lymphadenopathy. The causes of lymphadenopathy included benign follicular hyperplasia, tuberculous lymphadenitis, non-Hodgkin's lymphoma and lymphadenopathic Kaposi's sarcoma. Fite stains demonstrated acid-fast organisms within the cytoplasm of histiocytes in patients with mycobacterial infection. Bacterial cultures performed subsequently confirmed the cytologic diagnosis and allowed classification of the type of mycobacterium. They also reported the cytologic finding of Kaposi's sarcoma in one patient who presented with lymph node enlargement. The aspirate contained large fragments of spindle-shaped cells, which suggested the diagnosis.

LYMPHOMA

The diagnosis of lymphoma by needle aspiration biopsy cytology has long been a subject of debate. Although most investigators advocate needle aspiration biopsy of lymph nodes for the diagnosis of metastatic cancer, caution is advised when this method is used for the diagnosis of lymphoma. However, a review of the literature suggests that even though the final diagnosis usually depends on histologic examination of an excised lymph node, needle aspiration biopsy can provide answers to many important questions:

1. Is the lymph node enlargement due to hyperplasia or neoplasia?
2. If the process is malignant, is it lymphoma or metastatic cancer?
3. If the lesion is lymphoma, is it Hodgkin's or non-Hodgkin's lymphoma?

Further, in most cases, an experienced cytopathologist can subclassify the non-Hodgkin's lymphomas, although we agree with other authors[6,8,17,48] that needle aspiration biopsy does not always permit a precise categorization of non-Hodgkin's lymphomas according to the recognized histologic classifications. This drawback of needle aspiration biopsy is understandable when one realizes the size of the sample on which the cytologic diagnosis is being rendered. Although, in properly prepared and stained preparations and with experience, one may be able to differentiate the various cell types, the morphologic pattern (follicular or diffuse) still requires histologic verification. Recent studies have shown that material obtained by needle aspiration biopsy can be used for immunoperoxidase studies of lymphocyte surface and cytoplasmic markers, thereby adding another dimension to its usefulness in the diagnosis of lymphoproliferative disorders.[24]

Non-Hodgkin's Lymphoma

HISTOLOGIC CLASSIFICATION. For the past two decades, the classification of lymphomas has been a popular topic of controversy. A number of classifications have been proposed and modified during this period. The early ones were by Gall in 1955[49] and by Rappaport in 1966.[50] Rappaport's classification is based on the pattern of growth, diffuse or nodular, and on cytologic subtypes. Lymphomas are categorized as well differentiated or poorly differentiated, depending on the degree of the resemblance of the tumor cells to normal lymphocytes. Tumors composed of large cells are termed histiocytic. Rappaport's classification received wide acceptance, especially in the English-speaking countries, by clinicians and pathologists because of its easy reproducibility and good clinicopathologic correlation. The popularity of this classification is such that despite its deficiencies, it is still used today in a modified form.[51] Its main deficiencies are that it does not recognize the heterogeneous nature of lymphocytes and that the so-called histiocytic lymphomas are not neoplasms of histiocytes or macrophages but (as subsequent studies have shown), rather, are derived from transformed lymphocytes.

Recent advances relating to the origin and function of the lymphocytes have led to new classifications for non-Hodgkin's lymphomas. Both Lukes and Collins[52] and Lennert and colleagues[53] have put forward new classifications that are based on evidence of lymphocyte transformation and the B or T designation of lymphocytes.

TABLE 3.4. Classification of Non-Hodgkin's Lymphoma

Rappaport	Lennert	Lukes-Collins
		B-Cell Lymphomas
1. Well-differentiated lymphocytic	Lymphocytic Lymphoplasmacytoid	Small lymphocytic Plasmacytoid lymphocytic

2. Poorly differentiated lymphocytic
    Nodular
    Diffuse
	Centrocytic, small	Small cleaved follicular center cell
		    Follicular
		    Diffuse

3. Mixed histiocytic-lymphocytic
    Nodular
    Diffuse
	Centroblastic-centrocytic	

4.	Centrocytic, large	Large cleaved follicular center cell
		    Follicular
		    Diffuse

5. Histiocytic
    Nodular
    Diffuse
	Centroblastic	Large noncleaved follicular center cell
		    Follicular
		    Diffuse

6. Undifferentiated	Lymphoblastic	Small noncleaved follicular center cell
		    Diffuse
		    Burkitt's

7. Histiocytic	Immunoblastic	Immunoblastic sarcoma
		T-Cell Lymphomas
8. Well-differentiated lymphocytic	Lymphocytic (T-cell type)	Small-cell lymphocytic
9. Lymphoblastic	Lymphoblastic (convoluted type)	Convoluted cell
10. Histiocytic	T-zone lymphoma	Immunoblastic sarcoma
11.	Mycosis fungoides	Sézary-mycosis fungoides
12.		Null cell lymphoma
13. Histiocytic	Reticulosarcoma	Histiocytic

Studies have shown that the vast majority of non-Hodgkin's lymphomas are of B-cell origin. Lymphomas of T-cell origin involve lymph nodes or skin and most such tumors carry a poor prognosis. True neoplasms of histiocytic or macrophagic origin are extremely rare. Table 3.4 compares the three classifications.

Recently, the National Cancer Institute undertook a study of the various classifications of non-Hodgkin's lymphomas and devised a classification designed primarily for clinical usage.[54] This study classified non-Hodgkin's lymphomas into three major grades according to prognosis (Table 3.5).

CYTOLOGIC CLASSIFICATION. In the past, needle aspiration biopsy has been used largely for establishing a diagnosis of lymphoma and for differentiating such neoplasms from reactive lymphadenopathy and metastatic cancer. The suspicion or

TABLE 3.5. Non-Hodgkin's Lymphoma: National Cancer Institute Working Classification

Low Grade
   Malignant lymphoma, small lymphocytic
      Chronic lymphocytic leukemia
      Plasmacytoid
   Malignant lymphoma, follicular
      Predominantly small cleaved cells
      Mixed small cleaved and large cell
Intermediate Grade
   Malignant lymphoma, follicular
      Predominantly large cell
   Malignant lymphoma, diffuse
      Small cleaved cells
      Mixed small and large cells
      Large cleaved or noncleaved cell
High Grade
   Malignant lymphoma, large cell, immunoblastic
   Malignant lymphoma, lymphoblastic
   Malignant lymphoma, small noncleaved cell
      Burkitt's lymphoma

diagnosis of lymphoma by needle aspiration biopsy usually led to excision of a lymph node for histologic examination and classification. In 1974, Zajicek[13] proposed a cytologic classification (Table 3.6) that is based on the histologic guidelines proposed by Rappaport. Other investigators[8,12] have proposed cytologic classifications that divide the lymphomas into small, intermediate, large and mixed-cell types. These investigators, however, emphasize that when clinically possible, the cytologic diagnosis of primary nodal lymphoma be followed by histologic study of the excised lymph node. Koss and associates[48] have suggested that a simple morphologic classification based on cell size can account for most lymphomas and stressed that further categorization into subtypes is possible only on technically excellent aspirates examined by experienced observers. Koss and associates use the terminology of Lukes and Collins for their criteria for the cytologic diagnosis of lymphomas.

Recently, Orell and Skinner[11] have suggested that the classification of Lennert and colleagues is easily adaptable to cytology because it is based purely on cytologic criteria and not on pattern recognition. In a study of histologically confirmed cases

TABLE 3.6. Malignant Lymphoma: Cytologic Classification (Zajicek 1974)

Non-Hodgkin's lymphoma
   Lymphocytic
      Well differentiated
      Poorly differentiated
   Mixed lymphocytic-histiocytic
   Histiocytic
Hodgkin's lymphoma

in which needle aspiration biopsy was performed, there was full agreement between the cytologic and the histologic classifications in 44 of 53 cases. These authors are enthusiastic about using needle aspiration biopsy for the diagnosis of lymphoma.

CYTOLOGIC FEATURES. Aspirates from lymph nodes involved by lymphoma usually consist of one or two drops of gray, semisolid material. Although most aspirates contain blood, only a copious amount may interfere with interpretation. In well-prepared smears, neoplastic cells remain discrete and separate, although cells in clumps with overlapping of nuclei may be seen in unevenly spread smears. In our laboratory, the usual practice is to use alcohol to fix smears obtained by needle aspiration biopsy and to stain the slides with the Papanicolaou and hematoxylin and eosin methods. If two or more slides have been prepared, we keep the spares dry for subsequent use or special studies. We do not routinely use air-dried smears stained by the Romanowsky method.

Smears from patients with non-Hodgkin's lymphomas are usually cellular and examination under low magnification usually reveals a monomorphic or monotonous population of cells. Mixed-cell lymphomas are not common and careful attention to the cellular constituents and nuclear detail helps distinguish them from reactive hyperplasia. The observation of a few histiocytes and other inflammatory cells in an otherwise monomorphic smear does not rule out lymphoma. Such an appearance is commonly seen with rapidly growing lymphomas and most likely results from necrosis in the tumor. Some parts of the smear should not be evaluated. Areas in which the cells are clumped as a result of uneven spreading of the smear, areas that are improperly fixed or that have drying artifacts (usually seen at the edge) and areas in which there is streaking of chromatin due to trauma can contribute to interpretation errors and should be disregarded. After the initial screening to evaluate the cell population, attention should be directed to the finer cytologic features of individual cells. Cell size, cytoplasmic and nuclear characteristics and the presence or absence of nucleoli are helpful information for further categorizing lymphomas.

The follicular or diffuse pattern of a lymphoma cannot be determined on cytologic examination. The cytologic diagnosis is based purely on the morphologic characteristics of the lymphoreticular cells and not on the architectural pattern seen on histologic examination.

Small-Cell Lymphoma

In small-cell lymphomas, the hallmark of a smear is a monomorphic population of small cells (Fig. 3.18). The size of the cells depends on the type of small-cell lymphoma. In small-cell lymphocytic lymphoma, the neoplastic cells are slightly larger than resting lymphocytes. They have round, fairly uniform, dense nuclei with clumped chromatin. The cytoplasm is usually scanty and ill-defined. Nucleoli are usually not identifiable or are small and inconspicuous. In the plasmacytoid type, transitional forms occur and plasma cells may be present.

In the small, cleaved, follicular center cell type, the nucleus is larger than that seen in the lymphocytic variant and has been categorized by some investigators as intermediate in size. The nuclei are round and clefts can be seen in them (Fig. 3.19). The chromatin is coarse and granular and small nucleoli are visible. Some variation in

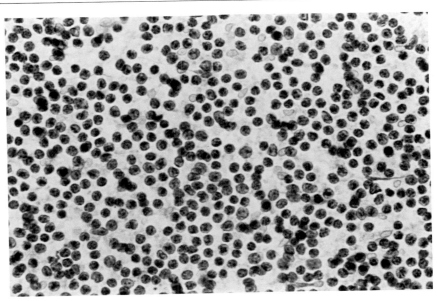

Fig. 3.18. Small-cell lymphocytic lymphoma. Cytology specimen contains a uniform population of small, round cells. Papanicolaou preparation. ×390.

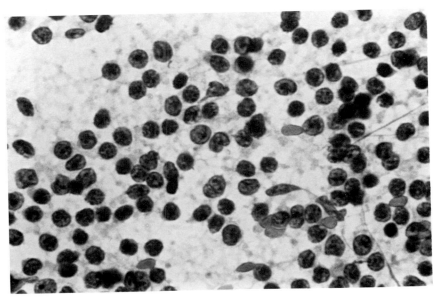

Fig. 3.19. Small, cleaved, follicular center cell lymphoma. Cytology specimen shows small clefts in the nuclei. Small nucleoli are also visible. Papanicolaou preparation. ×1000.

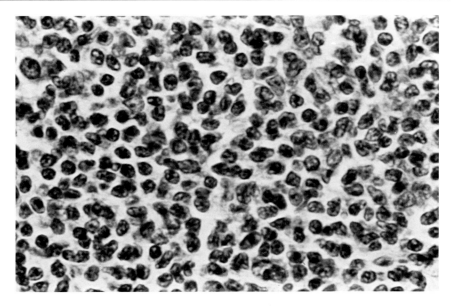

Fig. 3.20. Small, cleaved, follicular center cell lymphoma. Histology specimen shows the irregular nuclear outline. Hematoxylin and eosin preparation. ×625.

nuclear size is usually noted. The histologic appearance of such a lesion is shown in Figure 3.20.

Noncleaved, follicular center cell lymphoma is another type of small-cell lymphoma. A subtype that is common in African children was originally described by Burkitt in 1958.[55] This lesion is uncommon in North America and Europe. The cells of Burkitt's lymphoma have round nuclei that are about twice as large as those of resting lymphocytes and they contain coarse chromatin and one or more nucleoli (Figs. 3.21, 3.22 and 3.23). Tingible-body macrophages may be seen in the smears. Another type of small-cell lymphoma is convoluted cell lymphoblastic lymphoma, which is most common in children. Most such tumors are of T-cell origin, although a few B-cell variants have been described. Cytologic examination shows that the tumor cells are larger than resting lymphocytes and have round or irregular, lobulated or convoluted nuclei (Figs. 3.24 and 3.25). The chromatin is granular and the nucleoli are small.[48]

Large-Cell Lymphoma

The characteristic feature of large-cell lymphomas is the cell size. The nuclei may be three to four times as large as those of resting lymphocytes. These lymphomas are a heterogeneous group of tumors. Common examples include large, cleaved cell lymphoma, noncleaved cell lymphoma and immunoblastic sarcoma. Histiocytic lymphoma, an uncommon neoplasm, is another variant.

Aspirates from large, cleaved follicular center cell lymphomas contain large cells that have an ill-defined rim of cytoplasm around their nuclei (Fig. 3.26). The nuclei are usually large, but there is variation in size. The nuclei are round or oval and have

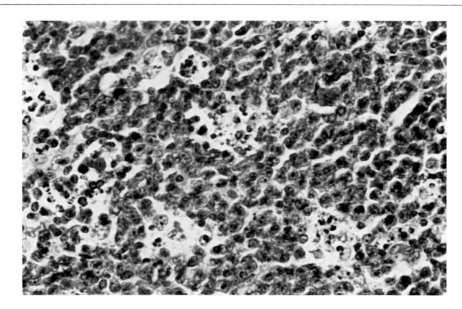

Fig. 3.21. Burkitt's lymphoma. Histology specimen contains monotonous, small, round cells coexisting with numerous tingible-body macrophages. Hematoxylin and eosin preparation. ×625.

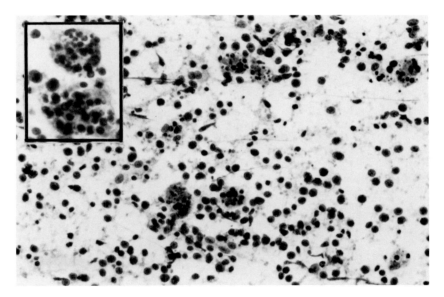

Fig. 3.22. Cytology specimen contains a monotonous population of small lymphocytes coexisting with tingible-body macrophages. Papanicolaou preparation. ×390. (*Inset,* ×625.)

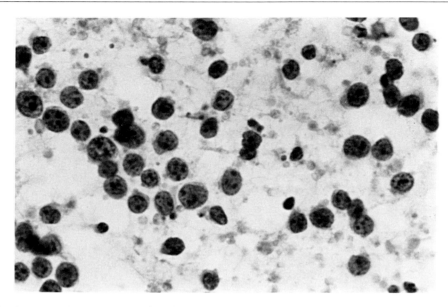

Fig. 3.23. High-power view of Burkitt's lymphoma cells. Papanicolaou preparation. ×1000.

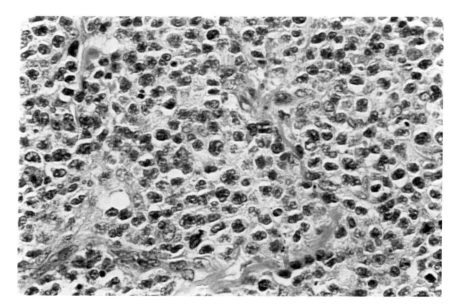

Fig. 3.24. Lobulated lymphoma. Histology specimen shows numerous convoluted or lobulated nuclei. Hematoxylin and eosin preparation. ×625.

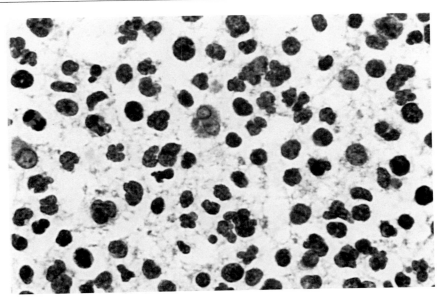

Fig. 3.25. Lobulated lymphoma. Cytology specimen. Papanicolaou preparation. ×625.

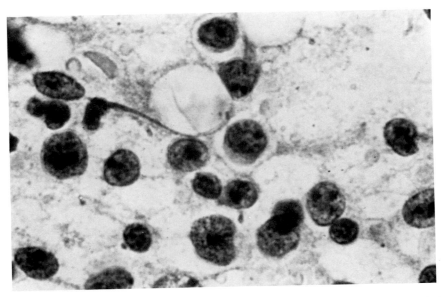

Fig. 3.26. Large, cleaved, follicular center cell lymphoma. Cytology specimen. Papanicolaou preparation. ×1500.

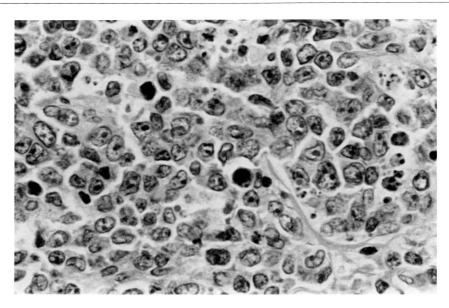

Fig. 3.27. Large, cleaved, follicular center cell lymphoma. Histology specimen shows large nuclei with clefts in the nuclear membrane. Hematoxylin and eosin preparation. × 1000.

irregular outlines due to clefts. The chromatin is coarsely granular and one or more large nucleoli are seen. A few tingible-body macrophages may be scattered among the tumor cells. The histologic appearance of a large, cleaved follicular center cell lymphoma is shown in Figure 3.27.

In large, noncleaved follicular center cell lymphoma, variation in cell size is again noted. The predominant cells are large and have round, noncleaved nuclei, coarsely granular chromatin and one or more prominent nucleoli (Fig. 3.28). Some nucleoli may be seen along the nuclear membrane. Mitotic figures are encountered and a few tingible-body macrophages may be seen in rapidly dividing tumors.

Immunoblastic sarcoma presents a characteristic picture on aspiration biopsy cytology, with large cells that have a narrow rim of ill-defined cytoplasm (Figs. 3.29, 3.30 and 3.31). Variation in cell size is noted. The nuclei are large and usually round, although irregular forms are occasionally seen. The chromatin is coarse and dispersed and the nuclei contain one or more prominent nucleoli. When there is only one nucleolus, it is usually centrally located. Plasmacytic differentiation may be seen in some tumor cells. Mitoses are frequent. The histologic appearance of this lesion is shown in Figure 3.32.

True histiocytic lymphoma is rare and probably constitutes less than 5 percent of all large-cell lymphomas.[56] Most such neoplasms are examples of so-called malignant histiocytosis. On cytologic examination, such tumors are found to consist of large cells that have an abundance of ill-defined cytoplasm and pleomorphic nuclei. Multinucleation is also encountered. Plasma cells, eosinophils and histiocytes may be seen in the background. The diagnosis relies on the detection of cytochemical and immunologic markers because such tumors can mimic some T-cell tumors, immunoblastic sarcoma and, occasionally, Hodgkin's lymphoma. Figures 3.33 and 3.34

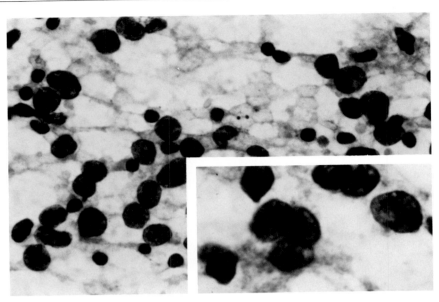

Fig. 3.28. Large, noncleaved, follicular center cell lymphoma. Cytology specimen. Papanicolaou preparation. × 1000. (*Inset*, × 1500).

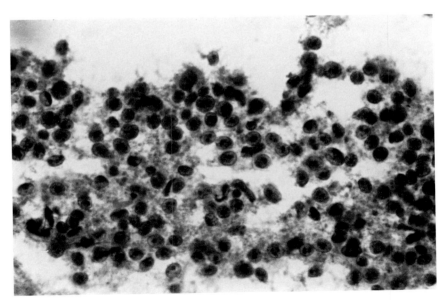

Fig. 3.29. Immunoblastic sarcoma. Cytology specimen contains a monotonous population of cells that have large, noncleaved nuclei and one or more nucleoli. Hematoxylin and eosin preparation. × 625.

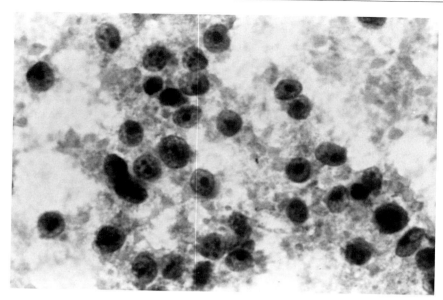

Fig. 3.30. Immunoblastic sarcoma cells. Hematoxylin and eosin preparation. × 1000.

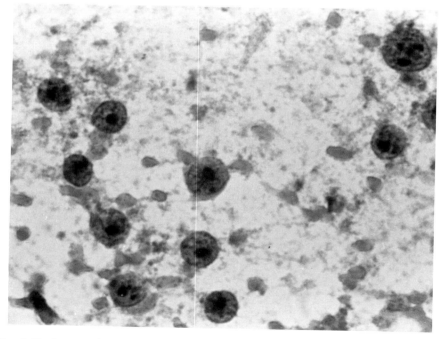

Fig. 3.31. Immunoblastic sarcoma cells. Hematoxylin and eosin preparation. × 1500.

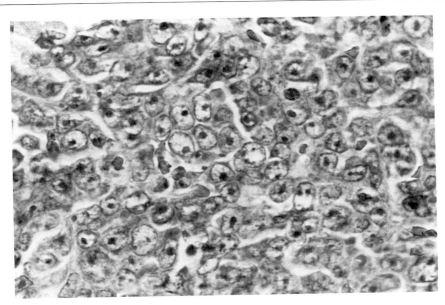

Fig. 3.32. Immunoblastic sarcoma. Histology specimen. Hematoxylin and eosin preparation. ×1000.

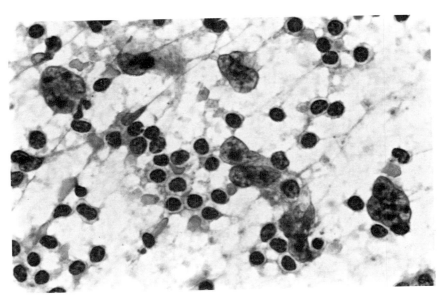

Fig. 3.33. A mixture of small and large cells. Cytology specimen shows the pleomorphic, convoluted nuclei of the latter. By immunocytochemistry, this lesion was diagnosed as a T-cell lymphoma. Papanicolaou preparation. ×1000.

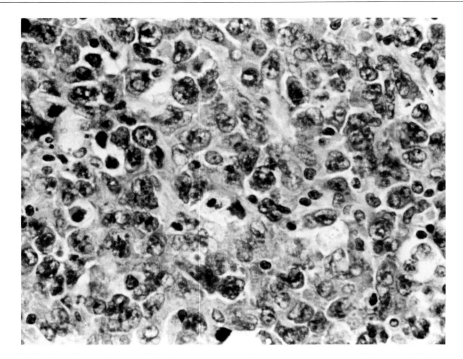

Fig. 3.34. T-cell lymphoma. Histology specimen shows large, pleomorphic nuclei. Hematoxylin and eosin preparation. × 625.

are from a patient with T-cell lymphoma diagnosed by immunocytochemical studies. The aspirate contained a pleomorphic cell population, with a large number of cells that had convoluted nuclei. The cytologic features of lymphoma are summarized in Table 3.7.

Mixed-Cell Lymphoma

In these tumors, small lymphocytes coexist with large lymphocytes and the diagnosis relies on the finding of almost equal proportions of small and large, cleaved lymphocytes in the aspirate. Large, noncleaved cells are present in varying proportions.

DIFFERENTIAL DIAGNOSIS. Conditions that must be considered in the differential diagnosis of non-Hodgkin's lymphoma include reactive lymphoid hyperplasia and metastatic undifferentiated or small-cell neoplasms. Differentiation of reactive lymphoid hyperplasia from lymphoma usually is not difficult and depends on the polymorphic nature of benign smears in contrast to the monomorphic picture in lymphoma. This subject was discussed on pages 125 to 129.

Metastatic small-cell tumors (e.g., small-cell carcinoma of the lungs, carcinoid and other neuroendocrine tumors, lobular carcinoma of the breasts, undifferentiated melanoma, Ewing's sarcoma, neuroblastoma and embryonal rhabdomyosarcoma) may mimic small-cell lymphomas. A number of tumors can mimic large-cell lymphomas; examples of such tumors are undifferentiated and poorly differentiated

TABLE 3.7. Common Types of Lymphoma: Summary of Cytologic Features

Cell Type	Morphologic Features of Aspirates	Type of Lymphoma
Lymphocyte, small	Nucleus slightly larger than that of resting lymphocyte; cells uniform, with round, dense nuclei and scanty cytoplasm; no nucleoli; plasmacytoid lymphocytes in plasmacytoid variant	Small lymphocytic chronic lymphocytic leukemia Plasmacytoid variant
Lymphocyte, intermediate	Nucleus larger than that of resting lymphocyte, round and cleaved; chromatin coarse and granular; nucleolus small	Small cleaved follicular center cell
	Nucleus about twice as large as that of resting lymphocyte, uniform and round; chromatin coarse and granular; nucleus not cleaved; one or more nucleoli; tingible-body macrophages in Burkitt's variant	Small noncleaved follicular center cell Burkitt's
Lymphocyte, large	Nucleus about three to four times as large as that of resting lymphocyte; cytoplasm variable and ill-defined; nucleus round or oval with irregular outlines due to clefts; chromatin coarsely granular; one or more large nucleoli; in noncleaved variant, nucleus round with no clefts; in immunoblastic sarcoma, nucleus round with one or more large, prominent nucleoli; cytoplasm has plasmacytoid differentiation; mitoses in all three types; few tingible-body macrophages may be seen	Large cleaved follicular center cell Large noncleaved follicular center cell Immunoblastic sarcoma
Lymphocyte, mixed	Nucleus small and cleaved or large and cleaved or noncleaved; chromatin coarsely granular; nucleolus small or prominent; mitoses seen	Small and large, mixed
Histiocyte	Large cell with pleomorphic nucleus; multinucleated cells seen; abundance of ill-defined cytoplasm; granular chromatin; nucleolus	Histiocytic
Reed-Sternberg	Mixed cell population; large, mononuclear Hodgkin's cells and binucleated or multilobated Reed-Sternberg cells; chromatin coarse; one or more prominent, pink nucleoli; histiocytes, plasma cells, eosinophils and lymphocytes in background	Hodgkin's

carcinomas, poorly differentiated melanoma and seminoma. The cytologic features of these neoplasms are discussed later in this chapter (see Tables 3.12 and 3.13). The history, clinical findings and the nonlymphoid character of the metastatic tumor cells help distinguish lymphoma from these neoplasms. In Romanowsky-stained preparations, the finding of lymphoglandular bodies helps greatly in recognizing the lymphoid nature of the aspirate.[8]

Akhtar and coworkers[22] have recently reported the use of electron microscopy in combination with needle aspiration biopsy for the diagnosis of round-cell malignant tumors of children. In their series, there were 29 lymphomas in 62 children with round-cell malignant tumors, consisting of neuroblastomas, Ewing's sarcomas, metastatic retinoblastomas, Wilms' tumors, rhabdomyosarcomas and a few unclassifiable tumors. In most cases, electron microscopy confirmed the cytologic impression and in a few cases allowed a definitive diagnosis.

Distinguishing among the various subtypes of lymphoma is a challenge for cytopathologists. However, careful attention to some of the tumor characteristics noted previously is helpful in making the diagnosis. On the basis of cell size, small-cell lymphomas can be differentiated from large-cell tumors. Careful attention to other features, particularly the characteristics of the nuclei (e.g., shape, cleaved or convoluted pattern and size of the nucleoli) helps further classifying the tumor. It must be recognized that a definitive diagnosis can be extremely difficult. Knowledge of the history and clinical findings, technically good preparations and experience on the part of the cytopathologist are prerequisites for an accurate diagnosis. Cytopathologists who perform lymph node aspirations may have an advantage over those who depend on clinicians for smears because the former are more likely to reaspirate if the first aspirate is not diagnostic. However, we believe that satisfactory results are always possible if there is good communication between the clinician and the cytopathologist. If the diagnosis is in doubt or if differentiation between B-cell and T-cell lymphoma is difficult, immunoperoxidase stains can be used on the aspirate.[24] The immunoperoxidase method is particularly helpful in differentiating metastatic neoplasms from lymphoma and reactive lymphadenitis from lymphoma and in determining the B-cell or T-cell origin of a lymphomatous process.

Hodgkin's Lymphoma

In contrast with non-Hodgkin's lymphoma, the Rye classification of Hodgkin's lymphoma[57] is relatively simple and widely accepted. The Rye classification is a modification of the original Lukes-Butler classification[58] that divides Hodgkin's lymphomas into four histologic types (Table 3.8). Reed-Sternberg cells and their mononuclear counterpart (often referred to as Hodgkin's cells) are considered neoplastic, whereas the other cellular components are regarded as benign and thought to represent an immune reaction to the neoplastic cells. The hallmark of the disease is Reed-Sternberg cells, without which the diagnosis cannot be made. However, because similar cells may occur in several other diseases,[59-62] Hodgkin's lymphoma can be diagnosed only when Reed-Sternberg cells are found in the appropriate cellular setting. The origin of Reed-Sternberg cells still remains unresolved, although recent studies have suggested that such cells are derived from the monocyte/macrophage cell line[63] or from reticular cells.[64] Lennert and associates[64] have suggested that

TABLE 3.8. Classifications of Hodgkin's Lymphoma

Lukes-Butler	Rye

Lymphocytic-histiocytic
    Nodular
    Diffuse
	Lymphocytic predominance

Nodular sclerosis	Nodular sclerosis
Mixed	Mixed cellularity
Diffuse fibrosis	Lymphocytic depletion
Reticular	

there may be two variants of Hodgkin's lymphoma, one derived from B-zone-specific dendritic cells and another derived from the T-zone-specific interdigitating reticular cells.

In the West, Hodgkin's lymphoma is the most common malignant neoplasm in young adults. The disease may involve a single lymph node or several nodes at different sites. The disease often involves the cervical and supraclavicular lymph nodes, making them easy targets for needle aspiration biopsy.

HISTOLOGIC FEATURES. In Hodgkin's lymphoma, there is a mixed population of cells, whereas in non-Hodgkin's lymphoma, there is a monomorphic population of cells. The relative proportions of neoplastic and nonneoplastic cells in Hodgkin's lymphoma vary and form the basis of the histologic subtypes.

The nonneoplastic cells are thought to be reactive and include small lymphocytes, plasma cells, eosinophils, neutrophils, histiocytes and fibroblasts. Epithelioid granulomas are encountered in approximately 10 percent of patients with Hodgkin's lymphoma.[65]

The neoplastic cells are the Hodgkin's cells and the Reed-Sternberg cells. Hodgkin's cells are large and have a large, oval, indented nucleus that appears vesicular and contains a prominent, round, eosinophilic nucleolus. Hodgkin's cells are considered precursors of Reed-Sternberg cells. A diagnosis of Hodgkin's lymphoma should not be based on the finding of Hodgkin's cells alone. The diagnosis relies on the observation of Reed-Sternberg cells. These large cells have an abundance of pale pink-staining cytoplasm. The nucleus of a Reed-Sternberg cell is large and multilobular and contains one or more large, circular, pink nucleoli that resemble inclusion bodies. The binucleated variant is sometimes referred to as a "mirror-image" or "owl-eye" cell. The chromatin is coarse with parachromatin clearing and a thick nuclear envelope. Electron microscopy shows that most cells have a single deeply cleaved nucleus, making the cell appear multilobular, or with two or more nuclei. In addition to such classical Reed-Sternberg cells, other forms that occur are helpful in identifying the various subtypes but cannot be used as the basis for the diagnosis. The lymphocytic and histiocytic variants of Reed-Sternberg cells have polylobular nuclei, which some authors compare to popcorn.[66] The lacunar type characteristically occurs in nodular sclerosing Hodgkin's lymphoma and has clear cytoplasm with lobular nuclei and small nucleoli.[58] Anaplastic Reed-Sternberg cells occur in the lymphocytic depletion type of Hodgkin's lymphoma and have pleomorphic, bizarre, polylobular nuclei with coarse chromatin and large, prominent nucleoli.

Lymphocytic Predominance

This variant of Hodgkin's lymphoma is usually evidenced by asymptomatic enlargement of lymph nodes (most commonly the cervical nodes) and carries the best prognosis of all the Hodgkin's lymphomas.[66] Characteristic features are Reed-Sternberg cells coexisting with small lymphocytes and solitary or small collections of histiocytes. Most of the Reed-Sternberg cells are of the L and H type and classical Reed-Sternberg cells are rarely encountered.

Nodular Sclerosis

Nodular sclerosis is the most common type of Hodgkin's lymphoma. The typical patient is a young woman with mediastinal or cervical lymphadenopathy. The prognosis of patients with nodular sclerosis variant of Hodgkin's lymphoma is good. The histologic pattern is one of bands of collagen separating nodules of lymphoid tissue that contain the lacunar type of Reed-Sternberg cell.[58] Typical Reed-Sternberg cells are seen but are few. A cellular phase of nodular sclerosis in which fibrosis is minimal also occurs.

Mixed Cellularity

About one-third of cases of Hodgkin's lymphoma fall in this category.[67] The cellular pattern, as the name indicates, is mixed, consisting of lymphocytes, eosinophils, plasma cells, histiocytes, neutrophils and classical Reed-Sternberg cells (Figs. 3.35 and 3.36).

Lymphocytic Depletion

This variant is an aggressive neoplasm that carries the worst prognosis of the four types. It occurs in elderly persons and is commonly associated with advanced disease. Histologic study shows that the nodes are not appreciably cellular and the parenchyma is replaced by fibrosis, with Reed-Sternberg cells usually showing anaplastic features,[58] and scattered lymphocytes. Foci of necrosis are usually observed.

CYTOLOGIC FEATURES. Hodgkin's lymphoma can be diagnosed on needle aspirates only if typical Reed-Sternberg cells are identified. If such cells are not seen, the appearance of the aspirates may be similar to that of normal lymph node aspirates or aspirates from cases of hyperplasia. Differentiation among the various subtypes is not possible and requires histologic study of the excised lymph node.

The cytologic appearance of aspirates is similar to the pattern seen on histologic examination. The aspirates are usually cellular, consisting largely of nonneoplastic lymphoid elements, including lymphocytes, plasma cells, eosinophils, neutrophils, histiocytes and fibroblasts in various proportions. The neoplastic cells are not numerous and a careful search is usually necessary to find the mononuclear Hodgkin's cells and the diagnostic Reed-Sternberg cells (Figs. 3.37 and 3.38). As was noted previously, these large cells have abundant cytoplasm. Their cell margins are not always well defined. The nuclei are large and round, oval or irregularly shaped. Binucleated, mirror-image, multinucleated and multilobular types can be identified.

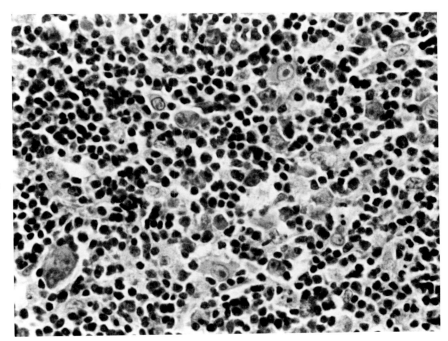

Fig. 3.35. Hodgkin's lymphoma, mixed cellularity type. Note the mononuclear Hodgkin's and Reed-Sternberg cells. Hematoxylin and eosin preparation. ×625.

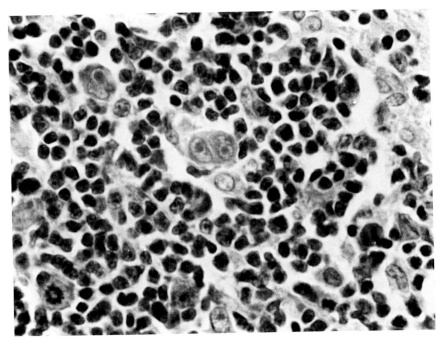

Fig. 3.36. Hodgkin's lymphoma. High-power view of Reed-Sternberg cells. Hematoxylin and eosin preparation. ×1000.

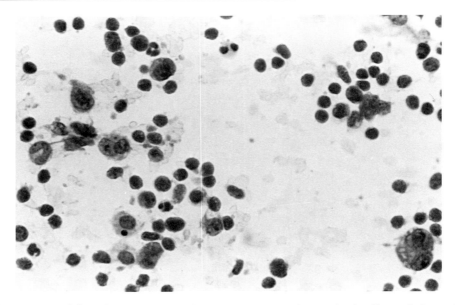

Fig. 3.37. Hodgkin's lymphoma. Cytology specimen contains a mixed cell population, with large, mononuclear Hodgkin's cells and Reed-Sternberg cells. Papanicolaou preparation. ×625.

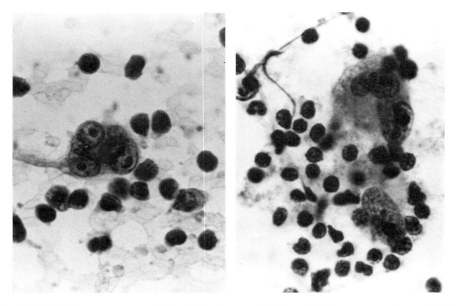

Fig. 3.38. High-power view of Reed-Sternberg cells. Papanicolaou preparation. ×1000.

The chromatin varies from fine to clumped, with aggregation at times along the nuclear membrane. Large, round or oval nucleoli that resemble inclusion bodies are characteristically seen in such cells. Even though Hodgkin's cells may also be encountered, the diagnosis relies on the finding of typical Reed-Sternberg cells. Mitoses may be seen in the mononuclear Hodgkin's cells. The cytologic features of Hodgkin's lymphoma visualized with Wright-Giemsa stain have been described in detail by Friedman and colleagues.[7] The cytologic features of Hodgkin's lymphoma are summarized in Table 3.7 and compared with those of non-Hodgkin's lymphoma. Aspirates from some cases of Hodgkin's lymphoma contain small clusters of histiocytic cells on a background of numerous lymphocytes. Histiocytic cells are usually detected in smears from patients with the lymphocytic predominance or mixed cellularity type of Hodgkin's lymphoma. Aspirates from cases of the nodular sclerosing type may contain few cellular elements, making the diagnosis difficult. The lymphocytic depletion type similarly may yield nondiagnostic material. Lymph nodes from patients undergoing treatment commonly have degenerative changes, necrosis or scarring, making the diagnosis difficult in such cases as well.

DIFFERENTIAL DIAGNOSIS. In the differential diagnosis, a number of disorders must be considered. The lymphocytic predominance type of Hodgkin's lymphoma may resemble small-cell lymphocytic lymphoma if Reed-Sternberg cells are not identified. The diffuse and mixed types of reactive lymphadenitis due to infectious mononucleosis or following vaccination and dermatopathic lymphadenitis may also pose problems in the differential diagnosis. In these conditions, there is a mixed cell population, consisting of numerous small lymphocytes, plasma cells, histiocytes, large, transformed lymphocytes and immunoblasts, which should be a clue to the diagnosis. Cells that resemble Reed-Sternberg cells may be encountered in patients with infectious mononucleosis[12,62] (Fig. 3.11, *inset*), toxoplasmosis,[62] post-vaccinial lymphadenitis or other malignant processes[61] and in those undergoing drug therapy.[59] If one finds a few such cells, caution is advisable. In such situations, the clinical findings and laboratory results should be taken into account in making the diagnosis. Only open excisional biopsy may provide definitive information.

Small loose groupings of elongated, histiocytic cells may be found in smears from patients with Hodgkin's lymphoma and such cells may be confused with those seen in granulomatous lymphadenitis. Distinction between these two processes depends on the identification of Reed-Sternberg cells. Aspirates from cases of the lymphocytic depletion type of Hodgkin's lymphoma may mimic the pattern seen in anaplastic carcinoma or histiocytic lymphoma and differentiation among these entities may be difficult.

DIAGNOSTIC PITFALLS IN LYMPHOMA

It is important to emphasize again that a diagnosis should not be attempted on unsatisfactory samples. Less than ideal preparations are often a cause of errors in interpretation and although one may be able to suspect a malignant process on examination of poorly prepared specimens, a definitive diagnosis is usually not possible in such cases. Areas in which the chromatin is streaked as a result of trauma should be disregarded in the examination of smears. Familiarity with aspirates from normal lymph nodes is essential if one is to avoid errors in the diagnosis of lympho-proliferative disorders. Confirmation of the cytologic diagnosis by excisional biopsy and histologic study is an important part of the learning process and should be done when a lymphoproliferative disorder is suspected. Experience can also be acquired by needling excised lymph nodes at the time of frozen section pathologic examination and the smears correlated with histologic sections.

Extensive necrosis and hyalinization may cause problems in interpretation and caution is advised. The cellular yield may not be sufficient to make a definitive diagnosis in some cases of lymphoma with hyalinization and when sclerosis is marked, as in the nodular sclerosis variant of Hodgkin's lymphoma. In the lymphocytic predominance variant, Reed-Sternberg cells may not be numerous and errors may occur. Moreover, the observation of epithelioid cell clusters may suggest a diagnosis of granulomatous lymphadenitis. Aspirates from cases of infectious mononucleosis and other disorders may contain cells that resemble Reed-Sternberg cell, increasing the possibility of misdiagnosis.

In non-Hodgkin's lymphoma, differentiation among the various subtypes may be difficult. Small-cell lymphocytic lymphoma (well-differentiated type of Rappaport) cannot be differentiated from chronic lymphocytic leukemia. Although tingible-body macrophages are usually found in reactive follicular hyperplasia, they may be seen in some large-cell lymphomas and Burkitt's lymphoma. Attention to the nuclear details in the surrounding cells should suggest the diagnosis because the nuclei in these lesions are unusually abnormal. Moreover, the mixed-cell pattern seen in reactive hyperplasia is lacking.

Differentiation of small-cell lymphomas from other small-cell tumors may be difficult. Similarly, some pleomorphic large-cell lymphomas can mimic undifferentiated carcinoma. Immunoperoxidase staining and electron microscopy can be performed on the aspirates in such cases. However, these special studies are not always available. In such situations, excision of the lymph node for histologic study is advisable.

RESULTS OF ASPIRATION BIOPSY CYTOLOGY IN LYMPHOMA

Despite the popularity of needle aspiration biopsy in recent years, only a few reports have attempted to document the accuracy of this technique in the diagnosis of malignant lymphoma. Loseke and Craver[9] in 1946 reported a diagnostic accuracy of 52 percent for Hodgkin's lymphoma. In a review of 101 patients, Morrison and associates[10] in 1952 reported a diagnostic accuracy of 83 percent for Hodgkin's lymphoma and 80 percent for non-Hodgkin's lymphoma. Subsequent reports have also noted the high accuracy of needle aspiration biopsy in the diagnosis of lymphoma.[5-7,11,13,17,68] We recently reviewed our experience with aspiration biopsy cytology of lymphomas.[12] Of 49 tumors, 42 were correctly diagnosed on needle aspiration biopsy (Table 3.9). The overall accuracy was 85.7 percent. Of the seven

TABLE 3.9. Aspiration Biopsy Cytology in Malignant Lymphoma

Pathologic Diagnosis	Number of Cases	Cytologic Diagnosis	Number of Cases
Non-Hodgkin's lymphoma		Non-Hodgkin's lymphoma	
Lymphocytic	23	Small cell, lymphocytic	19
Histiocytic	6	Large cell, lymphocytic	5
Hodgkin's lymphoma	15	Hodgkin's lymphoma	13
Chronic lymphocytic leukemia	4	Chronic lymphocytic leukemia	4
Waldenström's macro-globulinemia	1	Waldenström's macro-globulinemia	1
Total	49		42

false-negative cases, four were small-cell lymphocytic lymphomas and one was a large-cell lymphoma. The remaining two cases were Hodgkin's lymphomas. All the Hodgkin's lymphomas were of the nodular sclerosing type and the tumors contained relatively few neoplastic cells. All seven false-negative diagnoses were regarded as observer errors that were largely the result of inexperience during the early part of the study. There was one false-positive diagnosis in a patient with infectious mononucleosis. In this case, the observation of a few multinucleated cells that resembled Reed-Sternberg cells suggested a diagnosis of Hodgkin's lymphoma. Excision of the lymph node revealed reactive changes consistent with infectious mononucleosis.

METASTATIC NEOPLASMS

Lymph node enlargement is often the first clinical manifestation of metastasis of a malignant process. Metastases in the cervical lymph nodes are the presenting sign in about 25 to 50 percent of patients with cancer of the oral cavity, oropharynx, nasopharynx or thyroid.[69] Engzell and associates[15] studied 1101 cases of metastatic carcinoma involving the lymph nodes of the neck and found that the primary tumor was located above the clavicle in 47.5 percent of cases and below the clavicle in 48 percent; the site of the primary tumor could not be determined in 4.5 percent of cases. Ill-advised early excisional biopsy in the head and neck is known to complicate future surgical procedures.[70,71] Seeding of tumor cells into avascular planes and scarring are commonly noted after such biopsies. Needle aspiration biopsy provides an alternative to premature excisional biopsy for lesions that involve the lymph nodes of the head and neck.[72] This technique is especially helpful in the diagnosis of metastatic cancer involving the lymph nodes.[4-6,15,17,46] Because most lymph nodes of the head and neck are superficial, they are easily accessible for aspiration biopsy. Needle aspiration biopsy not only provides a cytologic diagnosis of metastatic cancer but also helps determine the type of the tumor cells and thus aids in predicting the site of the primary tumor.[15]

CLINICAL FEATURES. Most patients with metastatic cancer are between the ages of 50 and 80 years and male patients outnumber female patients. Often, only one

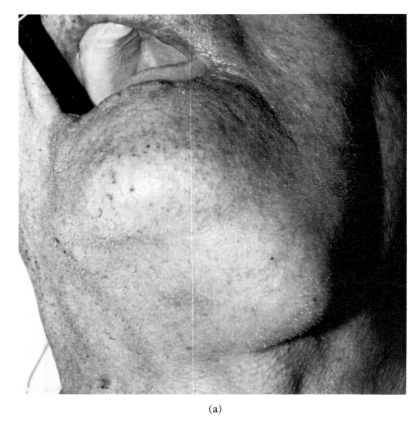

(a)

Fig. 3.39. (a) Submandibular lymph node enlargement the result of metastatic squamous cell carcinoma from a minute intraoral primary tumor involving the floor of the mouth (b) (arrows).

lymph node is palpable, although more than one node may be affected and bilateral involvement does occur. The location of the lymph node metastases may indicate the site of the primary lesion. The left supraclavicular lymph nodes commonly harbor metastases from carcinomas of the stomach, colon, lungs, breasts and prostate; the posterior cervical lymph nodes most commonly have metastases from nasopharyngeal carcinoma. Tumors of the skin of the upper part of the face, eyelids and temple area usually metastasize first to the preauricular and parotid nodes. The submandibular nodes are commonly involved by carcinoma of the lip, floor of the mouth and anterior part of the tongue and the submental nodes most often have metastases from carcinoma of the lip and anterior floor of the mouth (Fig. 3.39). Carcinomas of the palate, tonsils or lateral parts of the tongue tend to spread to the upper jugular lymph nodes, whereas carcinomas of the larynx and pharynx tend to metastasize first to the middle jugular nodes. Carcinomas of the thyroid usually spread to the lower and middle jugular lymph nodes and lateral supraclavicular nodes but can spread to the lymph nodes of the upper part of the neck, as shown in Figure 3.40.

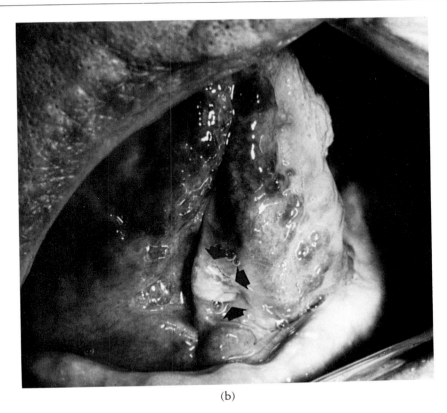

(b)

The work-up usually results in the localization of the primary tumor in the vast majority of cases. In 5 to 10 percent of cases, however, no primary tumor is found despite extensive investigation, including careful visualization, palpation and multiple endoscopy under general anesthesia.

Squamous cell carcinoma is the most common tumor that metastasizes to the lymph nodes of the head and neck. In one study, 40 percent of the tumors were squamous cell carcinomas, poorly differentiated carcinomas comprised 21 percent and the remaining 38 percent were adenocarcinomas.[15] Other primary tumors that arise in the head and neck, such as melanoma and carcinoma of the thyroid and salivary glands, also frequently metastasize to the cervical lymph nodes. Involvement of a single supraclavicular lymph node usually is the result of metastasis from a primary tumor below the clavicle, in most cases in the breasts, lungs, gastrointestinal tract or genital tract.

CYTOLOGIC FEATURES. Aspirates from involved lymph nodes of the neck usually consist of one or two drops of grayish, semisolid material. Some metastatic tumors are cystic. In metastatic papillary thyroid carcinoma, the fluid is clear or slightly murky and colorless or reddish brown. In well-differentiated squamous cell carcinoma, one or more milliliters of turbid yellow or puslike fluid may be obtained because the center of such a lesion often becomes partially necrotic.

The smears usually contain numerous tumor cells in most cases. Occasionally, the

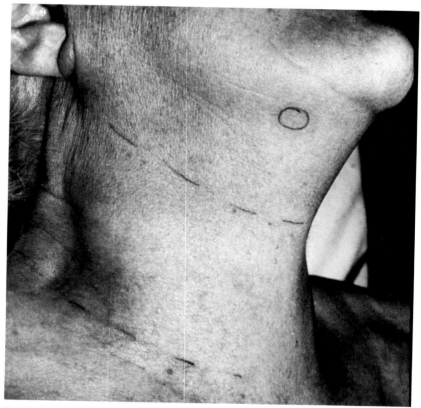

Fig. 3.40. Solitary metastasis in a lymph node of the upper part of the neck in an elderly woman with previous breast cancer. Aspiration biopsy cytology resulted in a diagnosis of papillary-follicular carcinoma metastatic from the thyroid.

lymphoid component may be abundant. The diagnosis of a malignant process is not difficult in most cases because cancer cells are easily recognizable. One may find solitary tumor cells or small loose groupings or large sheets and aggregates of neoplastic cells. Necrosis may be evident.

Squamous Cell Carcinoma

Squamous cell carcinoma in a node of the neck can be metastatic from the oral cavity, oropharynx, larynx, hypopharynx, nasal cavity, paranasal sinuses, nasopharynx or skin. Squamous cell carcinoma of the esophagus, trachea or bronchus can also metastasize to the lymph nodes of the neck. The histologic appearance of such metastases is usually similar to that of the primary lesion and may be keratinizing (Fig. 3.41), nonkeratinizing (Fig. 3.42), poorly differentiated, undifferentiated or anaplastic.

CYTOLOGIC FEATURES. Squamous cell carcinoma of a cervical lymph node is probably the easiest metastatic lesion to diagnose by aspiration biopsy cytology. The

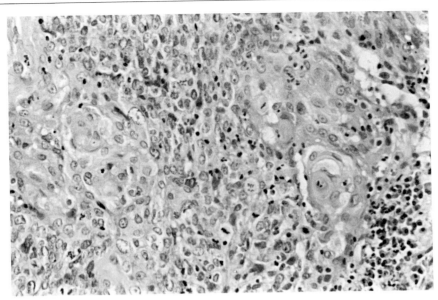

Fig. 3.41. Keratinizing squamous cell carcinoma. Hematoxylin and eosin preparation. ×390.

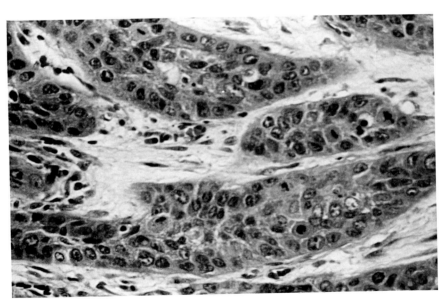

Fig. 3.42. Nonkeratinizing squamous cell carcinoma. Hematoxylin and eosin preparation. ×625.

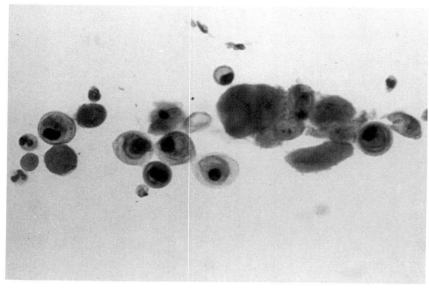

Fig. 3.43. Keratinizing squamous cell carcinoma metastatic to a lymph node of the neck. Cytology specimen. Papanicolaou preparation. ×625.

cytologic appearance varies with the degree of differentiation and the smears may consist of well-differentiated, keratinized tumor cells or completely undifferentiated, malignant cells.

In well-differentiated carcinoma, one sees solitary tumor cells and small loose groupings of tumor cells (Plate I.4). There are great variations in the size and shape of the tumor cells. The cytoplasm is usually abundant and pink to orangeophilic. Pearl formations and a bird's-eye pattern are usually observed. Fragments of keratinized cytoplasm (so-called ghost cells) may also be noted (Fig. 3.43). The keratinized cells have small, dark-staining, pyknotic nuclei and the nonkeratinized cells have large, round or oval nuclei. The chromatin of the nonkeratinized cells is coarse and granular and such cells have prominent nucleoli. Both cell types are usually identifiable in any given smear. In keratinized tumors, a giant-cell reaction to keratin may be evident in the aspirates (Fig. 3.44). In such cases, mononucleate, binucleate, and multinucleate histiocytes are encountered in the smears.

In the cystic variant, keratinized squames that have small, pyknotic nuclei are usually visible. It may be difficult to determine the malignant nature in cases of this variant because of the large amount of necrotic debris that can be present. In such cases, careful examination demonstrates small groupings of malignant cells. The clinical history is helpful in such cases and if there is a high clinical suspicion of cancer but the smear is not diagnostic, needle aspiration biopsy should be repeated.

In poorly differentiated tumors, or the nonkeratinizing type, solitary tumor cells or sheets and trabeculae of malignant cells may be observed (Fig. 3.45). The cell margins are indistinct and the nuclei overlap and contain coarsely granular chromatin and prominent nucleoli (Fig. 3.46). Mitoses are frequently seen.

In the anaplastic, giant-cell and spindle cell variants of squamous cell carcinoma,

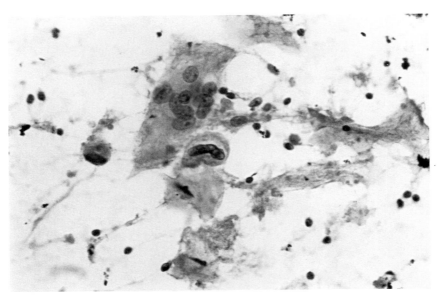

Fig. 3.44. Foreign-body giant-cell reaction to keratin in a case of well-differentiated squamous cell carcinoma. Papanicolaou preparation. ×390.

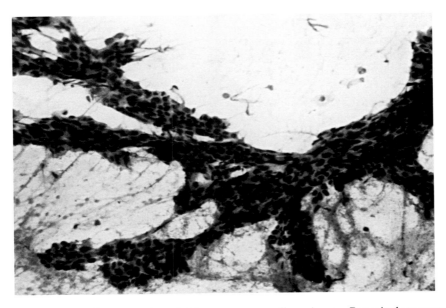

Fig. 3.45. Aspirate from a nonkeratinizing squamous cell carcinoma. Papanicolaou preparation. ×390.

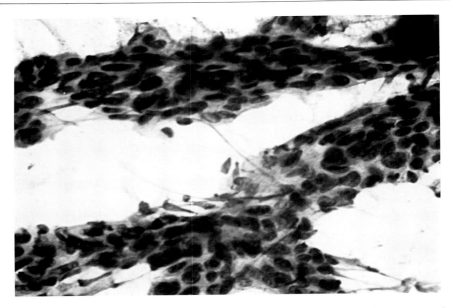

Fig. 3.46. High-power view of the cells shown in Figure 3.45. Papanicolaou preparation. ×625.

one sees small and large tumor cells that have abundant cytoplasm and many with two or more bizarre nuclei (Fig. 3.47). Spindle cells may also be observed. The squamous cell origin of such tumors may be difficult to ascertain on the basis of cytologic examination alone. The cytologic features of metastatic squamous cell carcinoma are summarized in Table 3.10.

DIFFERENTIAL DIAGNOSIS. The diagnosis of well-differentiated squamous cell carcinoma is usually straightforward. However, cystic metastases in lymph nodes of the lateral aspects of the neck must be differentiated from branchial cleft cysts.[73,74] If no

TABLE 3.10. Squamous Cell Carcinoma: Summary of Cytologic Features

Well Differentiated	*Poorly Differentiated*
Solitary and loose groupings of cells. Marked variation in cell size and shape. Round, oval, polygonal or spindle-shaped cells. Cytoplasm well defined, dense and eosinophilic. Keratinization. Nuclei small, round or oval and pyknotic in keratinized cells. Nuclei in other cells large with coarse chromatin and prominent nucleoli. Histiocytes and multinucleated giant cells may be seen. Necrotic and cystic.	Usually solitary cells, occasionally in groupings or sheets. Nuclear crowding. Smears more uniform in cell size and shape in comparison to well-differentiated tumors. Abundance of delicate cytoplasm with ill-defined margins. Keratinization rare. Nuclei large and pleomorphic with coarsely granular chromatin and large nucleoli. May be difficult to distinguish from poorly differentiated adenocarcinoma.

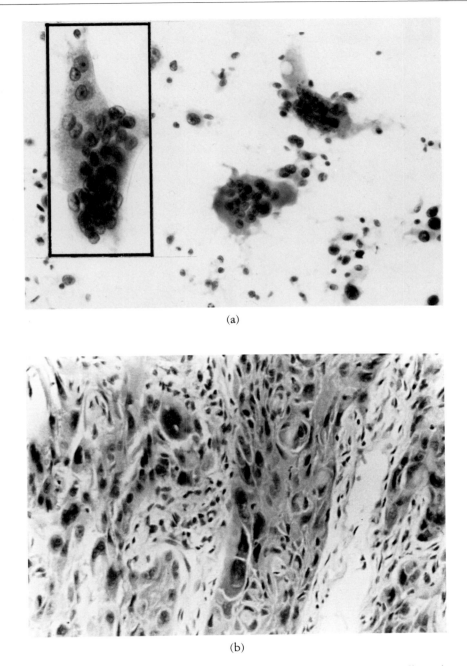

(a)

(b)

Fig. 3.47. (a) Aspirate from an anaplastic giant-cell variant of squamous cell carcinoma. Papanicolaou preparation. ×390. (*Inset*, ×625.) (b) Anaplastic giant-cell variant of squamous cell carcinoma. Histology specimen. Hematoxylin and eosin preparation. ×625.

malignant cells can be found, differentiation between these entities may be impossible. Most patients with metastatic cancer are more than 30 years of age, whereas most patients with congenital cysts are less than 30 years of age.[73] However, congenital cysts have been encountered in middle-age and elderly patients. Therefore, if a cystic lesion discovered on needle aspiration biopsy has no definite cytologic features of a malignant nature, reaspiration of residual tumor or a recurrent mass is mandatory. If the lesion is neoplastic, smears from the second aspirate usually contain clearly malignant cells, allowing one to make the diagnosis. Congenital cysts can be confused with metastatic squamous cell carcinoma. Diagnostic confusion usually occurs when branchial cleft cysts become infected. Atypia in the epithelial lining cells mimics a malignant process in such cases. (See pages 196 and 197 and Chapter 5.)

Anaplastic spindle and giant-cell variants of squamous cell carcinoma may mimic mesenchymal tumors and malignant melanoma. Similar cells are also seen in giant-cell tumors of the lungs, thyroid, pancreas and other organs. Differentiation among these entities can be difficult. (See pages 183 and 195.)

Poorly differentiated squamous cell carcinoma occasionally resembles poorly differentiated adenocarcinoma. In most cases, differences in the shape of the tumor cells and in their cytoplasmic and nuclear characteristics helps in making the correct diagnosis. However, differentiation may be impossible. The history and clinical findings may also be helpful in this regard.

Focal squamous differentiation in an otherwise undifferentiated tumor suggests poorly differentiated squamous cell carcinoma. However, a similar appearance may be seen in high-grade mucoepidermoid carcinoma, in which glandular differentiation may be difficult to identify on cytologic examination. This topic was discussed in Chapter 2.

Adenocarcinoma

Most adenocarcinomas that metastasize to the lymph nodes of the head or neck originate in the breasts, thyroid, salivary glands, gastrointestinal tract or lungs. Adenocarcinoma of the kidneys (Fig. 3.48), pancreas, ovaries, endometrium and prostate also metastasize to the lymph nodes of the neck.[13] About 5 to 20 percent of all carcinomas of the nose and paranasal sinuses are adenocarcinomas.[75] Most such neoplasms are adenoid cystic, arising from the minor salivary glands, although a distinctive tumor that resembles adenocarcinoma of the colon has been described.[76] The histologic appearance of metastatic adenocarcinoma of the lymph nodes of the neck is usually similar to that of the primary tumor. Carcinoma of the thyroid, most salivary gland neoplasms, clear-cell carcinoma of the kidneys, carcinoma of the breasts and some malignant tumors of the gastrointestinal and genital tracts have distinctive histologic features and such features may be clues to the site of the primary tumor. In other metastatic neoplasms, it may be impossible to determine the origin of the primary tumor on the basis of histologic examination.

CYTOLOGIC FEATURES. It is relatively easy to diagnose metastatic adenocarcinoma by aspiration biopsy cytology if there is evidence of glandular differentiation. If cytologic examination does not detect this feature, differentiation from poorly differentiated or undifferentiated squamous cell carcinoma and other neoplasms is

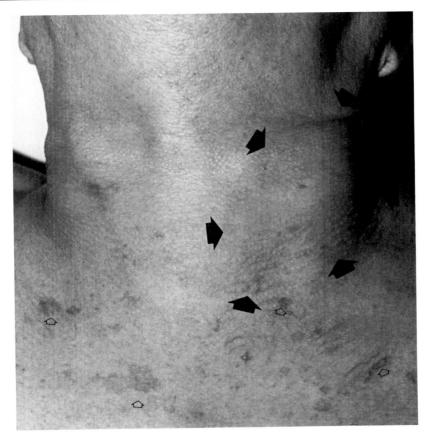

Fig. 3.48. Metastatic renal cell carcinoma of the lymph nodes of the left side of the neck and the left lobe of the thyroid. Note the dilated veins in the skin of the upper chest.

difficult. In well-differentiated variants, the aspirates consist of neoplastic cells in sheets, small groupings or ductlike or glandular structures (Figs. 3.49, 3.50, 3.51 and 3.52). Solitary tumor cells are also observed. The cells vary from cuboidal to columnar and have abundant cytoplasm. The cell borders appear well defined. Mucus may be detected inside cytoplasmic vacuoles or may be found outside the tumor cells in the background. With the Papanicolaou method, the mucus is translucent to pale pink, whereas with the Romanowsky methods, it stains purple to violet. The nuclei of adenocarcinoma cells are round or oval. Variation in nuclear size is not uncommon. Binucleate forms may also be identified. The chromatin is finely to coarsely granular. The cells of most such tumors have a single large nucleolus, but the cells of some well-differentiated tumors have an inconspicuous nucleolus or no nucleolus. Mitoses are usually observed.

Some adenocarcinomas have a distinctive cytologic appearance, enabling one to determine the histologic type. Papillary carcinoma consists of round or branching, three-dimensional groupings of tumor cells that are surrounded by a continuous, community type of border (Fig. 3.53). The peripheral layer of malignant cells may

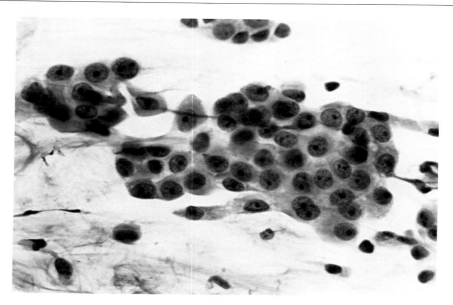

Fig. 3.49. Aspirate from a lymph node. Sheets of adenocarcinoma cells. The primary tumor was in the colon. Papanicolaou preparation. ×625.

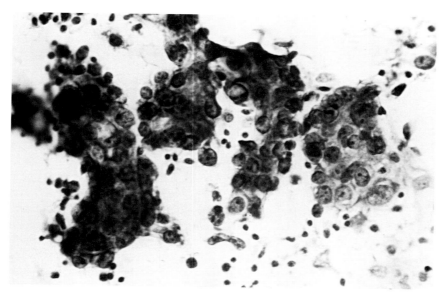

Fig. 3.50. Small groupings of cells in a glandular configuration. The primary tumor was in a breast. Papanicolaou preparation. ×625.

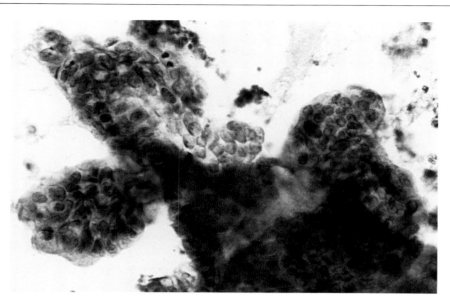

Fig. 3.51. Aspirate from a lymph node harboring a metastasis from an adenocarcinoma of the stomach. Note the common community border of the cellular fragments. Papanicolaou preparation. ×625.

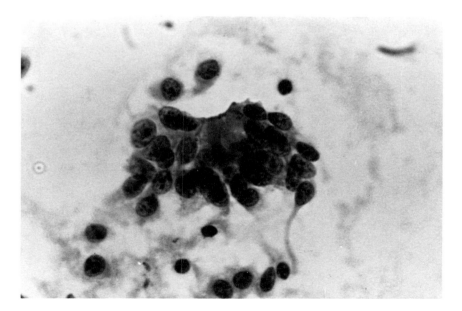

Fig. 3.52. A small fragment of tall, columnar, glandular lining cells shows pseudo-stratification of oval, malignant nuclei. The primary tumor was in the rectum. Papanicolaou preparation. ×1000.

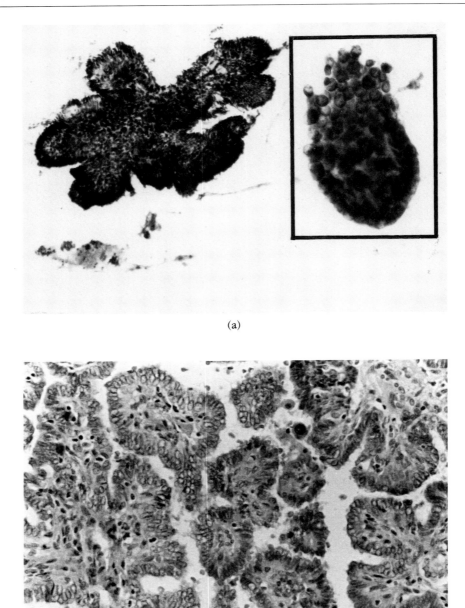

(a)

(b)

Fig. 3.53. (a) Aspirate from a papillary carcinoma of the thyroid metastatic to a lymph node of the neck. Note the three-dimensional papillary fragments. Papanicolaou preparation. ×150. (*Inset,* ×625.) (b) Papillary carcinoma. Histology specimen. Hematoxylin and eosin preparation. ×625.

appear cuboidal or columnar and lies at right angles to the other tumor cells in the cluster. Metastases in the cervical lymph nodes are not an uncommon manifestation of papillary carcinoma of the thyroid and, in rare cases, of papillary carcinoma of the ovaries. Psammoma bodies may be identified in carcinomas of the thyroid, ovaries, endometrium, pancreas, lungs and other organs.

Follicular carcinoma of the cervical lymph nodes consists of numerous tumor cells in small, follicle-like or rosette-like formations (Fig. 3.54). Colloid is usually not abundant. The nuclei are round and have fine, dispersed chromatin and small nucleoli. The cytoplasm is scanty and ill-defined. In Hürthle cell carcinoma, the tumor cells are dispersed. The cytoplasm is abundant and has a granular to dense quality (Fig. 3.55). With hematoxylin and eosin stain, the cytoplasm appears eosinophilic, although it has a greenish tinge with Papanicolaou stain. The tumor cells may have a small or large nucleus and prominent nucleoli. Binucleate forms are also encountered.

Adenoid cystic carcinoma and other primary carcinomas of the salivary glands may metastasize to the lymph nodes and the diagnosis in most cases is not difficult (see Chapter 2 for a discussion of the cytologic features of this neoplasm).

Signet-ring cell carcinoma consists of cells that have an eccentric nucleus and mucous vacuoles in the cytoplasm, usually suggesting mucus-secreting adenocarcinoma (Fig. 3.56), which commonly originates in the stomach, although similar cells may be seen in carcinomas of the colorectum and breasts. Low-grade mucoepidermoid tumors also contain groupings of goblet-like mucous cells; however, such cells are usually accompanied by intermediate and squamous cells. Colloid carcinomas metastatic from the breasts or gastrointestinal tract (Plate I.5) consist of small, ball-like clusters of tumor cells on a background of pale-staining mucus (Fig. 3.57). Aspirates from lymph nodes that harbor metastases from carcinoma of the breasts may contain cells in an Indian file arrangement (Fig. 3.58). However, one more often sees solid groupings of cells or strips of glandular epithelium (Fig. 3.59) aspirated intact from lymph nodes that harbor metastases. In addition, cytoplasmic vacuoles may be observed in some tumor cells in cases of infiltrating lobular carcinoma.

In adenocarcinoma metastatic from the prostate, a pattern reminiscent of carcinoma of the breasts may be seen, with solid groupings of cells. However, careful examination will also reveal glandular differentiation (Fig. 3.60). The cells of clear-cell carcinoma of the kidneys have an abundance of clear or granular cytoplasm and round, uniform nuclei that contain prominent nucleoli (Fig. 3.61). The cells may be in small groupings or in sheets that have well-defined borders.[48] Table 3.11 summarizes the cytologic features of metastatic adenocarcinoma.

DIFFERENTIAL DIAGNOSIS. In most cases, the diagnosis of metastatic adenocarcinoma is straightforward. However, the site of the primary tumor cannot always be determined by cytologic examination alone. Knowledge of the clinical findings and history and the cytologic features of the lymph node aspirate often narrow the search for the primary neoplasm. Poorly differentiated adenocarcinoma may be difficult to distinguish from poorly differentiated or undifferentiated squamous cell carcinoma. Careful investigation may provide a clue to the diagnosis. Vacuoles are not always an indication of glandular differentiation, sometimes reflecting cellular degeneration.

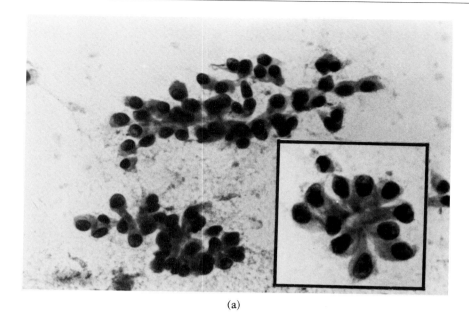

(a)

(b)

Fig. 3.54. (a) Aspirate from a follicular carcinoma of the thyroid metastatic to a lymph node of the neck. Note the follicle-like arrangement of the cells. Nucleoli are also visible. Papanicolaou preparation. ×625. (*Inset,* ×1000.) (b) Follicular carcinoma. Histology specimen shows small follicles, occasionally with colloid in their lumina. Hematoxylin and eosin preparation. ×390.

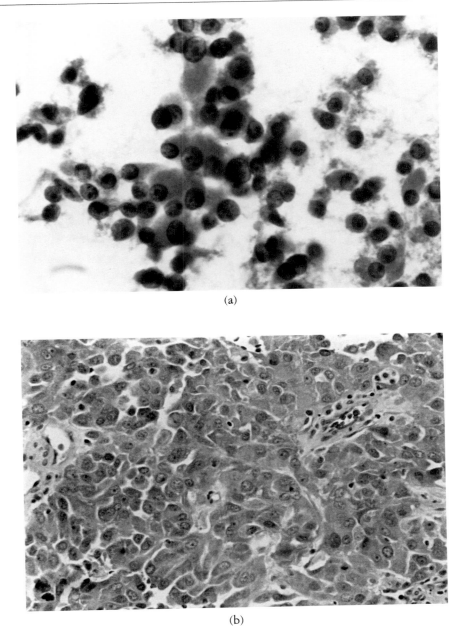

(a)

(b)

Fig. 3.55. (a) Aspirate from a Hürthle cell carcinoma metastatic to a lymph node of the neck. Note the dispersed cells that have an abundance of granular cytoplasm. Papanicolaou preparation. ×1000. (b) Hürthle cell carcinoma. Histology specimen. Hematoxylin and eosin preparation. ×390.

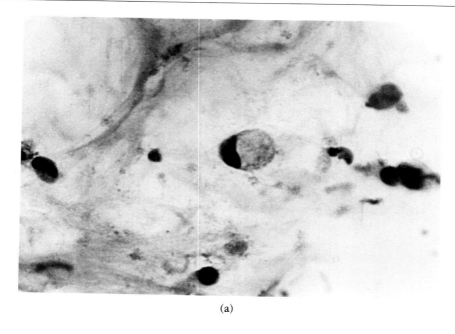

(a)

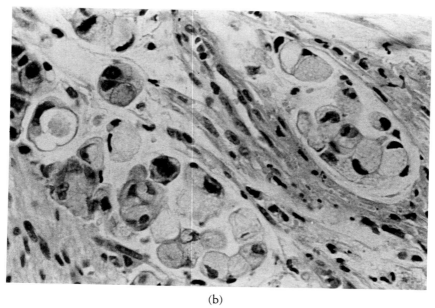

(b)

Fig. 3.56. (a) Aspirate from a signet-ring cell carcinoma metastatic to a supraclavicular lymph node. The primary tumor was in the cecum. Note the mucus-filled cytoplasm of the tumor cell, pushing the nucleus against the cell membrane. Papanicolaou preparation. ×1000. (b) Signet-ring cell adenocarcinoma of the cecum. Histology specimen. Hematoxylin and eosin preparation. ×625.

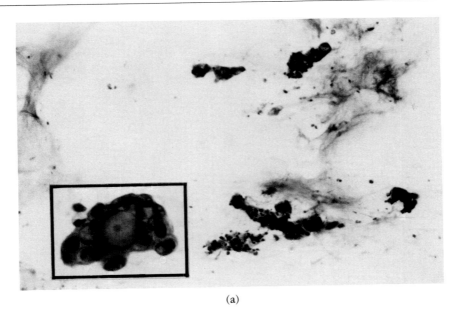

(a)

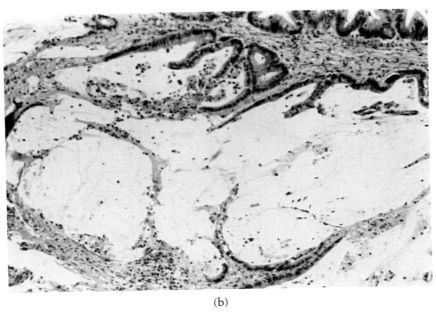

(b)

Fig. 3.57. (a) Aspirate from a colloid carcinoma of the rectum metastatic to a lymph node. Note the strands of mucus and the three-dimensional fragments of tumor cells. Papanicolaou preparation. ×150. (*Inset*, ×625.) (b) Colloid carcinoma. Note the lakes of mucus and the malignant, glandular epithelium. Hematoxylin and eosin preparation. ×150.

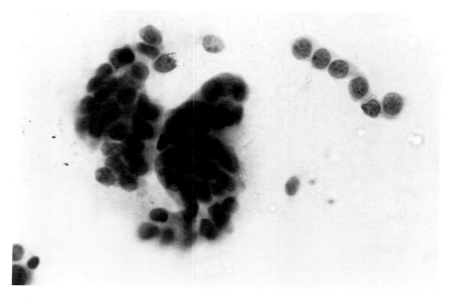

Fig. 3.58. Aspirate from a carcinoma of the breast metastatic to a lymph node. Note the small, glandular grouping of cells coexisting with a few cells in a single-file arrangement. Papanicolaou preparation. × 1000.

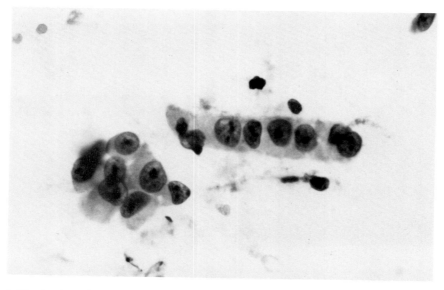

Fig. 3.59. Aspirate from an adenocarcinoma metastatic to a lymph node. The primary tumor was in a breast. Note the strips and small groupings of malignant, glandular cells. Papanicolaou preparation. × 1000.

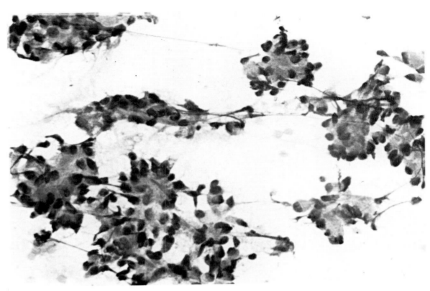

Fig. 3.60. Aspirate from an adenocarcinoma of the prostate metastatic to a lymph node. Note the numerous small acinar structures, reminiscent of the small glands seen in well-differentiated adenocarcinoma. Papanicolaou preparation. ×390.

Undifferentiated Carcinoma

Undifferentiated carcinoma arises in a variety of organs and frequently metastasizes to the cervical lymph nodes. Common examples include undifferentiated nasopharyngeal carcinoma, small-cell and large-cell undifferentiated carcinomas of the lungs, undifferentiated carcinoma of the salivary glands and undifferentiated carcinoma of the skin (Merkel cell tumor). Anaplastic giant-cell and spindle cell variants also occur and are discussed separately.

TABLE 3.11. Adenocarcinoma: Summary of Cytologic Features

Well Differentiated	Poorly Differentiated
Sheets, groupings and glandlike arrangement of cells. Solid papillary fragments may be seen. Solitary cuboidal or columnar cells also seen.	Solitary cells or small, loose groupings of cells. Nuclear overlapping and crowding. Solitary cells cuboidal of occasionally columnar.
Cytoplasm usually abundant and vacuolated with well-defined margins. Nucleus round or oval and fairly uniform in size with fine or coarse chromatin. One or more small or large nucleoli.	Cytoplasm scanty, delicate and ill-defined. Occasional vacuolation. Nucleus large and round or oval with coarsely granular chromatin. One or more usually large nucleoli.
Extracellular mucin may be seen.	In the absence of glandular differentiation, difficult to distinguish from poorly differentiated squamous cell carcinoma.

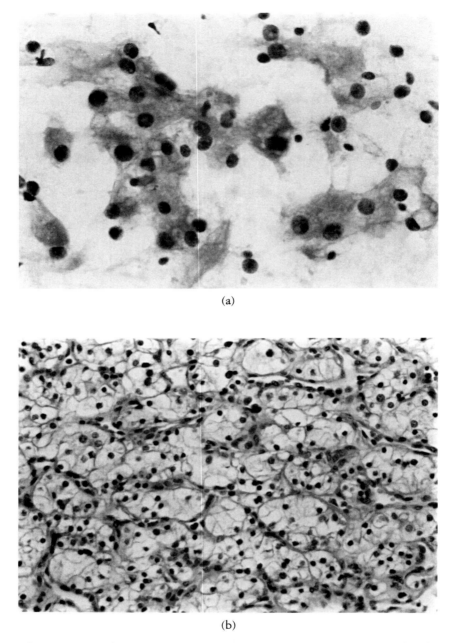

(a)

(b)

Fig. 3.61. (a) Aspirate from a metastasis from a renal cell carcinoma. Note the abundance of foamy cytoplasm and the round or oval nuclei that contain prominent nucleoli. Papanicolaou preparation. ×625. (b) Renal cell carcinoma, clear-cell type. Histology specimen. Hematoxylin and eosin preparation. ×390.

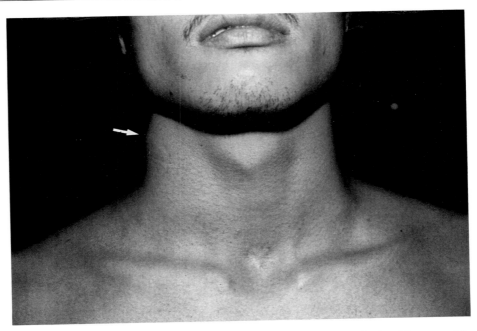

Fig. 3.62. Metastatic nasopharyngeal carcinoma, bilateral needle aspiration biopsy positive, of the lymph nodes of the posterior triangle in a young Oriental man. The involved node in the right side of the neck can be appreciated in the picture (arrow), and some fullness is visible on the left side of the neck.

CYTOLOGIC FEATURES. Aspirates from lymph nodes that harbor metastases from undifferentiated carcinoma are usually appreciably cellular. Solitary tumor cells and small, cohesive cell clusters may be observed. Necrosis is frequently noted and is manifested by small, pyknotic nuclei on a background of granular debris. Small-cell and large-cell types are seen. The cytoplasm is scanty and ill-defined in small-cell variants but usually plentiful in large-cell tumors. The chromatin is coarsely granular and may contain small or large nucleoli. Nuclear molding is commonly observed.

Nasopharyngeal Carcinoma

This unusual tumor arises from the epithelial cells of the nasopharynx. Metastases in the cervical lymph nodes are usually the first manifestation of such neoplasms (Fig. 3.62). Three histologic patterns have been described: keratinizing squamous cell carcinoma, nonkeratinizing carcinoma and undifferentiated carcinoma. The keratinizing type resembles the squamous cell carcinoma typically encountered in the upper aerodigestive tract. The nonkeratinizing type is similar to transitional cell carcinoma. The undifferentiated type, or lymphoepithelioma, consists of undifferentiated tumor cells admixed with lymphoid cells (Fig. 3.63).

CYTOLOGIC FEATURES. In lymphoepithelioma, the tumor cell nuclei are large and vesicular and round or oval and contain a prominent nucleolus. The tumor cells occur in masses or sheets or as solitary cells. Cytologic study shows that most smears

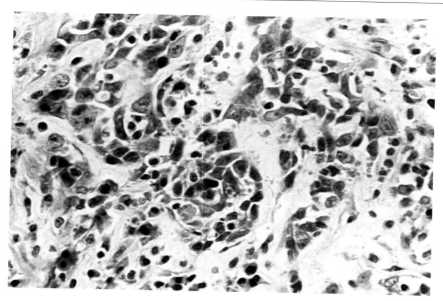

Fig. 3.63. Lymphoepithelioma metastatic to a posterior cervical lymph node. Histology specimen. Hematoxylin and eosin preparation. ×625.

consist of undifferentiated carcinoma cells and lymphoid cells in variable proportions (Fig. 3.64). The lymphocytes are usually mature and small. The epithelial cells occur as solitary cells or in small, cohesive clusters. The cytoplasm is ill-defined. The nuclei are round or oval and contain finely granular chromatin and prominent nucleoli.

The keratinizing and nonkeratinizing types have features similar to squamous cell carcinoma of other parts of the body. Lymphoid cells are usually not found in the smears from such neoplasms, unless they are lymphocytes from a lymph node that harbors a metastasis.

Small-Cell Undifferentiated Carcinoma

Small-cell carcinoma of lungs may metastasize to the supraclavicular lymph nodes. Needle aspirates from involved lymph nodes are usually diagnostic and thus obviate excisional biopsy. There are two types of small-cell undifferentiated carcinoma, the oat cell type and the intermediate cell type. These two types can be differentiated on the basis of cell size on cytologic study.

CYTOLOGIC FEATURES. In the oat cell type, the tumor cells have round or oval nuclei about twice the size of a nucleus of a normal lymphocyte. The cytoplasm is difficult to see in the cellular samples. The tumor cells are mostly solitary, although small, loose groupings are also observed (Fig. 3.65). Nuclear molding is usually noted in the cell groupings. The chromatin is fine and nucleoli are not identifiable. In the intermediate cell type, the tumor cells occur in small groupings and as solitary cells. The tumor cells are larger than those of the oat cell variety and have a slightly greater quantity of ill-defined cytoplasm (Fig. 3.66). The tumor cell nuclei are round

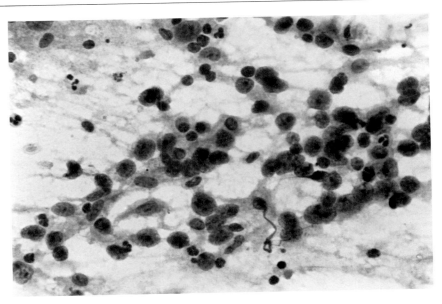

Fig. 3.64. Lymphoepithelioma. Aspirate from an enlarged posterior cervical lymph node. Note the admixture of undifferentiated tumor cells, lymphocytes and plasma cells. Papanicolaou preparation. ×625.

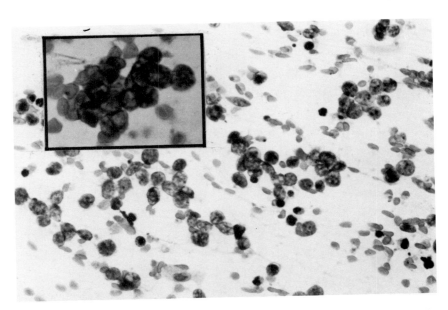

Fig. 3.65. Small-cell undifferentiated carcinoma metastatic to a supraclavicular lymph node. Note the nuclear molding, which is better seen in the inset. Papanicolaou preparation. ×625. (*Inset*, ×1000.)

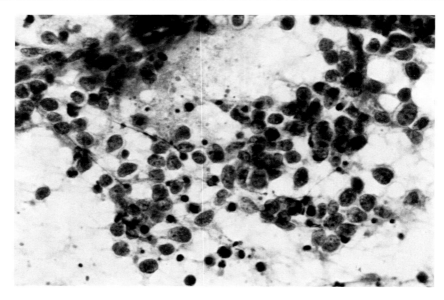

Fig. 3.66. Small-cell undifferentiated carcinoma, intermediate cell type. Small, dark-staining, necrotic cells are seen in the background. Papanicolaou preparation. ×625.

or oval and have coarser chromatin; small nucleoli can be identified in well-preserved cells. Nuclear molding is noted. In both tumor cell types, degenerative cells with small, pyknotic nuclei are usually associated with tumor cells that have large nuclei. A streaking artifact that results from crushing of the chromatin is commonly observed in small-cell undifferentiated carcinomas.

Large-Cell Undifferentiated Carcinoma

This tumor is composed of large, undifferentiated carcinoma cells in solid masses. Areas of necrosis are commonly observed. Large-cell undifferentiated carcinomas of the lungs occasionally have squamous or glandular differentiation. Cytologic examination shows that the smears are cellular, consisting of solitary tumor cells and small groupings of such cells. The tumor cells are large and round or oval (Fig. 3.67). The cytoplasm may be scanty or abundant. The cell margins are distinct. Most tumor cells have a large nucleus that contains coarsely granular chromatin. Binucleate forms also occur. One or more large nucleoli are observed. Mitoses are frequently seen.

Merkel Cell Tumor

This tumor is also known as neuroendocrine carcinoma, small-cell neuroepithelial tumor and cutaneous apudoma. It is an undifferentiated carcinoma of the skin that consists of tumor cells that contain electron-dense core granules similar to those found in epidermal Merkel's cells. Such tumors commonly occur on the lips (Fig. 3.68) or face (see Fig. 7.1) and have a reddish, raised, smooth surface. Histologic examination demonstrates that such tumors are composed of small, uniform, undif-

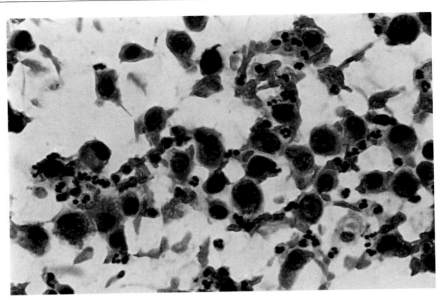

Fig. 3.67. Aspirate from a large-cell undifferentiated carcinoma. The primary tumor was in a lung. Note the solitary cells that have abundant cytoplasm and large, round nuclei. Papanicolaou preparation. ×625.

ferentiated cells in the dermis and subcutaneous tissues, with the epidermis uninvolved (Fig. 3.69). Cytoplasmic granules can be demonstrated by Grimelius' stain. Metastases in the lymph nodes of the neck are not uncommon and distant visceral metastases are also encountered. Differentiation from other small-cell tumors may be difficult on light microscopy. In addition to knowledge of the history and clinical findings, immunoperoxidase staining and electron microscopy may be required to arrive at the diagnosis. Cytologic study shows that the aspirates are extremely cellular, consisting of uniform, undifferentiated tumor cells that occur as solitary cells or in loose groupings.[77] The cytoplasm is scanty and ill-defined. The tumor cell nuclei are round or oval and about twice the size of a nucleus of a normal lymphocyte (Fig. 3.70). The chromatin is finely granular and one or more small nucleoli are seen. Mitotic figures are noted.

Giant-Cell and Spindle Cell Variants of Undifferentiated Carcinoma

These tumors commonly arise in the lungs and thyroid. Pleomorphic giant-cell variants of malignant melanoma and squamous cell carcinoma also occur.

Tumors of the lungs and thyroid are highly malignant and are composed of polygonal, spindle-shaped and pleomorphic giant cells (Fig. 3.71). The neoplastic cells have one or more nuclei. The chromatin is coarse and there are prominent nucleoli. The tumor cells have abundant cytoplasm. Mitoses are frequently observed. Necrosis is commonly encountered.

Giant-cell and spindle cell variants of squamous cell carcinoma are rarely reported. We recently studied a case of metastatic squamous cell carcinoma of the

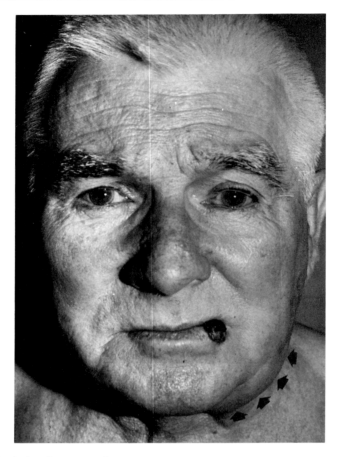

Fig. 3.68. Merkel cell tumor of the lip presenting as a needle aspiration biopsy-positive enlargement of the left submandibular lymph node (arrows). (Photograph courtesy of Dr. S. D. Archibald.)

larynx that was found to contain numerous malignant, pleomorphic, giant and spindle cells on aspiration biopsy cytology (Fig. 3.47). Solitary tumor cells and cohesive clusters were observed. The tumor cells were of various sizes and shapes. Large, bizarre neoplastic cells had two or more nuclei. Small, polygonal or spindle-shaped cells were also seen. The cytoplasm was abundant, dense and basophilic. The chromatin was granular and prominent nucleoli were observed. A similar case has recently been reported by Schautz and associates.[78]

The anaplastic giant-cell variant of malignant melanoma is described on page 192.

DIFFERENTIAL DIAGNOSIS. Poorly differentiated adenocarcinoma and squamous cell carcinoma may resemble large-cell undifferentiated carcinoma and distinction among these entities is difficult. Poorly differentiated malignant melanoma, seminoma and large-cell lymphoma may also be difficult to differentiate. The differential diagnosis of large-cell undifferentiated carcinoma is summarized in Table 3.12.

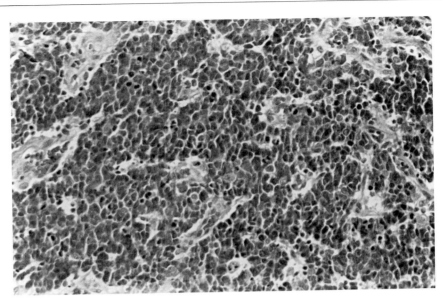

Fig. 3.69. Merkel cell tumor. Histology specimen. The tumor is composed of small, undifferentiated cells. Hematoxylin and eosin preparation. ×390.

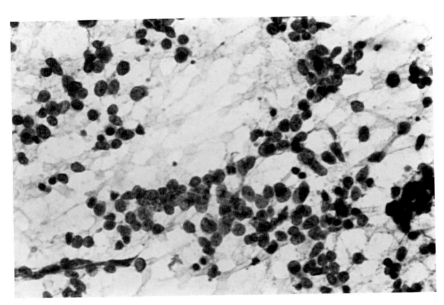

Fig. 3.70. Aspirate from a Merkel cell tumor metastatic to a submandibular lymph node. Small, undifferentiated tumor cells are seen. Papanicolaou preparation. ×625.

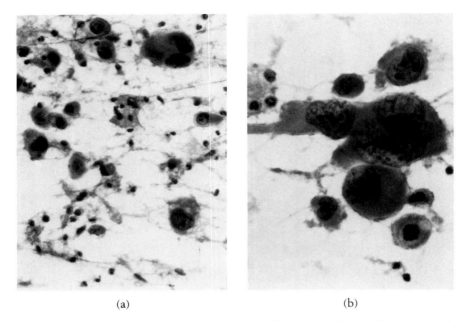

(a)   (b)

Fig. 3.71. Giant-cell carcinoma. Note the pleomorphic nature of the cells in this aspirate. The primary tumor was in a lung. Papanicolaou preparation. (a) ×390, (b) ×625.

The differential diagnosis of small-cell undifferentiated tumors includes nasopharyngeal carcinoma, small-cell carcinoma of the lungs, Merkel cell carcinoma, carcinoid tumor and other apudomas, undifferentiated malignant melanoma, small-cell lymphoma, neuroblastoma, Ewing's sarcoma and embryonal rhabdomyosarcoma. Other small-cell tumors, for example, metastatic retinoblastoma and Wilms' tumor, also should be considered in the differential diagnosis. Other, less common tumors that may cause difficulty in the diagnosis include small-cell malignant tumor of the thoracopulmonary region of childhood,[79] the so-called Askin's tumor and neuroectodermal tumor of bone.[80] The cytologic features of common undifferentiated small-cell tumors are summarized in Table 3.13. It is important to emphasize that aspirates from undifferentiated malignant tumors should be interpreted with knowledge of the history and clinical findings and, if possible, radiologic and other laboratory data. The age of the patient, the location of the tumor and, especially, knowledge of previous surgical procedures or other methods of treatment are essential information that can help minimize diagnostic errors.

Malignant Melanoma

Malignant melanoma accounts for approximately 1 percent of all cancers in the United States. The skin is the site of the primary lesion in nearly 85 percent of cases of malignant melanoma. In the head and neck, the skin of the face, ears, neck and scalp are the most common sites of origin of this neoplasm. Malignant melanoma also arises in the mucosae of the oral cavity, nose, paranasal sinuses and orbits. In rare instances, this tumor develops in the esophagus or trachea. Metastases commonly occur in the lymph nodes of the head and neck (Fig. 3.72) and may be the

TABLE 3.12. Differential Diagnosis of Large-Cell Undifferentiated Carcinoma

Tumor Type	Cellular Arrangement	Cell Size and Shape	Cytoplasm	Nucleus	Nucleolus	Special Features
Poorly differentiated adenocarcinoma	Solitary cells and cohesive clusters	Large, oval or round	Scanty, ill-defined margins, occasionally vacuolated	Large, round or oval, central or eccentric; chromatin coarsely granular; nuclear molding; occasionally two or more nuclei	Large, one or more	Look for glandular differentiation
Poorly differentiated squamous cell carcinoma	Solitary cells and loose groupings	Large, round to polygonal	Scanty, ill-defined margins	Large, round or oval; chromatin coarsely granular; pyknotic; occasionally two or more nuclei	Large, single	Look for keratinization
Malignant melanoma	Usually solitary cells; in undifferentiated variant, loose groupings	Variable in size, round or oval, spindle and pleomorphic bizarre forms	Usually abundant, dense, undifferentiated variant scanty and ill-defined	Large, round or oval, eccentric; chromatin coarsely granular; frequently two or more nuclei	Large, single	Pigment in cytoplasm
Seminoma	Solitary cells and occasional loose groupings	Large, round or oval	Fragile and ill-defined	Large, round; chromatin finely granular; mitosis +++	Variable in size, one or more	Nuclear pleomorphism; pale-staining cellular debris and lymphocytes in background
Large cell, lymphoma	Solitary cells	Large, round, monomorphic	Narrow rim to ill-defined	Large, round, smooth or clefted; chromatin finely granular	Large, one or more	Solitary cells; no nuclear molding
Large-cell undifferentiated carcinoma	Solitary cells and occasional loose groupings	Large, round or oval	Scanty, ill-defined, delicate, occasionally better defined and granular	Large, round or oval, one or more; chromatin coarsely granular; nuclear molding; mitosis ++	Large, one or more	

TABLE 3.13. Differential Diagnosis of Small-Cell Undifferentiated Carcinoma

Tumor Type	Cellular Arrangement	Cell Size and Shape	Cytoplasm	Nucleus	Nucleolus	Special Features
Nasopharyngeal carcinoma	Solitary cells and loose groupings	Small or medium-sized, round or oval	Scanty, delicate	Small, round or oval, single; finely granular chromatin; nuclear molding	Variable in size, one or more	Mixture of lymphocytes and epithelial tumor cells
Small-cell carcinoma, lung	Solitary cells and loose groupings	Small or medium-sized, round or oval	Ill-defined or absent	Small, round to fusiform; chromatin fine to coarsely granular; nuclear molding; mitoses rare	Usually absent or tiny	Degenerated, pyknotic nuclei in background
Merkel cell carcinoma	Solitary cells and loose groupings	Small, round or oval	Absent or ill-defined	Small, round or oval; chromatin finely dispersed; nuclear molding; mitoses +++	Small, more than one	Nucleoli adjacent to nuclear membrane; degenerated, pyknotic nuclei
Carcinoid tumor	Solitary cells and loose groupings; occasionally organoid pattern	Small, round or oval	Variable; when abundant, margins well-defined, granular to opaque	Small, round or oval; chromatin fine; no nuclear molding; mitoses uncommon	Usually absent or small	Monomorphic population of cells

188

Undifferentiated malignant melanoma	Solitary cells and cohesive clusters	Small or medium-sized, round or oval	Scanty to ill-defined	Small, round or oval; chromatin coarsely granular; nuclear molding; mitoses ++	Variable, usually single	Melanin usually absent
Small-cell lymphoma	Solitary cells	Small or medium-sized, round	Absent or narrow rim	Small, round or cleaved; chromatin finely granular; no nuclear molding; mitoses +	Absent or small	Monomorphic smear, solitary cells
Neuroblastoma	Solitary cells and groupings and sheets; rosettes in well-differentiated tumors	Small, round or oval	Scanty to ill-defined; fine, fibrillar processes in center of rosettes	Small, round or oval; chromatin coarsely granular; nuclear molding	Absent or small, peripherally located	Homer-Wright rosettes and neurofibrils
Ewing's sarcoma	Solitary cells and groupings and sheets; pseudo-rosettes and perivascular palisading	Small, round or oval	Scanty in groupings, better defined in solitary cells; wisps interconnecting cells in monolayers	Small, round or oval; chromatin finely granular; nuclear molding uncommon; mitoses +	Small, one or two	Periodic acid-Schiff-positive, diastase-digestible granules in cytoplasm; background granular, fibrillar, proteinaceous
Embryonal rhabdomyosarcoma	Solitary cells and small groupings	Small or round, medium-sized	Usually scanty; rhabdomyoblasts have eosinophilic cytoplasm	Small, round or oval; variation more marked; chromatin coarsely granular; mitoses ++	Small, single	Rhabdomyoblasts

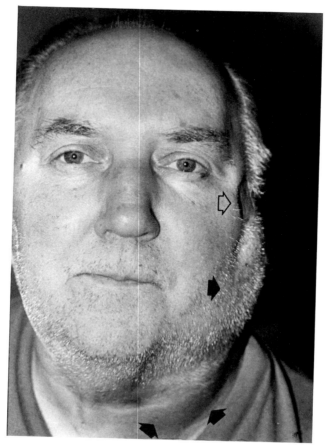

Fig. 3.72. Malignant melanoma metastatic to the lymph nodes of the left side of the neck. Open arrow shows the site of a previous skin graft.

presenting feature of this neoplasm. Aspiration biopsy cytology is a simple, practical method for diagnosing metastatic malignant melanoma.

CYTOLOGIC FEATURES. The aspirates are unusually cellular, consisting mostly of solitary tumor cells and, occasionally, of loose groupings, cohesive clusters or tissue-like fragments. Monolayer sheets are encountered infrequently. Red blood cells, lymphocytes and neutrophils are usually visible in the background. Macrophages with ingested melanin pigment in the cytoplasm are also seen. Necrosis is occasionally observed. There are wide variations in the size and shape of the tumor cells, their nuclear features, staining characteristics and pigment distribution. Our experience is based on a study of 45 needle aspirates from 22 patients with metastatic malignant melanoma. Our findings are essentially similar to those of Woyke and associates.[81] We have also found four morphologic types of melanoma cells in the smears (Table 3.14). Although all four morphologic types may coexist, there usually is one dominant pattern.

TABLE 3.14. Malignant Melanoma: Average Percentages of Cell Types in 45 Aspirates

Number of Aspirates	Cell Type (average percentage of 300 cells)			
	Epithelioid	Spindle Shaped	Giant	Undifferentiated
32	80–99		1–20	
5	85–98	1–10	1–5	
2	1–5	95–99		
2	50–60		40–50	
4				100

The epithelioid type of melanoma (Plate I.6) consists of small, round, oval or polygonal, solitary cells that have dense, eosinophilic cytoplasm (Fig. 3.73). The cytoplasm may have a hyaline-like quality. The cell margins are distinct. The tumor cell nuclei are round or oval and usually located eccentrically. The chromatin is coarsely granular. The tumor cell nuclei contain one or more large nucleoli. Binucleated cells are usually seen in the smears. A few giant cells are also encountered. A bird's-eye, or "cell-in-cell," arrangement of tumor cells is occasionally noted.

The spindle type of melanoma consists of elongated cells that have slender, bipolar, cytoplasmic processes. Aspirates contain solitary tumor cells and small and large groupings of such cells (Fig. 3.74). The tumor cells have one or more oval or fusiform nuclei. The chromatin is finely granular and small nucleoli are usually seen. Occasionally, the chromatin is coarse and the nucleoli are large. The epithelioid-type cells are usually admixed with a small number of spindle forms.

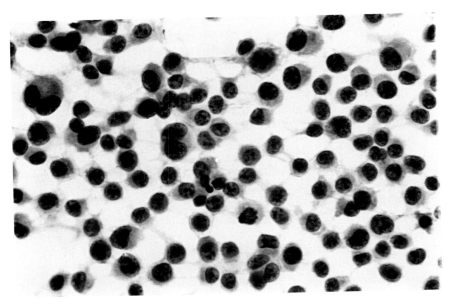

Fig. 3.73. Aspirate from a malignant melanoma, epithelioid type. Dense cytoplasm, eccentric locations of the nuclei, binucleation and coarse chromatin are well visualized. Papanicolaou preparation. ×390.

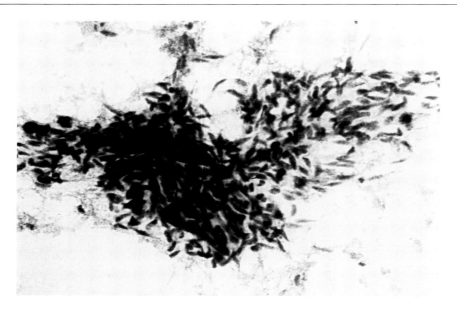

Fig. 3.74. Aspirate from a spindle cell melanoma consists largely of spindle-shaped cells. In the absence of a previous pathologic diagnosis, a definitive cytologic diagnosis would be impossible on the basis of such a smear. Papanicolaou preparation. ×390.

The undifferentiated type of malignant melanoma is composed of small, round or oval cells that are about two to three times the size of a mature lymphocyte. Solitary tumor cells are encountered along with small cohesive clusters and large, tissue-like fragments (Fig. 3.75). The cytoplasm is scanty and ill-defined. The chromatin is fine and evenly distributed. The nucleoli are small and inconspicuous.

The giant-cell variant consists of large, bizarre, multinucleated, solitary cells (Fig. 3.76). There is marked variation in cell size, with some cells measuring several hundred micrometers in diameter. The cytoplasm is abundant and has a hyaline-like or glassy appearance. The tumor cell nuclei contain one or more eccentrically located nuclei, giving such cells a characteristic appearance. The chromatin is coarsely granular and large nucleoli are usually observed. Large nuclear vacuoles are seen.

Table 3.15 summarizes the cytologic features of malignant melanoma and gives their relative frequencies of occurrence. In our experience, melanin is seen in about 25 percent of malignant melanomas on cytologic examination. The melanin is found not only in the tumor cell cytoplasm but also in macrophages and extracellularly. It takes the form of fine to coarse, light to dark brown granules. In most cases, the pigment is found only by careful search, although some tumors are so heavily pigmented that virtually all the tumor cells contain pigment (Plate II.1). In smears with scanty pigmentation, the slides can be decolorized and restained by the Masson-Fontana method. With this stain, melanin appears black and is easily recognized (Fig. 3.77). Nucleoli are identifiable in most cases.

Mitotic figures are not uncommonly seen and can be found in most smears if a careful search is undertaken. Intranuclear cytoplasmic vacuoles are less frequently

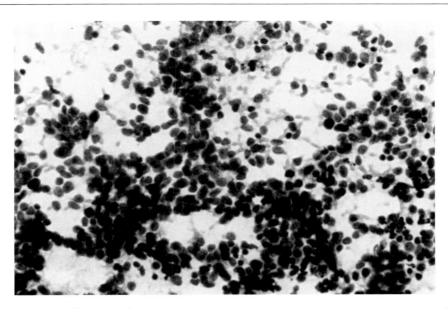

Fig. 3.75. Undifferentiated malignant melanoma. The tumor is composed of small, round or oval, undifferentiated cells. Papanicolaou preparation. ×390.

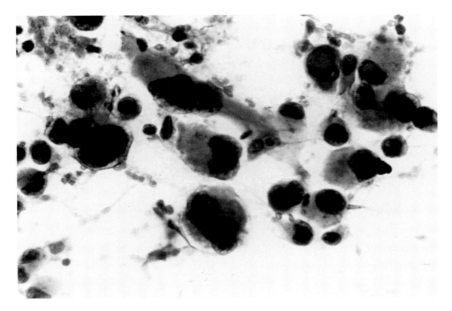

Fig. 3.76. Aspirate from an anaplastic malignant melanoma, giant-cell variant, metastatic to a cervical lymph node. Papanicolaou preparation. ×625.

TABLE 3.15. Malignant Melanoma: Cytologic Features and Their Relative Frequencies of Occurrence in 45 Aspirates

	Cytologic Feature														
	Melanin Pigment						Nucleoli		Mitotic Figures		Intra-nuclear Vacuoles		Binucle-ation		Multi-nucleation	
	Tumor Cells		Macro-phages		Extra-cellular											
Relative Frequency	No.	Percent	No.	Percent	No.	Percent	No.	Percent	No.	Percent	No.	Percent	No.	Percent	No.	Percent
Frequent	2	4.4	1	2.2	1	2.2	21	46.6	0	0	3	6.7	8	17.8	4	8.9
Rare	7	15.6	5	11.1	2	4.4	16	35.6	8	17.8	3	6.7	22	48.9	4	8.9
Occasional	3	6.7	3	6.7	7	15.6	8	17.8	19	42.2	11	24.4	11	24.4	21	46.6
Not seen	33	73.3	36	80.0	35	77.8	0	0.0	18	40.0	28	62.2	4	8.9	16	35.6

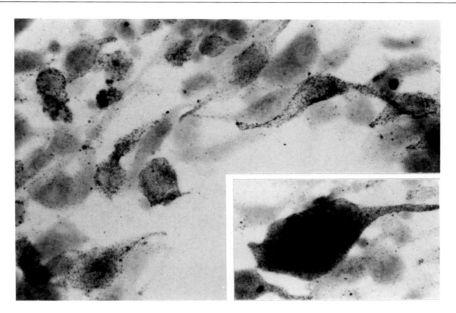

Fig. 3.77. Masson-Fontana stain shows melanin in malignant melanoma cells. ×625. (*Inset,* ×1000.)

encountered and are most common in the giant-cell and epithelioid types of malignant melanoma. We have not seen them in the undifferentiated type. The cytologic features of malignant melanoma are summarized in Table 3.16.

DIFFERENTIAL DIAGNOSIS. The diagnostic feature of malignant melanoma is melanin. However, even if melanin is not detected, this neoplasm can be diagnosed on the basis of the cytologic features described previously. The finding of dissociated cells that have one or more eccentrically located nuclei, dense cytoplasm and nuclear vacuoles suggests the diagnosis. However, the spindle cell type may be difficult to differentiate from mesenchymal tumors if melanin cannot be detected. The undifferentiated type may be difficult to distinguish from other undifferentiated malignant tumors, as was noted previously. The giant-cell variant resembles other giant-cell tumors and a definitive diagnosis of this neoplasm may be difficult if there are no suggestive findings in the history. However, the giant cells are usually admixed with a large number of solitary epithelioid-type tumor cells that have eccentrically

TABLE 3.16. **Malignant Melanoma: Summary of Cytologic Features**

Solitary cells, occasional loose groupings in spindle and undifferentiated types.
Round, polygonal, spindle-shaped and giant, bizarre forms.
Cytoplasm abundant, eosinophilic, dense and well defined in epithelial and giant-cell types.
One or more round or oval, eccentrically located nuclei. Nucleolus prominent. Intranuclear vacuoles and mitoses usually seen.
Melanin pigment.

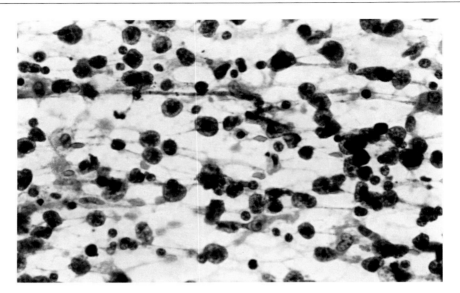

Fig. 3.78. Aspirate from a seminoma metastatic to a cervical lymph node. Two cell types are clearly recognized. The chromatin of the tumor cells is coarse and there are prominent nucleoli. Papanicolaou preparation. ×625.

located nuclei and an abundance of glassy cytoplasm, a finding that points to the diagnosis. In our cases of giant-cell malignant melanoma, melanin was not identified.

Seminoma

Seminoma may metastasize widely and patients may present with enlarged cervical lymph nodes. The tumor cells are usually solitary but may occur in loose groupings in poorly differentiated cases. The large, round or oval tumor cells have fragile cytoplasm, which may be absent in some aspirates. The tumor cells have large, round nuclei that contain finely or moderately granular chromatin (Fig. 3.78). Most tumor cell nuclei contain one or more nucleoli of variable size. Mitoses are not infrequently observed. Admixed with the tumor cells are numerous mature lymphocytes. Histiocytes and giant cells are occasionally seen in the smears. The histologic appearance of a seminoma is shown in Figure 3.79.

DIAGNOSTIC PITFALLS IN METASTATIC NEOPLASMS

Some of the pitfalls discussed in the section on lymphomas apply equally to aspiration biopsy cytology of metastatic carcinomas. Satisfactory, well-prepared smears and experience in interpretation of cellular samples are prerequisites if misinterpretation is to be avoided. Postradiation fibrosis and scarring may be the cause of scanty material and responsible for misdiagnosis. Extensive necrosis in a lymph node may

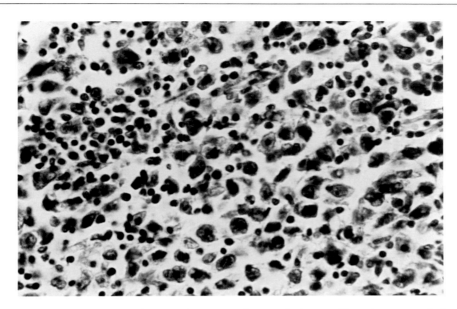

Fig. 3.79. Seminoma. Histology specimen contains an admixture of lymphocytes and plasma cells coexisting with large, primitive germ cells. Hematoxylin and eosin preparation. × 625.

also result in a poor cell yield, making the diagnosis difficult. Other masses in the neck can mimic enlarged lymph nodes. The diagnosis of congenital cysts is usually straightforward, although, as was noted previously, such cysts are occasionally mistaken for cystic squamous carcinoma (for further discussion, see Chapter 5). On the other hand, metastatic, cystic, squamous cell carcinomas may be mistaken for a benign cyst. Metastatic, cystic, papillary carcinoma of the thyroid may be overlooked on aspiration biopsy cytology if only cystic fluid without the characteristic cells is obtained. Similarly, small carcinomas that arise in thyroglossal cysts may also escape detection. As was emphasized previously, if a residual mass is felt after aspiration, the lesion should be reneedled or excised.

Lesions of the salivary glands, such as Warthin's tumor and lymphoepithelial lesion, may be confused with reactive lymph nodes, lymphoma or even metastatic carcinoma. In both lesions, the admixture of epithelial and lymphoid cells should help in differentiating these entities from reactive hyperplasia and lymphoma. The atypia seen in the oncocytic cells of Warthin's tumor should not be regarded as evidence of a malignant process and this tumor also should not be confused with metastatic carcinoma. Similarly, atypical Hürthle cells in a smear from Hashimoto's thyroiditis may be misinterpreted as carcinoma metastatic to the cervical lymph nodes.[48] Skin appendage tumors can resemble small lymph nodes and may be misinterpreted as poorly differentiated squamous cell carcinoma.[13] Needle aspirates from carotid body tumors may be mistaken for metastatic carcinoma or neural tumors.[13] The first carotid body tumor that we examined cytologically was incorrectly diagnosed as metastatic carcinoma. The wide variation in the size of the tumor cells and the large, hyperchromatic nuclei suggested a malignant process. This topic is discussed in detail in Chapter 6.

TABLE 3.17. Anatomic Distribution of 516 Lymph Node Aspirates

Site	Positive	Negative	Total
Lymph nodes of head and neck	294	181	475
Lymph nodes of other sites	26	15	41
Total	320 (62%)	196 (38%)	516

The difficulty of diagnosing various undifferentiated malignant tumors has already been noted. Similarly, spindle cell and pleomorphic giant-cell variants may also pose problems in the differential diagnosis. The recognition of a malignant process is not difficult in such cases; however, if there is no suggestive history, the site of the primary lesion may be difficult to determine by cytologic examination alone.

RESULTS OF ASPIRATION BIOPSY CYTOLOGY IN METASTATIC NEOPLASMS

Five hundred fifty patients who presented with lymphadenopathy during a seven-year period in our institution were investigated by needle aspiration biopsy as the initial step in the diagnostic work-up. Thirty-four patients (6 percent) were excluded from the study because their specimens were unsatisfactory or because they were lost to follow-up. Needle aspiration biopsy in 475 (92 percent) of the remaining 516 patients was performed on enlarged lymph nodes of the neck (Table 3.17). In 320 cases (62 percent), the biopsy samples were reported as positive; in the other 196 cases (38 percent), the samples were negative. The overall diagnostic accuracy was 98 percent. There were eight false-negative and two false-positive diagnoses. The cytologic tumor types are listed in Table 3.18.

TABLE 3.18. Metastatic Carcinoma in Lymph Nodes: Cytologic Diagnosis

Tumor Type	Number of Cases
Squamous cell carcinoma	197
Adenocarcinoma	48
Undifferentiated carcinoma	28
Malignant melanoma	21
Merkel cell carcinoma	3
Nasopharyngeal carcinoma	5
Malignant paraganglioma	2
Acinic cell carcinoma	2
Seminoma	3
Renal cell carcinoma	2
Adenocarcinoma expleomorphic adenoma	1
Total	312

Three aspirates each from patients with metastatic small cell carcinoma and from those with squamous cell carcinoma were read as negative. One aspirate each from a patient with malignant melanoma and from one with adenocarcinoma were reported as negative for metastatic tumor. Three false-negative diagnoses were interpretation errors and five were sampling errors.

Of the two false-positive diagnoses, one occurred in a patient with a histologically confirmed branchial cleft cyst whose smears contained atypical, malignant-looking squamous cells. The other false-positive diagnosis occurred in a patient with a carotid body tumor that was misdiagnosed as metastatic carcinoma. Both false-positive diagnoses were interpretation errors. Other investigators[5,6,15,46,82] have also reported a diagnostic accuracy in excess of 90 percent for aspiration biopsy cytology.

COMPLICATIONS OF NEEDLE ASPIRATION BIOPSY OF LYMPH NODES

Complications of needle aspiration biopsy of lymph nodes are rare. We have not experienced any complications. Frable[6] reported the formation of a small hematoma immediately after aspiration of a submandibular lymph node; the hematoma disappeared soon afterward. Fine-needle aspiration biopsy also does not cause much distortion of lymph node architecture and thus does not interfere with subsequent histologic study of excised lymph nodes.[83]

REFERENCES

1. Greig EDW, Gray ACH: Note on the lymphatic glands in sleeping sickness. *Brit Med J* 1:1252, 1904.

2. Guthrie CG: Gland puncture as a diagnostic measure. *Bull Johns Hopkins Hosp* 32:266–269, 1921.

3. Martin HE, Ellis EB: Biopsy by needle puncture and aspiration. *Ann Surg* 92:169–181, 1930.

4. Stewart FW: The diagnosis of tumors by aspiration biopsy. *Amer J Pathol* 9:801–812, 1933.

5. Cordoza PL: The cytologic diagnosis of lymph node punctures. *Acta Cytol* 8:194–205, 1964.

6. Frable WJ: *Thin Needle Aspiration Biopsy*. Philadelphia, Saunders, 1983, pp. 74–118.

7. Friedman M, Kim U, Shimaoka K, et al: Appraisal of aspiration cytology in management of Hodgkin's disease. *Cancer (Philadelphia)* 45:1635–1663, 1980.

8. Khoory MS: Disease of lymph node and spleen, in Linsk JA, Sixten F (eds): *Clinical Aspiration Cytology*. Philadelphia, Lippincott, 1983, pp 297–317.

9. Loseke L, Craver LF: The diagnosis of Hodgkin's disease by aspiration biopsy. *Blood* 1:76–82, 1946.

10. Morrison M, Samvick AA, Rubinstein J, et al: Lymph node aspiration. Clinical and hematological observations in 101 patients. *Amer J Clin Pathol* 22:255–262, 1952.

11. Orell SR, Skinner JM: The typing of non-Hodgkin's lymphomas using fine needle aspiration cytology. *Pathology* 14:389–394, 1982.

12. Qizilbash AH, Elavathil LJ, Chen V, et al: Aspiration biopsy cytology of lymph nodes in malignant lymphoma. *Diagn Cytopathol* 1:18–22, 1985.

13. Zajicek J: Aspiration biopsy cytology, Part 1, cytology of supradiaphragmatic organs. *Monogr Clin Cytol* 4:90–124, 1974.

14. Betsill WL Jr, Hajdu SI: Percutaneous aspiration biopsy of lymph nodes. *Amer J Clin Pathol* 73:471–479, 1980.

15. Engzell U, Jakobsson PA, Sigurdson A, et al: Aspiration biopsy of metastatic carcinoma in lymph nodes of the neck. A review of 1011 consecutive cases. *Acta Oto-Laryngol* 72:138–147, 1971.

16. Kaur S: Fine needle aspiration of lymph nodes in leprosy. A study of bacteriologic and morphologic indices. *Int J Lepr* 45:369–372, 1977.

17. Kline TS, Kannan V, Kline IK: Lymphadenopathy and aspiration biopsy cytology. Review of 376 superficial nodes. *Cancer (Philadelphia)* 54:1076–1081, 1984.

18. Ramzy I, Rone R, Schultenover SJ, et al: Lymph node aspiration biopsy. Diagnostic reliability and limitations. An analysis of 350 cases. *Diagn Cytopathol* 1:39–45, 1985.

19. Aruss JE, Scanlon EF, Christ MA: Aspiration cytology of head and neck masses. *Amer J Surg* 136:342–347, 1978.

20. Bailey TM, Akhtar M, Ali MA: Fine needle aspiration biopsy in the diagnosis of tuberculosis. *Acta Cytol* 29:732–736, 1985.

21. Pollock PG, Meyers DS, Frable WJ, et al: rapid diagnosis of actinomycosis by thin needle aspiration biopsy. *Amer J Clin Pathol* 70:27–30, 1978.

22. Akhtar M, Ali MA, Sabbah R, et al: Fine needle aspiration biopsy. Diagnosis of round cell malignant tumors of childhood. A combined light and electron microscopic approach. *Cancer (Philadelphia)* 55:1805–1817, 1985.

23. Domagali W, Cross LG: Confirmation of surfaces of human cancer cells obtained by fine needle aspiration biopsy. A comparative light microscopic and scanning electron microscopic study. *Acta Cytol* 24:427–434, 1980.

24. Levitt S, Chang L, DuPuis MH, et al: Fine needle aspiration diagnosis of malignant lymphoma with confirmation by immunoperoxidase staining. *Acta Cytol* 29:895–902, 1985.

25. Diamond LW, Nathwani BN, Rappaport H: Flow cytometry in the diagnosis and classification of malignant lymphoma and leukemia. *Cancer (Philadelphia)* 50:1122–1135, 1982.

26. Sallstrom JS, Juhlin R, Stenkvist B: Membrane properties of lymphatic cells in fine needle biopsies of lymphomas. I. Cap formation after exposure to fluorescein conjugated concanavalin A. *Acta Cytol* 18:392–398, 1974.

27. Lennert K, Stein H, Kaiseling E: Cytological and functional criteria for the classification of malignant lymphomata. *Brit J Cancer* 31:29–43, 1975.

28. Lukes RJ, Collins RD: New approaches to the classification of the lymphomata. *Brit J. Cancer* 31(Suppl 1):1–28, 1975.

29. Soderstrom N: The free cytoplasmic fragments of lymphoglandular tissue (lymphoglandular bodies). *Scand J Haematol* 5:138–152, 1968.

30. Butler JJ: Non-neoplastic lesions of lymph nodes of man to be differentiated from lymphomas. *Natl Cancer Inst Monogr* 32:233–255, 1969.

31. Dorfman RF, Warnke R: Lymphadenopathy simulating the malignant lymphomas. *Hum Pathol* 5:519–550, 1974.

32. Rosai J, Dorfman RF: Sinus histiocytosis with massive lymphadenopathy; a pseudolymphomatous benign disorder. *Cancer (Philadelphia)* 30:1174–1188, 1972.

33. Lukes RL, Tindle BH: Immunoblastic lymphadenopathy. *N Engl J Med* 292:1–8, 1975.

34. Gray GF Jr, Kimball AC, Kean PH: The posterior cervical lymph node in toxoplasmosis. *Am J Pathol* 69:349–358, 1972.

35. Miglets AW, Viall JH, Kataria VYP: Sarcoidosis of the head and neck. *Laryngoscope* 87:2038–2048, 1977.

36. Naji AF, Cabonelle B, Barker HJ: Cat scratch disease. *Amer J Clin Pathol* 38:513–521, 1962.

37. Rajwanshi A, Bhambhani S, Das DK: Fine needle aspiration cytology diagnosis of tuberculosis. *Diagn Cytopathol* 3:13–16, 1987.

38. Salyer KE, Voheler TP, Dorman GW: Surgical management of cervical adenitis due to atypical mycobacterium in children. *J Amer Med Assoc* 204:1037–1040, 1968.

39. Silverman JF: Fine needle aspiration cytology of cat scratch disease. *Acta Cytol* 29:542–547, 1985.

40. Smith EB, Custer RP: The histopathology of lymphogranuloma venereum. *J Urol* 63:546–563, 1980.

41. Turk JL, Waters MFR: Immunological significance of changes in lymph nodes across the leprosy spectrum. *Clin Exp Immunol* 8:363–376, 1971.

42. Turner RR, Wright DJM: Lymphadenopathy in early syphilis. *J Pathol* 110:305–308, 1973.

43. Frable AM, Frable WJ: Fine needle aspiration biopsy in the diagnosis of sarcoid of the head and neck. *Acta Cytol* 28:175–177, 1984.

44. Christ ML, Seltes-Kennedy M: Fine needle aspiration cytology of toxoplasmic lymphadenitis. *Acta Cytol* 26:425–428, 1982.

45. Kaur F: Fine needle aspiration of lymph nodes in leprosy. A study of bacteriologic and morphologic indices. *Int J Lepr* 45:369–372, 1977.

46. Shultenover SJ, Ramsay I, Page CP, et al: Needle aspiration biopsy: Role and limitations in surgical decision making. *Amer J Clin Pathol* 82:405–410, 1984.

47. Bottles K, Cohen MB, Brodie H, et al: Fine needle aspiration cytology of lymphadenopathy in homosexual males. *Diagn Cytopathol* 2:31–35, 1986.

48. Koss LG, Woyke S, Olszewski W: *Aspiration Biopsy. Cytologic Interpretation and Histologic Bases.* New York, Igaku-Shoin, 1984, pp. 105–153.

49. Gall EA: Enigmas in lymphoma reticulum cell sarcoma and mycosis fungoides. *Minn Med* 38:674–681, 1955.

50. Rappaport H: Tumours of the hematopoietic system, in *Atlas of Tumour Pathology,* second series. Washington, DC, Armed Forces Institute of Pathology, 1966, pp 9–15.

51. Nathwani BN: A critical analysis of the classification of non-Hodgkin's lymphomas. *Cancer (Philadelphia)* 44:347–348, 1979.

52. Lukes RJ, Collins RD: New approaches to the classification of the lymphomata. *Br J Cancer* 31(Suppl 1):1–28, 1975.

53. Lennert K, Mohri N, Stein N, et al: The histopathology of malignant lymphoma. *Brit J Haematol* 31(Suppl 1):193–203, 1975.

54. National Cancer Institute sponsored study of classification of non-Hodgkin's lymphomas. Summary and description of working formulation for clinical usage. The non-Hodgkin's lymphoma pathologic classification project. *Cancer (Philadelphia)* 49:2112–2135, 1982.

55. Burkitt D: A sarcoma involving the jaws in African children. I. A clinical syndrome. *Brit J Surg* 46:218–233, 1958.

56. Berard CW, Jaffe E, Braylan RC, et al: Immunologic aspects and pathology of the malignant lymphomas. *Cancer (Philadelphia)* 42:911–921, 1978.

57. Lukes RJ, Craver LS, Hall TC, et al: Report of the nomenclature committee. *Cancer Res* 26:1311, 1966.

58. Lukes RJ, Butler JJ: The pathology and nomenclature of Hodgkin's disease. *Cancer Res* 26:1063–1081, 1966.

59. Doyle AP, Heelstom HR: Mesantoin lymphadenopathy morphologically simulating Hodgkin's disease. *Ann Intern Med* 59:363–368, 1963.

60. Hartsock RJ: Post vaccinial lymphadenitis. *Cancer (Philadelphia)* 21:632–649, 1968.

61. Strum BS, Park KG, Rappaport H: Observation of cells resembling Sternberg-Reed cells in conditions other than Hodgkin's disease. *Cancer (Philadelphia)* 26:176–190, 1970.

62. Tindle BH, Parker JW, Lukes RJ: "Reed-Sternberg cells" in infectious mononucleosis. *Amer J Clin Pathol* 58:607–617, 1972.

63. Payne SE, Wright DH, Jones KJM, et al: The macrophage origin of Reed-Sternberg cells. An immunohistochemical study. *J Clin Pathol* 35:159–166, 1982.

64. Lennert K, Kaiserling E, Muller-Hermelink HK: Malignant lymphoma. Models of differentiation and cooperation of lymphoreticular cells, in Clarkson B, Marks PA, Till JE (eds): *Differentiation of Normal and Neoplastic Hematopoietic Cells,* Book B. Cold Spring Harbor, NY, Cold Spring Harbor Laboratory, 1978, vol 5, pp 897–913.

65. Sacks EL, Donaldson SS, Gordon J, et al: Epithelioid granulomas assocated with Hodgkin's disease. *Cancer (Philadelphia)* 41:562–567, 1978.

66. Neiman RF: Current problems in the histopathologic diagnosis and classification of Hodgkin's disease. *Pathol Annu* 13(II):289–328, 1978.

67. Berard CW, Thomas LB, Axtell LM, et al: The relationship of histopathological subtype to clinical state of Hodgkin's disease at diagnosis. *Cancer Res* 31:1776–1785, 1971.

68. Bloch M: Comparative study of lymph node cytology by puncture and histopathology. *Acta Cytol* 11:139–144, 1967.

69. Lindberg R: Distribution of cervical lymph node metastases from squamous cell carcinoma of the upper respiratory and digestive tracts. *Cancer (Philadelphia)* 29:1446–1449, 1972.

70. MacComb WS: Diagnosis and treatment of metastatic cervical cancerous nodes from an unknown primary site. *Amer J Surg* 124:441–449, 1972.

71. Martin H: Untimely lymph node biopsy. *Amer J Surg* 102:17–18, 1961.

72. Young JEM, Archibald SD, Shier KJ: Needle aspiration cytologic biopsy in head and neck masses. *Amer J Surg* 142:484–489, 1981.

73. Engzell U, Zajicek J: Aspiration biopsy of tumours of the neck. I. Aspiration biopsy and cytologic findings in 100 cases of congenital cysts. *Acta Cytol* 14:51–57, 1970.

74. Micheau C, Cachin Y, Caillou B: Cystic metastases in the neck revealing occult carcinoma of the tonsil. *Cancer (Philadelphia)* 33:228–233, 1974.

75. Batsakis JG, Holtz F, Super RH: Adenocarcinoma of nasal and paranasal cavities. *Arch Otolaryngol* 77:625–633, 1963.

76. Salassa JR, McDonald TJ, Weiland LH: "Colonic type" adenocarcinoma of the nasal cavity and paranasal sinuses. *Otolaryngol Head Neck Surg* 88:133–135, 1980.

77. Pettinato G, Dechiara A, Insabato L, et al: Neuroendocrine (Merkel cell) carcinoma of

the skin. Fine needle aspiration cytology and clinical pathologic study of a case. *Acta Cytol* 28:283–289, 1984.

78. Schautz HD, Ramsay I, Tio FO, et al: Metastatic spindle-cell carcinoma. Cytologic features and differential diagnosis. *Acta Cytol* 29:435–441, 1985.

79. Askin FB, Rosai T, Sibley RK, et al: Malignant small cell tumour of the thoracopulmonary region in childhood. A distinctive clinicopathologic entity of uncertain histogenesis. *Cancer (Philadelphia)* 43:2438–2451, 1979.

80. Jaffe R, Agostini RM, Santamaria M, et al: The neuroectodermal tumour of bone. *Amer J Surg Pathol* 8:885–898, 1984.

81. Woyke S, Domagala W, Czerniak B, et al: Fine needle aspiration cytology of malignant melanoma. *Acta Cytol* 24:529–538, 1980.

82. Zajdela A, Ennuyer A, Bataini P, et al: Valeur du diagnostique cytologie des adenopathies par ponction aspiration. Confrontation cyto-histologique de 1756 ca. *Bull Cancer* 63:327–340, 1976.

83. Behm FG, O'Dowd GJ, Frable WJ: Fine needle aspiration effects on benign lymph node histology. *Amer J Clin Pathol* 82:195–198, 1984.

COLOR PLATES

Plate I.1. Pleomorphic adenoma of a parotid gland. Note the eosinophilic, mesenchymal fragment that contains myoepithelial cells. Hematoxylin and eosin preparation. ×50.

Plate I.2. Low-grade mucoepidermoid carcinoma of a submandibular gland. Intermediate and mucus-containing cells are seen. Papanicolaou preparation. ×120.

Plate I.3. Adenoid cystic carcinoma of a parotid gland. Shown is the characteristic pattern of mucous cylinders overlying basaloid tumor cells. Papanicolaou preparation. ×120.

Plate I.4. Keratinizing squamous cell carcinoma metastatic to a cervical lymph node. Papanicolaou preparation. ×200.

Plate I.5. Colloid (mucinous) adenocarcinoma metastatic to a supraclavicular lymph node. Papanicolaou preparation. ×120.

Plate I.6. Malignant melanoma, epithelioid cell type, metastatic to an intraparotid lymph node. Golden-brown pigment is visible in one tumor cell. Hematoxylin and eosin preparation. ×300.

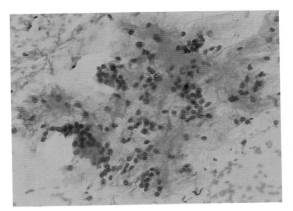

Plate I.1.

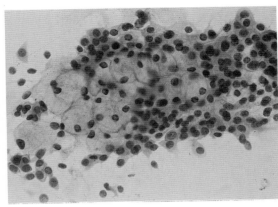

Plate I.2.

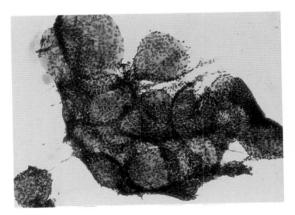

Plate I.3.

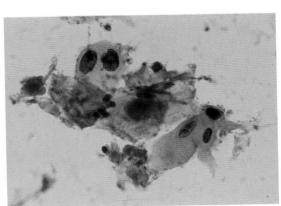

Plate I.4.

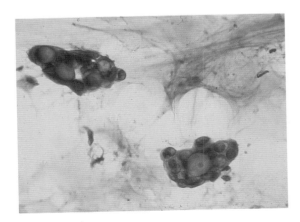

Plate I.5.

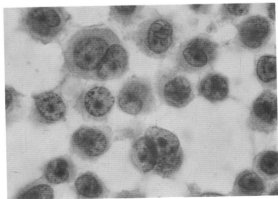

Plate I.6.

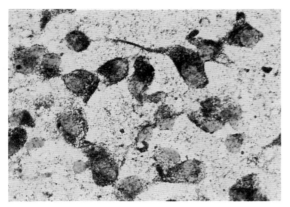

Plate II.1.

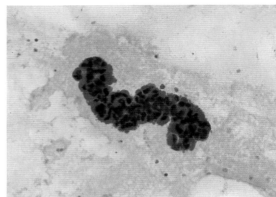

Plate II.2.

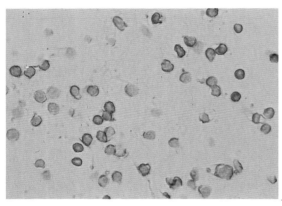

Plate II.3.

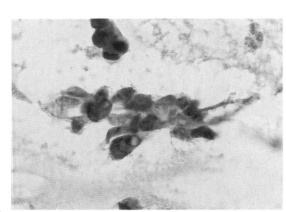

Plate II.4.

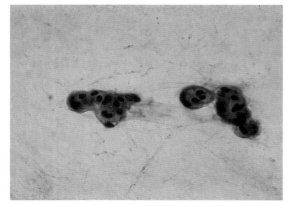

Plate II.5. (a)

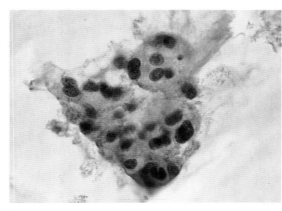

Plate II.5. (b)

Plate II.1. Malignant melanoma. Heavily pigmented tumor cells. Masson-Fontana preparation. ×200.

Plate II.2. Sebaceous carcinoma. A group of tumor cells demonstrating intra-cytoplasmic lipid. Oil red O preparation. ×200.

Plate II.3. Non-Hodgkin's lymphoma, small cell type. The cells stain positively for leucocyte common antigen. ×200.

Plate II.4. Metastatic prostatic adenocarcinoma in a neck node. Positive intracytoplasmic staining of tumor cells for prostate-specific acid phosphatase. ×200.

Plate II.5. Recurrent chordoma presenting as a neck mass. (a) Positive staining of tumour cells for neuron-specific enolase. ×120. (b) Positive staining of tumour cells for S-100 protein. ×200.

4

Soft-Tissue Tumors

INTRODUCTION

Approximately 10 to 15 percent of soft-tissue, or mesenchymal, tumors occur in the head and neck.[1] Most such tumors arise in the adipose tissue, fibrous connective tissue, endothelium of the blood and lymphatic vessels, muscles and nerves. They either are localized to the soft tissues of the head and neck or may involve the orbits, the lymph nodes or paranasal sinuses or the thyroid or salivary glands. Benign and malignant neoplasms occur. In addition, a number of reparative processes, for example, proliferative myositis, nodular fasciitis and fibromatosis, occur and mimic soft-tissue neoplasms. Although aspiration biopsy cytology has been successfully used for the diagnosis of epithelial neoplasms, its application for the diagnosis of mesenchymal tumors and reparative processes has not received the same degree of attention. There has been relatively little attention in this regard for many reasons, including the lack of experience on the part of cytopathologists, the infrequent occurrence of soft-tissue tumors and the existence of a number of tumor types, making accurate diagnosis difficult. Although several case reports have appeared on needle aspiration biopsy of benign and malignant soft-tissue tumors and reparative processes,[2-24] the literature contains only a few large series.[25-29] A number of textbooks on needle aspiration biopsy contain detailed descriptions of the cytologic features of soft-tissue neoplasms.[30-32]

Needle aspiration biopsy plays an important part in the diagnosis and management of soft-tissue tumors. It is useful in the following circumstances:

1. In the distinction between benign neoplastic or reparative processes and malignant tumors. With experience, benign processes can be differentiated from malignant lesions in most cases.
2. In the diagnosis of primary sarcomas and in the differentiation of such tumors from malignant lymphoma, metastatic carcinoma and melanoma. Primary sarcomas can be readily differentiated from metastatic carcinomas, but it may be difficult to differentiate small-cell sarcomas from small-cell lymphomas and carcinomas. Moreover, a definitive diagnosis of primary soft-tissue sarcomas may also

205

be difficult. In some cases, one can render an accurate cytologic diagnosis, but in other cases, one may be able only to classify the sarcoma as spindle, pleomorphic or round cell in type. The history, including the age of the patient and the site of the lesion, is helpful in the correct interpretation of aspirates.

3. In the diagnosis of recurrent or metastatic mesenchymal neoplasms. In cases in which there is a history of sarcoma, needle aspiration biopsy has an important role in confirming a clinical suspicion of recurrence or metastasis. The smears can be compared with previous histologic slides and the diagnosis confirmed. The aspirates from metastatic tumors usually resemble those from the primary neoplasms, although metastatic tumors are occasionally less differentiated than the primary lesions.

Pathologic Classification

Soft-tissue tumors are superficial or deep. Most superficial lesions are easily palpable and originate in the dermis, subcutis or fascia. Most such tumors are benign. Lesions situated deep to the fascia, especially those that involve muscle, are usually malignant. Table 4.1 lists common benign and malignant soft-tissue tumors and tumorlike lesions of the head and neck. The histogenesis of most such tumors is known, although there is a miscellaneous group of tumors, benign and malignant, in which the cell of origin is disputed or unknown.

General Cytologic Features of Needle Aspirates

Aspirates from soft-tissue tumors usually consist of one or two drops of semisolid material, the gross features of which vary with the tumor type. There is usually some blood in the aspirates. Aspirates from myxoid tumors have a gelatinous appearance, whereas those from lipomas consist of a small drop of material that contains fat globules. Scanty material is obtained from certain benign tumors, for example, fibromatoses, and from fibrotic lesions. Aspirates from vascular tumors may consist predominantly of blood, with a scanty amount of solid tumor particles. Malignant tumors tend to be more cellular consisting of blood admixed with numerous tiny particles of tumor tissue. On the basis of the cytologic features of the smears, one is able to differentiate benign from malignant lesions in most cases. However, the accurate classification of some soft-tissue tumors is difficult. Identification as spindle, pleomorphic or small, round-cell type may be all that one can accomplish. The cytologic features of some of the soft-tissue tumors listed in Table 4.1 will be briefly described and illustrated.

TUMORS OF ADIPOSE TISSUE

Lipoma

Lipomas are benign tumors that are composed of mature fat cells. They occur in all parts of the body, with approximately 10 to 15 percent found in the head or neck. The posterior triangle of the neck is a common site for lipomas. Other relatively

TABLE 4.1. Benign and Malignant Soft-Tissue Tumors and Tumor-Like Lesions of the Head and Neck

Benign	Malignant
Tumors of Adipose Tissue	
Lipoma	Liposarcoma
Tumors and Tumor-Like Lesions of Fibrous Tissue	
Nodular Fasciitis	Fibrosarcoma
Fibromatosis	
Fibrohistiocytic Tumors	
Fibrous histiocytoma	Fibrous histiocytoma
Dermatofibrosarcoma protuberans	Giant-cell tumor of soft tissue
Tumors of Smooth Muscle	
Leiomyoma	Leiomyosarcoma
Tumors of Striated Muscle	
Rhabdomyoma	Rhabdomyosarcoma
Tumors of Peripheral Nerves	
Neurilemoma	Neurofibrosarcoma
Neurofibroma	
Tumors of the Sympathetic Nervous System	
Ganglioneuroma	Neuroblastoma
Tumors of Blood and Lymphatic Vessels	
Angioma	Angiosarcoma
Hemangiopericytoma	
Lymphangioma	Lymphangiosarcoma
Tumors of Synovium	Synovial sarcoma
Miscellaneous Tumors	
Granular cell tumor	Granular cell tumor
Myxoma	Alveolar soft-part sarcoma
	Epithelioid sarcoma
	Extraskeletal chondrosarcoma
	Extraskeletal Ewing's sarcoma

frequent sites include the face, scalp, nasal cavity, paranasal sinuses, nasopharynx and hypopharynx and oral cavity.[33] Lipomas have also been described in the parotid glands.[34] Most patients with such tumors are asymptomatic and present with a solitary soft, well-circumscribed, movable, nontender mass, usually less than 5.0 centimeters in diameter. Lipomas are most common in middle and old age, although lipoblastomas and hibernomas arise in infancy and childhood. Women have lipomas more frequently than do men. Some patients have more than one lipoma. Pleomorphic lipomas,[35] spindle cell lipomas[36] and lipoblastomas[37] may be confused with liposarcoma. Tumors derived from brown fat are referred to as hibernomas.[38]

On gross inspection, lipomas appear lobulated and most of them have a yellow coloration. Hibernomas, on the other hand, are tan to brown.

HISTOLOGIC FEATURES. Histologic examination shows that lipomas are typically composed of mature fat cells that contain a single large lipid vacuole that pushes the

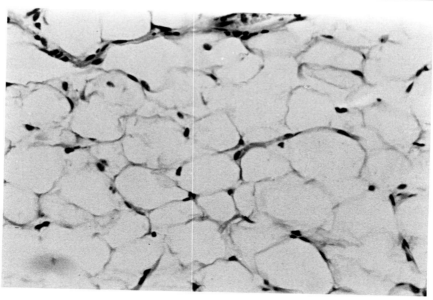

Fig. 4.1. Lipoma. Histology specimen from a lesion composed of mature fat cells. Hematoxylin and eosin preparation. × 390.

nucleus peripherally against the cell membrane (Fig. 4.1). Hibernomas have a characteristic appearance, being composed of large, polygonal cells that have prominent cell borders and small, centrally or eccentrically located nuclei.[38] The cytoplasm contains numerous small vacuoles of fat (Fig. 4.2). In the pleomorphic[35] and spindle cell types,[36] mature fat cells and elongated spindle cells are admixed with thick bands of collagen. Multinucleated giant cells that have peripherally located nuclei, the so-called floret cells, are seen in the pleomorphic type of lipoma.[35] In lipoblastoma, the tumor cells are in varying stages of maturation, ranging from small lipoblasts to spindle cells and mature lipocytes.[37]

CYTOLOGIC FEATURES. The cytologic appearance of lipomas is similar to their histologic appearance. The smears typically consist of small or large cohesive aggregates of mature fat cells that have prominent cell borders and small, round or oval nuclei (Fig. 4.3). The nucleus may be located centrally or peripherally along the cell border. Nuclear atypia is not seen. In the pleomorphic and spindle cell types, in addition to mature fat cells, spindle cells and cells with atypia coexist with multinucleated floret cells.[32] In lipoblastoma, one would expect to find mature and primitive lipoblasts in variable proportions. In hibernoma, the tumor cells are large and their cytoplasm is granular, containing small, uniform vacuoles (Fig. 4.4).

DIFFERENTIAL DIAGNOSIS. Because lipomas are composed of mature fat cells, the observation of small aggregates of fat cells in a smear is not always evidence of a lipoma. Fat cells from subcutaneous tissue or other tissues cannot be distinguished from lipoma cells on aspiration biopsy cytology. The spindle cell and pleomorphic variants of lipoma must be differentiated from liposarcoma. Differentiation on the

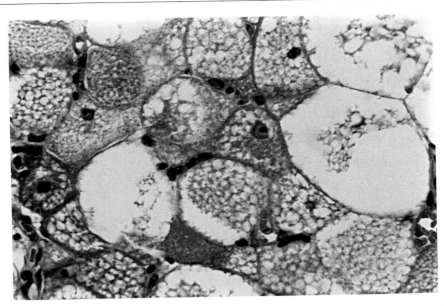

Fig. 4.2. Hibernoma. Histology specimen contains tumor cells that have the characteristic small vacuoles of fat in the cytoplasm. Hematoxylin and eosin preparation. ×625.

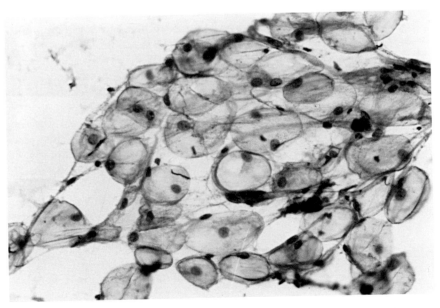

Fig. 4.3. Aspirate from a lipoma. Cohesive groups of mature fat cells. Papanicolaou preparation. ×390.

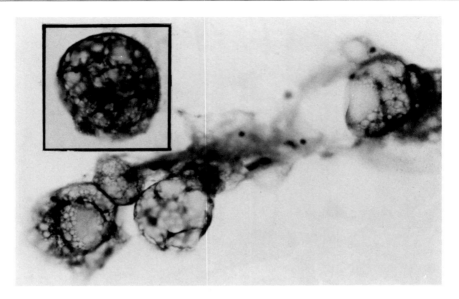

Fig. 4.4. Aspirate from a hibernoma. Note the numerous small vacuoles in the cytoplasm of the tumor cells. Papanicolaou preparation. ×625. (*Inset,* ×1000.)

basis of cytologic examination alone may be impossible. The site of the lesion and the clinical findings should be taken into consideration when atypical spindle and mature fat cells are observed. Spindle cell and pleomorphic lipomas are usually superficial, whereas liposarcomas are intramuscular or deeply located. Differentiation of lipoblastomas from liposarcomas on the basis of cytologic features is equally difficult. The age of the patient must be taken into consideration in such cases. Liposarcomas in infants or young children are exceedingly rare. Hibernoma may be confused with rhabdomyoma or granular cell tumor. In rhabdomyoma, the cells are polygonal, but the cytoplasm is dense and granular. Vacuolation of the cytoplasm may be observed, but this feature results from glycogen, an observation that can be confirmed with periodic acid-Schiff staining. Cross striations may be visible. In addition, elongated forms may be seen. In granular cell tumors, the cytoplasm is granular and eosinophilic. Moreover, the cell borders are usually not as prominent as those of lipoma cells.

Liposarcoma

Liposarcoma is one of the most common soft-tissue sarcomas. Unlike lipomas, this tumor occurs in deep tissues. Although liposarcomas commonly arise in the legs and retroperitoneum, they also occur in the head and neck,[33,39,40] most often involving the neck. Such tumors usually grow slowly and patients present with an enlarging mass in the neck. Most patients are in their fourth decade or older. As was noted previously, liposarcomas are rarely encountered in infants or young children.

Most tumors of the head and neck are less than 10.0 centimeters in greatest dimension. On gross inspection, such tumors vary from soft, yellow, lipoma-like,

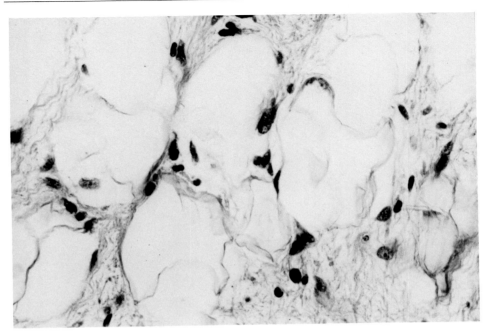

Fig. 4.5. Well-differentiated liposarcoma. Histology specimen. Hematoxylin and eosin preparation. ×625.

well-demarcated lesions to firm, gray lesions that have areas of hemorrhage or necrosis. Myxoid variants are commonly encountered.

HISTOLOGIC FEATURES. Well-differentiated, myxoid, round-cell, pleomorphic and mixed cell types have been described.[41] Well-differentiated liposarcomas resemble the common and pleomorphic types of lipoma (Fig. 4.5). They myxoid type is probably the most common variant of liposarcoma (Fig. 4.6). Myxoid liposarcomas contain not only lipoblasts but also a delicate, branching, vascular network on a myxomatous background. Round-cell tumors are composed of small, round cells that have an epithelioid appearance. Vacuoles may be observed. Pleomorphic tumors, as their name implies, are composed of large, bizarre cells that have one or more nuclei. Small lipoblasts are usually seen. In about one-fourth of such tumors, two or more of the histologic patterns may coexist. In such cases, the tumor is referred to as a mixed liposarcoma.

CYTOLOGIC FEATURES. The smears usually consist of tumor cells and fat globules[32] (Fig. 4.7). Solitary tumor cells and small groupings of such cells are encountered. The diagnosis relies on the observation in the smear of small or large single or multiple lipoblasts (Fig. 4.8). The tumor cell nuclei are located centrally or eccentrically and are round or oval. The chromatin is finely granular and the nucleoli may be small or large. Signet-ring-type lipoblasts may also be observed. In myxoid liposarcoma, a capillary network similar to that seen in histologic sections may be visible in the aspirates.[32] The background of the smear is myxoid (Fig. 4.9) and is

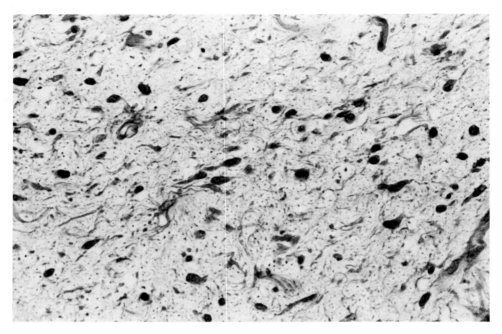

Fig. 4.6. Myxoid liposarcoma. Histology specimen. Hematoxylin and eosin preparation. ×625. (Courtesy of Dr G.K.Nguyen.)

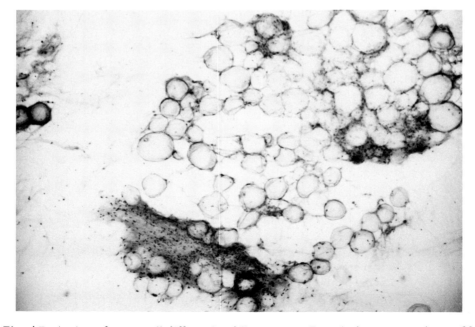

Fig. 4.7. Aspirate from a well-differentiated liposarcoma. Papanicolaou preparation. ×50.

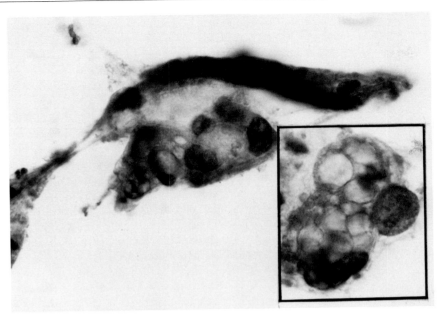

Fig. 4.8. High-power view of multivacuolated lipoblasts. Papanicolaou preparation. ×625. (*Inset,* ×390.)

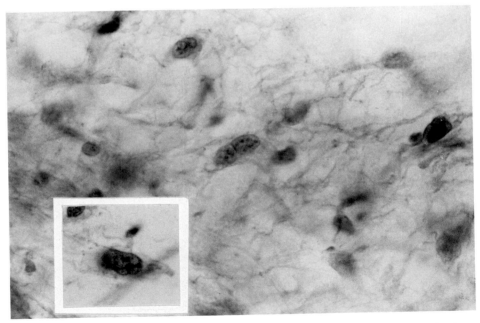

Fig. 4.9. Aspirate from a myxoid liposarcoma. Nuclear changes are best seen in the inset. Papanicolaou preparation. ×625. (*Inset,* ×1000.) (Courtesy of Dr G.K.Nguyen.)

best seen with May-Grünwald-Giemsa stain. Round-cell tumors are composed of small, round cells that have scanty cytoplasm. Atypical lipoblasts are also encountered. The morphologic features of the various types of liposarcoma have been described by Willems.[32] In spindle cell liposarcoma, elongated cells in loose groupings coexist with atypical lipoblasts. The pleomorphic variant consists of large, bizarre tumor cells, spindle cells and atypical lipoblasts.

DIFFERENTIAL DIAGNOSIS. The diagnosis can be made only if atypical lipoblasts are observed. Differentiation of lipoma-like liposarcomas from the common type of lipoma may be difficult. Similarly, spindle cell and pleomorphic liposarcomas may mimic spindle cell and pleomorphic lipomas as well as other spindle cell types of soft-tissue sarcoma, including malignant fibrous histiocytoma. Myxoid liposarcomas may be difficult to distinguish from myxomas and other soft-tissue tumors that have myxoid areas, including myxoid chondrosarcoma. Round-cell liposarcomas mimic other small round-cell tumors and differentiation from other similar-appearing tumors is not possible unless the atypical lipoblasts are found.

TUMORS AND TUMOR-LIKE LESIONS OF FIBROUS TISSUE

Nodular Fasciitis

This reactive lesion usually arises from the superficial fascia but occasionally arises from the deep fascia. The overlying subcutaneous fat and underlying muscle may be involved. The most common sites for such lesions are the arms and trunk. Nodular fasciitis also has been reported in the head and neck.[42] Most patients are between 20 and 40 years of age and present with a rapidly enlarging, tender, movable mass.

On gross inspection, the lesion is usually less than 5.0 centimeters in diameter, firm and gray to yellow.

HISTOLOGIC FEATURES. Histologic examination demonstrates that nodular fasciitis is composed of proliferating oval to elongating myofibroblasts on a myxoid stroma admixed with small blood vessels and lymphocytes. Multinucleated giant cells may be seen. Mitoses are plentiful.

CYTOLOGIC FEATURES. The cytologic features of nodular fasciitis have been well documented.[5,32,43] The aspirates may be cellular or sparse, depending on the degree of fibrosis. The oval or elongated, spindle-shaped myofibroblasts occur as solitary cells or in loose groupings. Some of them have slender, bipolar cytoplasmic processes. In well-preserved preparations, the cell borders are clearly outlined. The nuclei are oval or elongated and contain finely granular chromatin and small nucleoli. Mitoses are observed. In addition, lymphocytes, plasma cells, histiocytes and multinucleated giant cells may be seen. The background material appears granular or may be fibrillar to myxoid.

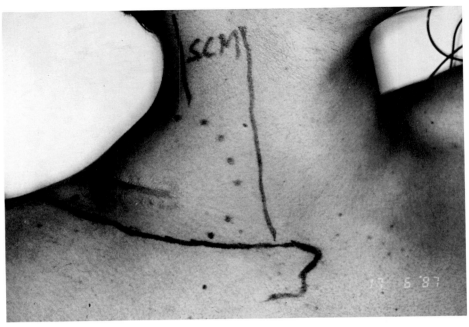

Fig. 4.10. Large desmoid of the neck in a 17-year-old boy. Needle aspiration biopsy suggested a fibrous tumor. A radical resection of the mass was performed, preserving the brachial plexus, which was surrounded by the tumor.

Fibromatosis

This heterogeneous group of benign fibroproliferative lesions may be localized or diffuse. Familial cases have been reported. Fibromatosis occurs at all ages and involves different areas of the body. The adult (extraabdominal desmoid) or juvenile (fibromatosis colli, congenital fibromatosis) variants of fibromatosis may occur in the head or neck.[44-46] Approximately 10 to 20 percent of cases of fibromatosis involve the head or neck. The clinical findings depend on the site of the lesion; involvement of the neck usually is manifested by a painless mass (Fig. 4.10). Ulceration of the overlying skin may be an accompanying feature. A patient may have one or more such lesions of variable size.

On gross inspection, fibromatosis appears circumscribed even though such lesions are infiltrative. The cut surface is firm and has a gray to pink, whorled appearance.

HISTOLOGIC FEATURES. Histologic study shows that such tumors consist of bundles of elongated or fusiform fibroblasts admixed with a variable amount of collagen (Fig. 4.11). The nuclei are oval or elongated and uniform. Mitoses are infrequently seen. Infiltration into adjacent structures is a common feature of fibromatosis that makes complete excision in the head and neck difficult. Without complete excision, recurrence takes place. Metastasis has not been reported, however.

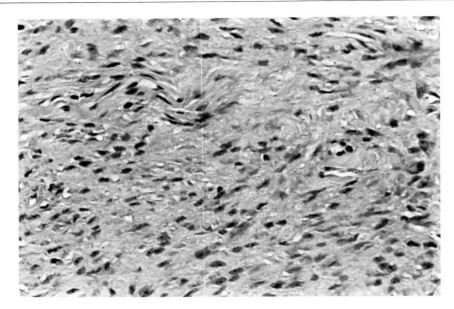

Fig. 4.11 Fibromatosis. Histology specimen from a lesion composed of elongated fibroblasts. Hematoxylin and eosin preparation. × 390.

CYTOLOGIC FEATURES. Needle aspiration biopsy in the numerous variants of fibromatosis yields scanty cellular material admixed with blood. Solitary tumor cells and loose groupings of such cells are observed.[32] The spindle-shaped cells have ill-defined cell borders (Fig. 4.12). The nuclei are ovoid or elongated and contain finely granular chromatin and small nucleoli. In the background, blood and granular or fibrillar, pale-staining material is visible. A definitive diagnosis of fibromatosis usually cannot be made on cytologic grounds alone because many soft-tissue lesions, benign or malignant, can have a similar cytologic appearance. The age of the patient, the history and the clinical findings must be taken into account in making the diagnosis.

Fibrosarcoma

At one time, fibrosarcoma was regarded as the most common malignant soft-tissue tumor. However, it probably accounts for less than one-fourth of all malignant soft-tissue lesions. Although most such tumors occur in the superficial soft tissues of the legs and trunk, fibrosarcomas have also been reported in the soft tissues of the neck and in other structures of the head and neck.[47] Fibrosarcomas occur at all ages but are most common between 20 and 50 years of age. The two sexes are equally affected. The clinical findings depend on the site of the lesion and its size. Fibrosarcomas of the neck present as gradually enlarging, painless lumps. When the nose or paranasal sinuses are involved, the presenting complaint is pain, bleeding or obstruction. Fibrosarcomas may be infiltrative or well circumscribed. Some fibrosarcomas are polypoid, especially those of the oral cavity, nose or paranasal sinuses. Ulcer-

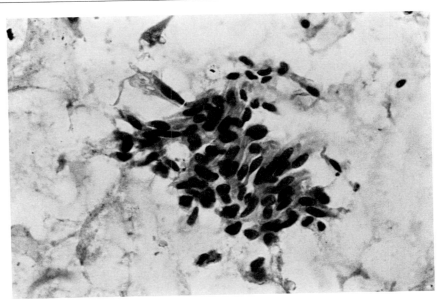

Fig. 4.12. Aspirate from the lesion shown in Figure 4.11. Note the loose grouping of spindle-shaped cells. Papanicolaou preparation. ×625.

ation of the overlying epithelium or skin may be an accompanying feature. Fibrosarcomas are rarely larger than 10.0 centimeters in greatest dimension.

HISTOLOGIC FEATURES. Histologic examination reveals that such tumors are composed of uniform, spindle-shaped cells in interlacing bundles or in a herringbone pattern (Fig. 4.13). Collagen and reticular fibers can be visualized. Mitoses are frequently seen, in contrast to the fibromatoses, in which mitoses are infrequently observed. Lymph node metastases are an uncommon feature. Fibrosarcomas usually spread via the bloodstream.

CYTOLOGIC FEATURES. In most cases, the cytologic features of fibrosarcoma are similar to those of fibromatosis. The smears may consist of solitary tumor cells or a few loose groupings of such cells. In poorly differentiated tumors, the aspirates are more cellular and the tumor cell nuclei are larger than nuclei of normal fibroblasts and oval or spindle shaped (Fig. 4.14). The chromatin is finely to coarsely granular and prominent nucleoli are usually not seen. Atypia is more marked in poorly differentiated than in well-differentiated fibrosarcoma. Differentiation of well-differentiated fibrosarcoma from other tumors and tumor-like lesions of fibrous tissue may be difficult.

DIFFERENTIAL DIAGNOSIS. All the fibrous tissue lesions described previously may appear similar on needle aspiration biopsy and a definitive cytologic diagnosis may not be possible. Spindle-shaped myofibroblasts and other inflammatory cells, including multinucleated giant cells, should be clues to a diagnosis of nodular fasciitis. In

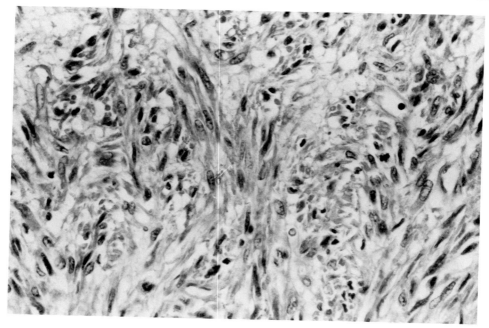

Fig. 4.13. Fibrosarcoma. Histology specimen from an infiltrative lesion composed of spindle-shaped cells. Hematoxylin and eosin preparation. ×390.

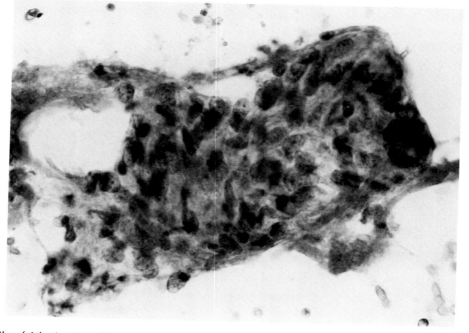

Fig. 4.14. Aspirate from the lesion shown in Figure 4.13. Papanicolaou preparation. ×625.

most cases, well-differentiated fibrosarcoma cannot be differentiated from the various fibromatoses or from some fibrous histiocytic tumors. In poorly differentiated fibrosarcoma, a diagnosis of spindle cell sarcoma can be made, but differentiation from other malignant spindle cell soft-tissue tumors (e.g., synovial sarcoma, leiomyosarcoma and neurofibrosarcoma) may be impossible.

FIBROUS HISTIOCYTIC TUMORS

This heterogeneous group of benign and malignant tumors is believed to have a common histiocytic origin, based on the tissue culture studies of Ozzello and colleagues.[48] These investigators showed that even though there are many morphologic variants of fibrous histiocytic tumor, all the variants have a common cell of origin, namely, a histiocyte that can transform into a fibroblast and produce collagen. Recent studies performed with the aid of electron microscopy, however, suggest that the cell of origin is a primitive mesenchymal cell that can differentiate into a histiocyte or a fibroblast.[49] Myofibroblasts are also seen in such lesions. Most benign variants occur in the dermis or subcutaneous tissue, whereas malignant fibrous histiocytomas occur deeply, involving the soft tissues of the neck, nose or paranasal sinuses, larynx, orbits or other structures.[50-52] Less than 5 percent of malignant fibrous histiocytomas occur in the head or neck; most such lesions occur in the limbs or retroperitoneum.[53] The clinical findings are similar to those encountered with other soft-tissue tumors of these regions. The clinical signs and symptoms vary with the site of the lesion. A tumor of the neck, for example, may present as an enlarging mass (Fig. 4.15), whereas involvement of the nose or paranasal sinuses may be associated with pain, bleeding and obstruction. Proptosis and diplopia are encountered with orbital lesions.

Benign Fibrous Histiocytoma

HISTOLOGIC FEATURES. These well-circumscribed nodules are tan to yellow on cut surface. Histologic study shows that such tumors are composed of interlacing bundles of spindle-shaped cells in a cartwheel pattern. Most such lesions contain collagen as well as lipid and hemosiderin-laden histiocytes.

CYTOLOGIC FEATURES. The aspirates consist of large cohesive clusters of stellate and spindle-shaped cells. Few solitary cells are seen. Some tumor cells have scanty cytoplasm, whereas others have abundant cytoplasm and usually well-defined cell borders. The nuclei are round or oval and contain fine, evenly distributed chromatin and small nucleoli.

Malignant Fibrous Histiocytoma

HISTOLOGIC FEATURES. Such tumors are gray and have yellow areas. The histologic appearance varies from a fibrosarcomatous pattern to one that is storiform or pleomorphic (Fig. 4.16). In the fibrosarcomatous and storiform variants, the tumor

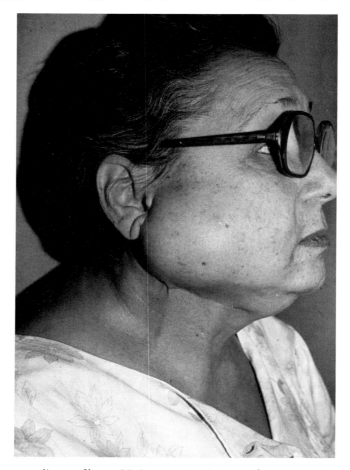

Fig. 4.15. Large malignant fibrous histiocytoma in the parotid space invading the mandible.

cells are spindle shaped or fusiform, whereas in the pleomorphic type, numerous multinucleated giant cells coexist with polygonal and spindle-shaped cells. Myxoid[54] and giant-cell[55,56] variants have also been described (Fig. 4.17).

CYTOLOGIC FEATURES. The aspirates usually contain a large number of cells.[32] The cytologic appearance depends on the predominant histologic pattern. In the spindle cell variant, elongated, fusiform and stellate cells predominate, whereas in the pleomorphic type, numerous bizarre, polygonal and giant cells (Fig. 4.18) coexist with spindle cells. The spindle cells usually occur in cohesive clusters, whereas the polygonal and giant cells are solitary.[32] The tumor cell nuclei are round, ovoid or irregularly shaped and contain coarsely granular chromatin. Multinucleation is a feature of the giant cells. The nucleoli vary in size and shape. Mitoses are also noted. In the myxoid variant, in addition to the cellular constitutents described previously, a fibrillar, myxoid substance is visible in the background[32] (Fig. 4.19). In the giant-cell variant, gigantic, osteoclastic-type tumor cells coexist with small, mononuclear, stellate or spindle-shaped cells.[56]

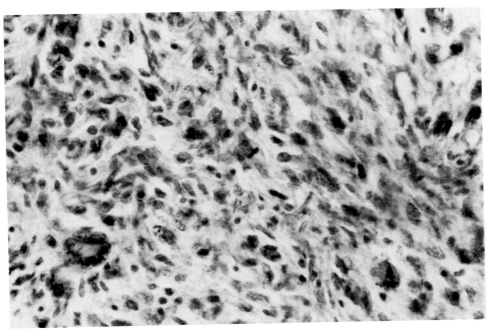

Fig. 4.16. Malignant fibrous histiocytoma. Note the spindle-shaped cells coexisting with multinucleated giant cells. Hematoxylin and eosin preparation. ×390. (Courtesy of Dr G.K.Nguyen.)

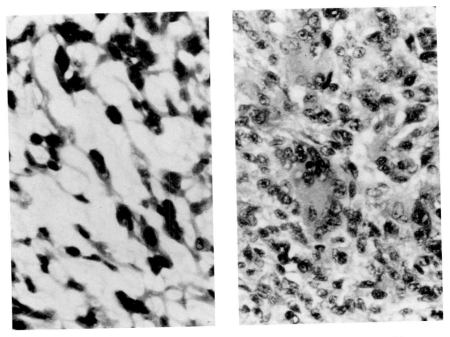

Fig. 4.17. Malignant fibrous histiocytoma, myxoid variant. Note the myxoid appearance (*left*). Elsewhere, the tumor appeared more solid, being composed of spindle and multinucleated giant cells (*right*). Hematoxylin and eosin preparation. ×390. (Courtesy of Dr G.K.Nguyen.)

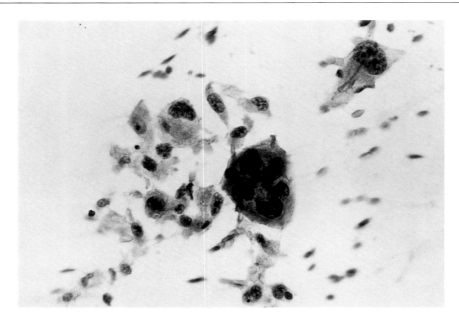

Fig. 4.18. Aspirate from a malignant fibrous histiocytoma. Note the stellate and bizarre, multinucleated tumor cells. Papanicolaou preparation. × 625. (Courtesy of Dr G.K. Nguyen.)

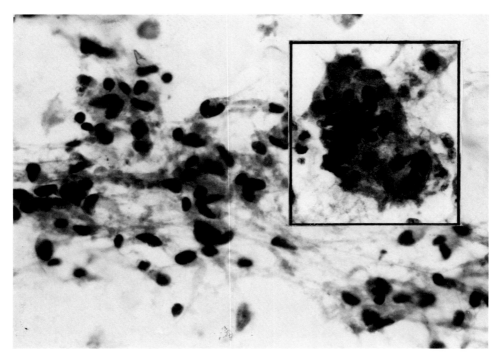

Fig. 4.19. Aspirate from a malignant fibrous histiocytoma, myxoid variant. Note the fibrillar, myxoid material in the background. Inset shows a multinucleated giant cell. Papanicolaou preparation. × 390. (Courtesy of Dr G.K. Nguyen.)

DIFFERENTIAL DIAGNOSIS. It may be difficult to differentiate benign fibrous histiocytomas from other spindle cell tumors, particularly fibroblastic lesions. Benign histiocytoma cells generally have a uniform appearance and lack the nuclear pleomorphism seen in malignant tumors. As with fibroblastic tumors, differentiation of benign fibrous histiocytomas from well-differentiated malignant tumors may be difficult.

It may be difficult to differentiate malignant fibrous histiocytomas, especially those in which a spindle or storiform pattern predominates, from other spindle cell sarcomas. Occasionally, spindle cell carcinomas and melanomas also mimic malignant fibrous histiocytoma. The giant-cell variant cannot be distinguished from other giant-cell tumors, including extraskeletal osteosarcoma.[32] Myxoid variants may be confused with myxoid liposarcoma, myxoid chondrosarcoma, myxoma and chordoma. In myxoid liposarcoma, atypical lipoblasts coexisting with branching capillaries are a clue to the diagnosis. In myxoid chondrosarcoma, spindle-shaped mesenchymal cells and chondroblasts are found on a myxoid background.[24] Myxomas usually consist of spindle-shaped or stellate cells on a myxomatous background. Vacuolation of the cells may be observed.[32] In chordoma, physaliphorous cells are encountered. The vacuoles contain mucin, which can be demonstrated by special stains. Extracellular mucin is also noted in the background.[14] Spindle cells are usually not seen.

TUMORS OF SMOOTH MUSCLE

Leiomyoma

This benign tumor of smooth muscle is encountered most often in the uterus. A few cases have been reported in the head and neck, most commonly in the cervical segment of the esophagus.[57] Other sites include the skin, lips, tongue and oral and nasal cavities.[58,59] Most leiomyomas present as asymptomatic masses. Lesions of the skin may be painful. Leiomyomas of the cervical portion of the esophagus may be associated with dysphagia. Leiomyoma occurs at all ages. The tumors are well circumscribed and usually measure less than 3.0 centimeters in diameter.

HISTOLOGIC FEATURES. They are composed of spindle-shaped cells in interlacing bundles. The tumor cell nuclei are ovoid. Epithelioid variants have also been reported.[60]

CYTOLOGIC FEATURES. The aspirates contain few cells, most of which are in cohesive clusters; solitary cells are infrequently seen. The tumor cells are elongated and have delicate cytoplasm and elongated, cigar-shaped nuclei. The chromatin is finely granular and the nucleoli are inconspicuous or absent.

Leiomyosarcoma

Like their benign counterparts, most leiomyosarcomas occur in the uterus and gastrointestinal tract. Less than 5 percent of such tumors arise in the head or neck, most of which occur in the nasal cavity and paranasal sinuses,[61] skin[62] or esophagus.[63] The

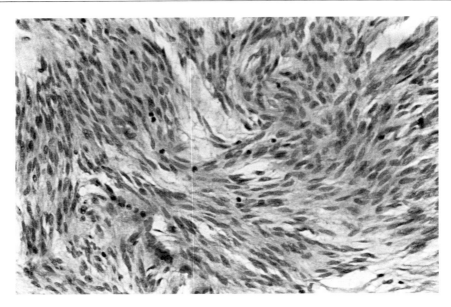

Fig. 4.20. Leiomyosarcoma. Bundles of elongated cells have cigar-shaped nuclei. Hematoxylin and eosin preparation. × 390.

clinical findings vary with the site of the tumor. Nasal and paranasal tumors may cause obstruction, pain and bleeding. Lesions of the skin and subcutaneous tissue may be ulcerated and are sometimes associated with pain. Tumors of the oral cavity or esophagus may present as masses, or the presenting complaints may be dysphagia, weight loss and vomiting. Most patients are middle-aged or elderly. Leiomyosarcoma has a slight predilection for the male sex. On gross inspection, leiomyosarcomas appear circumscribed and are gray to pink with a smooth or trabeculated cut surface. Hemorrhage and necrosis are common features of such tumors, especially large ones.

HISTOLOGIC FEATURES. Histologic study demonstrates that leiomyosarcomas are composed of bundles of spindle-shaped cells. The tumor cells have eosinophilic cytoplasm and elongated, cigar-shaped nuclei (Fig. 4.20). Palisading of nuclei may be observed. Mitoses vary from case to case. Some tumors are unusually vascular, whereas others are composed of epithelioid or polygonal cells.

CYTOLOGIC FEATURES. The aspirates may be appreciably cellular or contain few cells. Most of the tumor cells are in cohesive clusters, but solitary cells may be encountered as well. The cytoplasm is delicate and the cell borders are ill-defined. The ovoid or cigar-shaped tumor cell nuclei contain finely granular chromatin (Fig. 4.21). Small nucleoli are visible. In poorly differentiated tumors, nuclear variability and pleomorphism are marked.

DIFFERENTIAL DIAGNOSIS. The differential diagnosis of benign and malignant tumors of smooth muscle includes other spindle cell soft-tissue tumors. If nuclear

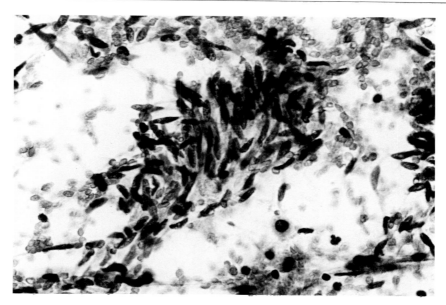

Fig. 4.21. Aspirate from the lesion shown in Figure 4.20. Note the cohesive clusters of elongated cells. Papanicolaou preparation. ×625.

atypia cannot be detected, differentiation of leiomyoma from well-differentiated leiomyosarcoma may be difficult. In fibrosarcoma, neurofibrosarcoma, rhabdomyosarcoma, synovial sarcoma and malignant fibrous histiocytoma, the smears may consist only of spindle-shaped cells, thereby making cytologic differentiation and a definitive diagnosis impossible. In such cases, the tumor is usually reported as spindle cell sarcoma and removed for histologic examination.

TUMORS OF STRIATED MUSCLE

Rhabdomyoma

Rhabdomyoma is a rare tumor that arises in striated muscle. The head and neck are not uncommon sites for such neoplasms. Most patients with rhabdomyomas are asymptomatic and present with a slowly growing mass, usually subcutaneous. Adult and fetal types have been described. The adult variant occurs in the elderly, more often in men than in women. These well-circumscribed tumors are usually less than 5 centimeters in diameter.

HISTOLOGIC FEATURES. Histologic examination shows that they are composed of large, polygonal cells that have eosinophilic cytoplasm and one or two round nuclei that contain prominent nucleoli. The cytoplasm may be vacuolated as a result of glycogen. Cross striations and crystalline deposits may be seen in the cells.

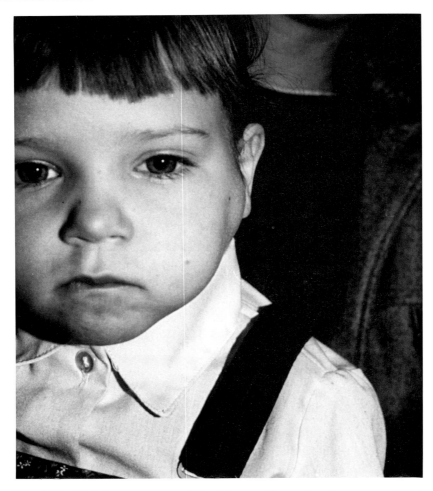

Fig. 4.22. Rhabdomyosarcoma of the left parotid area in a three-year-old girl.

CYTOLOGIC FEATURES. The aspirates contain scanty cellular material. Solitary tumor cells and loose groupings of such cells may be seen. The characteristic cytologic pattern consists of large, polygonal or elongated cells that have an abundance of dense, granular, eosinophilic cytoplasm.[32] Small vacuoles are visible in some cells. The nuclei appear uniform and are round or oval.

Rhabdomyosarcoma

Rhabdomyosarcoma is not an uncommon tumor; approximately one-third of such tumors occur in the head or neck.[64] Most patients are less than 15 years of age[65] (Fig. 4.22). The juvenile types, which usually involve the head or neck, include embryonal rhabdomyosarcoma, alveolar rhabdomyosarcoma and sarcoma botryoides. The

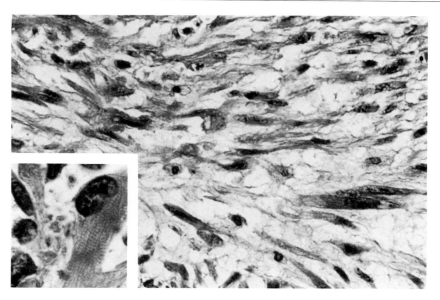

Fig. 4.23. Pleomorphic rhabdomyosarcoma composed of spindle-shaped cells. Inset shows cross striations. Hematoxylin and eosin preparation. ×625. (*Inset,* ×1000.)

adult, or pleomorphic, type more often affects the limbs and the trunk. Most cases of the adult form occur between 30 and 60 years of age. About 5 percent of pleomorphic rhabdomyosarcomas occur in the head or neck.[64] About 45 percent of juvenile tumors involve structures of the head or neck, including the orbits.[64] The embryonal variant is probably the most common juvenile form.

Adult, or pleomorphic, tumors commonly involve skeletal muscle and on gross inspection are soft, gray to pink lesions that have areas of hemorrhage and necrosis.

HISTOLOGIC FEATURES. Histologic study demonstrates that such tumors are composed of spindle-shaped cells (Fig. 4.23) admixed with large, round, strap-shaped or racket-shaped rhabdomyoblasts; the racket-shaped rhabdomyoblasts have their nuclei at the expanded end. Multinucleated cells are also observed. The diagnosis relies on the finding of longitudinal and cross striations in the abundant, eosinophilic cytoplasm. If this feature is not observed, differentiation from malignant fibrous histiocytoma may be difficult.

The embryonal type is composed of spindle-shaped cells and small, round cells that have eosinophilic cytoplasm and round or oval nuclei. Cross striations can be visualized in some cells. Mitoses are easily found. The stroma is edematous and myxoid. In alveolar rhabdomyosarcoma, histologic examination shows alveolar spaces lined by small, round cells that have small, round or oval, hyperchromatic nuclei. Mitoses are a common feature. Small cells that have a similar appearance lie free in the centers of the spaces. The cytoplasm is scanty and pink.

The botryoid variant differs from the other types on gross inspection. It arises from mucosal surfaces and tends to be polypoid, lobulated and myxoid, resembling a bunch of grapes. The characteristic feature of this variant is a highly cellular sub-epithelial zone, referred to as the cambium layer.[64] Spindle-shaped and small, round rhabdomyoblasts are more easily demonstrated in this layer than in the edematous, less cellular parts of such tumors.

All three variants invade adjacent tissues and are capable of metastasizing via the lymphatic system and bloodstream. The alveolar type metastasizes to the lymph nodes at an early stage and may be manifested by enlargement of a lymph node of the neck on presentation.

CYTOLOGIC FEATURES. The aspirates usually consist of solitary tumor cells or small loose groupings of such cells. In the pleomorphic type, the smears consist of spindle-shaped and pleomorphic tumor cells coexisting with round, strap-shaped or racket-shaped cells (Figs. 4.24 and 4.25). The cytoplasm is abundant and eosinophilic. The cytoplasm may appear dense, but cross striations are difficult to find on cytologic examination. The tumor cell nuclei vary from round to elongated and contain coarsely granular chromatin and large nucleoli. Mitoses are frequently encountered. In the juvenile variants, the smears consist of numerous round or plump, spindle-shaped cells. The round or ovoid nuclei are located centrally or eccentrically and contain granular chromatin and small nucleoli. In most tumor cells, the cytoplasm is scanty, ill-defined and pale. However, a few large cells that have an abundance of dense, eosinophilic cytoplasm can be found. These cells are rhab-domyoblasts and are a necessary finding for a definitive diagnosis in most cases. The nuclei of rhabdomyoblasts may be located eccentrically. Binucleated and multinu-cleated forms may be seen. Cross striations are usually not observed.

DIFFERENTIAL DIAGNOSIS. The pleomorphic variant must be differentiated from other spindle cell and pleomorphic tumors, including malignant fibrous histiocy-toma, pleomorphic liposarcoma, fibrosarcoma, leiomyosarcoma, neurogenic sar-coma and synovial sarcoma. Differentiation from the various spindle cell sarcomas may be difficult and a diagnosis of spindle cell or pleomorphic sarcoma may have to be made in such cases. Spindle cell melanoma and squamous cell carcinoma may also cause difficulty in the diagnosis. Small-cell rhabdomyosarcoma must be differ-entiated from other small-cell tumors, including lymphoma, neuroblastoma, Ewing's sarcoma, nasopharyngeal carcinoma, small-cell carcinoma of the lungs, carcinoid tumors and other apudomas, undifferentiated malignant melanoma and Merkel cell carcinoma. The differential diagnosis of these tumors is summarized in Table 3.13. The age of the patient, the site of the lesion and other pertinent information in the history may be helpful in making the diagnosis. Differentiation from other small-cell tumors is not always possible and other investigations may be necessary for making the diagnosis. The immunoperoxidase method is being used with increasing fre-quency and can be applied to cytology specimens with advantage.[66-68] Electron microscopy is also helpful in differentiating needle aspirates from small-cell tumors.[69] Nonetheless, even with all the techniques described so far, a definitive diagnosis sometimes must await histologic study of the excised tumor. In such instances, it is prudent to take small samples of fresh tumor tissue at the time of surgical intervention in the event that immunoperoxidase and ultrastructural studies become necessary.

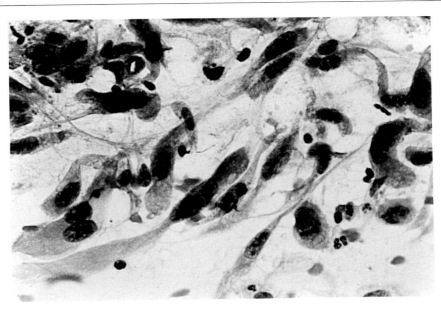

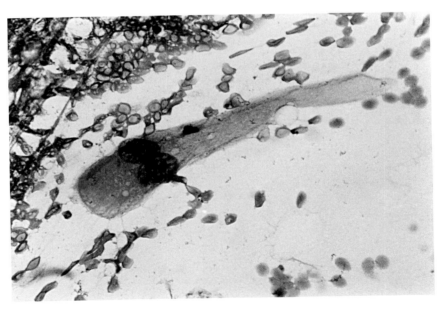

Figs. 4.24 and 4.25. Aspirate from the lesion shown in Figure 4.23. Note the pleomorphic tumor cells. Papanicolaou preparation. ×625.

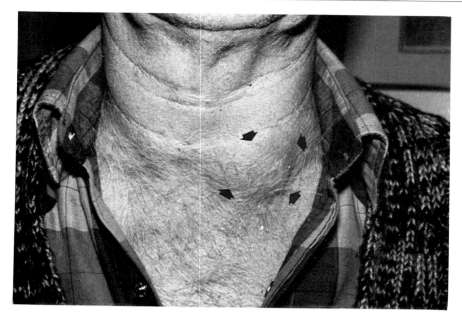

Fig. 4.26. Neurilemoma (arrows) of the left brachial plexus.

TUMORS OF PERIPHERAL NERVES

Neurilemoma (schwannoma)

Neurilemoma is a benign, encapsulated tumor of Schwann cell origin. Such tumors occur anywhere, but because of the large number of nerves in the head and neck, neurilemomas frequently arise in these regions.[9] About 45 percent of neurilemomas occur in the head and neck, most arising in the lateral aspects of the neck.[70] Such tumors occur more often in women than in men and most cases occur between 30 and 60 years of age. The clinical findings depend on the site of the tumor. Most neurilemomas of the neck, for example, are asymptomatic masses (Fig. 4.26), whereas tumors of the oral cavity or nose may be associated with difficulty eating or breathing. Figure 4.27 shows a neurilemoma of the vagus nerve that measured 1.5 centimeters in greatest dimension.

Most such tumors are less than 5.0 centimeters in greatest dimension at the time of diagnosis. On gross inspection, one sees a gray cut surface with hemorrhagic areas and myxoid or cystic areas.

HISTOLOGIC FEATURES. On microscopy, compactly arranged spindle cells (Antoni type A) are found to be admixed with myxoid areas (Antonia type B) (Fig. 4.28). Palisading nuclei result in the formation of Verocay bodies. Hyalinized variants are referred to as ancient schwannomas.

CYTOLOGIC FEATURES. Needle aspiration biopsy of neurilemomas may be painful. The aspirates usually consist of small or large, irregularly shaped clusters of cells.

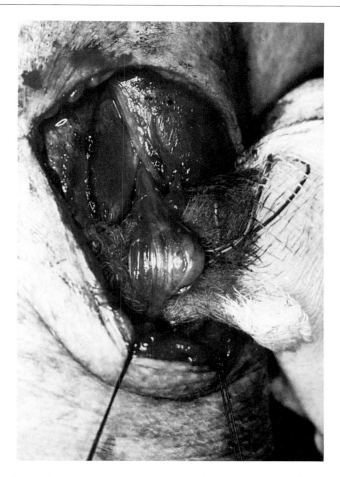

Fig. 4.27. Small neurilemoma of the vagus nerve. Note the splaying of the nerve fibers. No vocal cord weakness was observed after a nerve-preserving resection.

Few solitary tumor cells are seen. Interlacing, swirling fascicles of spindle-shaped cells are observed[9] (Fig. 4.29). Small clumps of myxoid, Antoni type-B tissue may also be encountered. The spindle-shaped tumor cells have indistinct cell borders because of the clumping of the cells. The elongated nuclei may appear uniform or be slightly pleomorphic. The chromatin is finely granular and nucleoli are usually not seen. Mitoses also are not observed. The smears occasionally contain Verocay bodies, which consist of a central core of fibrillar substance lying between two rows of palisaded nuclei.[21]

Neurofibroma

Neurofibromas may be solitary or multiple and are often a component of vonRecklinghausen's disease (Fig. 4.30). Neurofibromas may involve the skin and subcutaneous tissue, develop along nerve trunks or arise in the viscera. Like neurilemomas,

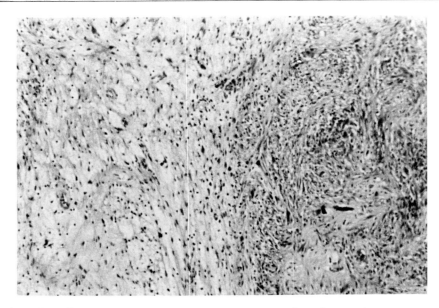

Fig. 4.28. Neurilemoma. Histology specimen contains spindle and myxoid areas. Hematoxylin and eosin preparation. ×150.

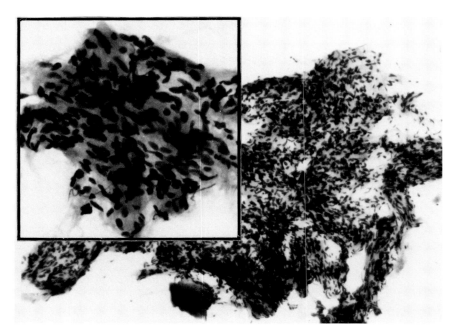

Fig. 4.29. Aspirate from the lesion shown in Figure 4.28. Note the bundles of spindle-shaped cells. Inset shows a fragment that corresponds to Antoni type-A areas of the biopsy specimen. Papanicolaou preparation. ×150. (*Inset,* ×390.)

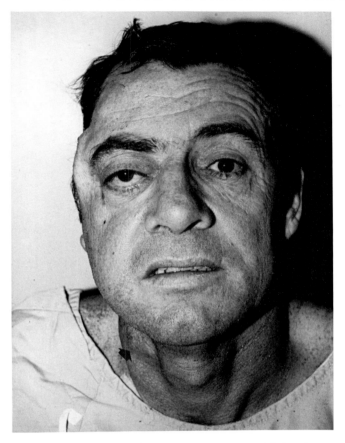

Fig. 4.30. Neurofibromatosis of the orbit, causing proptosis, with involvement of right side of the face and neck (arrow), confirmed by needle aspiration biopsy.

neurofibromas commonly occur in the head and neck and may be manifested by a mass in the neck.

HISTOLOGIC FEATURES. Microscopy shows that such tumors are not encapsulated and are composed of axons and Schwann cells. The interstitial matrix is myxoid or fibrous, containing mast cells.

CYTOLOGIC FEATURES. The aspirates usually consist of irregular tissue groups and dissociated cells. The cells are spindle shaped and the cell borders in the tissue fragments are poorly defined. The ovoid or elongated nuclei contain finely granular chromatin and inconspicuous nucleoli. Pale-staining, fibrillar material may be visible in the background.

Neurofibrosarcoma

Neurofibrosarcoma is not uncommonly associated with vonRecklinghausen's disease. Some tumors are encountered sporadically, however.[9] The neck is more often

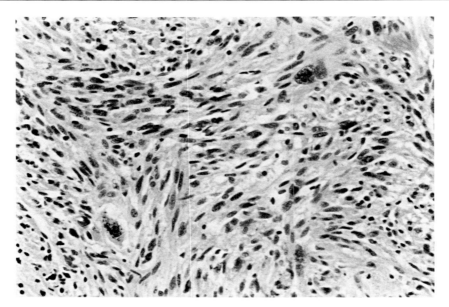

Fig. 4.31. Neurofibrosarcoma. Note the cellular spindle cell appearance of the tumor with a few large, bizarre nuclei. Hematoxylin and eosin preparation. ×390.

involved than is the head. We recently reported the cytologic features of a solitary malignant schwannoma of the inferior alveolar nerve.[9] Such tumors usually are asymptomatic masses but may be associated with pain and weakness of the muscles.

On gross inspection, neurofibrosarcomas are round to fusiform. Such tumors are large, most being greater than 5.0 centimeters in diameter. The cut surface is gray to tan. Cystic degeneration and hemorrhage are not uncommon features of neurofibrosarcomas.

HISTOLOGIC FEATURES. Histologic examination demonstrates that such tumors are composed of spindle-shaped cells tightly packed in interlacing fascicles. Wavy collagen fibers are admixed with the tumor cells (Fig. 4.31).

CYTOLOGIC FEATURES. Needle aspiration biopsy yields small loose groupings of tumor cells and solitary cells. The tumor cells are elongated or spindle shaped and have indistinct cytoplasm. The tumor cell nuclei are large and ovoid or elongated and contain coarsely granular to clumped chromatin (Fig. 4.32). Nucleoli are present. Binucleated and multinucleated cells may be observed[9] (Fig. 4.32, *inset*). Necrotic debris may be visible in the background.

DIFFERENTIAL DIAGNOSIS. Other benign and malignant spindle cell tumors must be considered in the differential diagnosis of nerve sheath tumors. Verocay bodies are usually regarded as pathognomonic of neurilemoma. Even when Verocay bodies are not seen, the observation of Antoni type-A and type-B tissues in the aspirate suggests the diagnosis. However, if only spindle cells are found, differentiation from fibromatosis, leiomyoma and benign fibrous histiocytoma may be difficult. Although

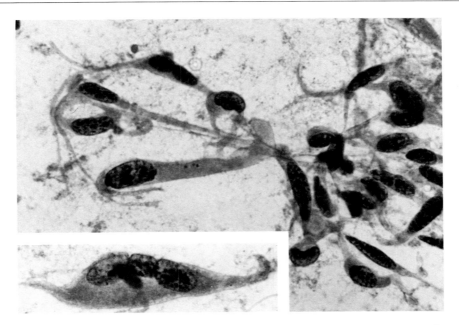

Fig. 4.32. Aspirate from the lesion shown in Figure 4.31. Inset shows a multinucleated tumor cell. Papanicolaou preparation. ×625.

the malignant nature of the process may be identifiable on the basis of nuclear features, a definitive diagnosis may have to await histologic study. Immunoperoxidase staining for S-100 protein may provide a clue to the diagnosis.[9]

TUMORS OF THE SYMPATHETIC NERVOUS SYSTEM

Ganglioneuroma, Neuroblastoma and Ganglioneuroblastoma

These tumors usually arise from the ganglia of the sympathetic nervous system. Tumors composed of mature neural elements are referred to as ganglioneuromas, whereas those composed of primitive neuroblasts are called neuroblastomas. A ganglioneuroblastoma contains mature and immature neural elements. Relatively few neuroblastomas arise in the head and neck; most such tumors occur in the adrenal glands.[71] Tumors of the head and neck most commonly arise from the sympathetic chain[72] or the ganglion nodosum of the vagus nerve[73] and are manifested as neck masses. The urine of patients may contain elevated levels of catecholamine metabolites.

HISTOLOGIC FEATURES. Ganglioneuromas usually occur in young adults and are rarely encountered before two years of age. On gross inspection, such tumors are

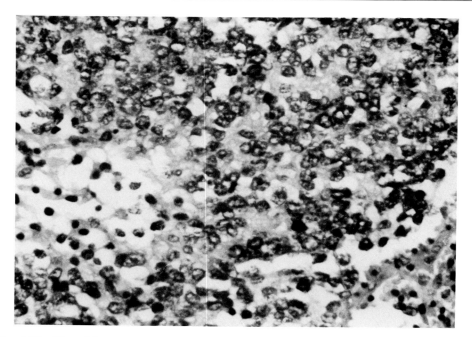

Fig. 4.33. Neuroblastoma. The tumor is composed of small, round cells and areas of necrosis. Hematoxylin and eosin preparation. ×390. (Courtesy of Dr G.K.Nguyen.)

firm and gray to yellow. Histologic study shows that they consist of ganglion cells, nerve fibers and connective tissue elements. Neuroblastomas, on the other hand, often occur in the first few years of life and are rarely encountered in late childhood or adult life. On gross inspection, such tumors are soft and gray and have areas of necrosis and hemorrhage. Microscopy demonstrates that they are composed of small, round cells that have scanty cytoplasm. Rosettes are seen in approximately one-third of cases (Fig. 4.33). Delicate neurofibers fill the centers of the rosettes. Histologic study shows that ganglioneuroblastomas contain small, round, primitive neuroblasts and large ganglion cells. Such tumors commonly occur in older children and adolescents.

CYTOLOGIC FEATURES. The aspirates from all three types of lesions contain an abundance of cellular material. The smears from neuroblastomas contain small, round cells that are slightly larger then lymphocytes (Fig. 4.34). The cytoplasm is scanty and fragile. In well-differentiated tumors, one observes rosettes with peripherally located nuclei and a central syncytium of cytoplasm that has a fine fibrillar appearance[15] (Fig. 4.35). The nuclei are round or oval and contain finely granular chromatin. Minute nucleoli are seen in some cells. In poorly differentiated tumors, rosettes may not be identifiable. The cells of such tumors have more irregularity of nuclear size and shape. Nuclear molding is observed. The tumor cell nuclei contain coarsely granular chromatin and one or more nucleoli. Mitoses are seen and binucleated cells are occasionally encountered. The aspirates from ganglioneuromas consist of clusters of oval or spindle-shaped cells and a few large ganglion cells that

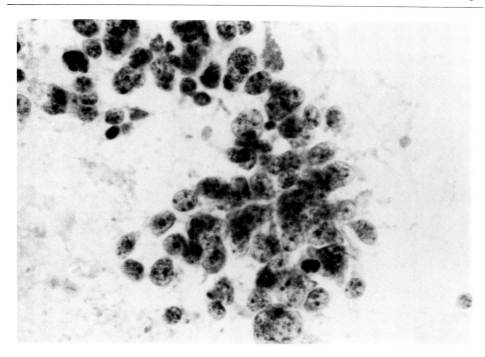

Fig. 4.34. Aspirate from a neuroblastoma composed of small, round cells that have scanty cytoplasm. Papanicolaou preparation. ×625. (Courtesy of Dr G.K.Nguyen.)

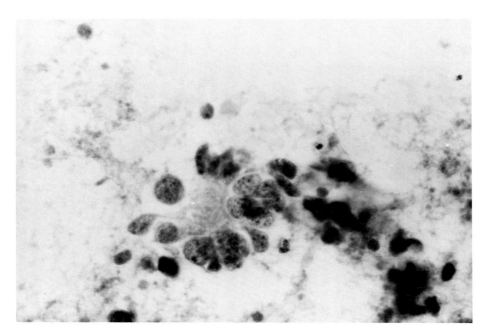

Fig. 4.35. Rosette-like arrangement of small, round tumor cells. Papanicolaou preparation. ×625. (Courtesy of Dr G.K.Nguyen.)

have abundant cytoplasm, round or oval, eccentrically located nuclei and prominent nucleoli. In the absence of ganglion cells, a definitive diagnosis cannot be made. In ganglioneuroblastoma, the aspirate contains small, round cells admixed with large ganglion cells. If this biphasic pattern is not observed, a diagnosis of ganglioneuroblastoma cannot be made. Amorphous, fibrillar material is encountered in the aspirates from neuroblastomas, ganglioneuromas and ganglioneuroblastomas. With the Bodian method, delicate, silver-positive fibers are identified within this amorphous material.[15]

DIFFERENTIAL DIAGNOSIS. A number of small-cell mesenchymal and epithelial tumors must be considered in the differential diagnosis of neuroblastoma. The differential diagnosis of such tumors is summarized in Table 3.13. Electron microscopy may provide a clue to the diagnosis in difficult cases. Enzyme histochemistry may also be helpful in the differentiation of neuroblastomas from other tumors. In a recent report, Miller and colleagues[15] using material obtained by needle aspiration biopsy and embedded in plastic demonstrated a reaction to acid phosphatase in cells of neuroblastomas but not in cells from childhood leukemias and lymphomas. Moreover, no reaction was seen in two cases of embryonal rhabdomyosarcoma.

Olfactory Neuroblastoma

This tumor arises from the olfactory epithelium and occurs in all age groups. Such tumors involve the superior turbinate of the nasal fossa and may extend into the sinuses. Olfactory neuroblastomas are soft and polypoid and usually cause nasal obstruction, epistaxis and pain. Histologic and cytologic studies demonstrate that such tumors are composed of cells that are small but larger than lymphocytes and have scanty cytoplasm. The appearance of the cells is similar to that of the cells of neuroblastomas that arise elsewhere. The cytologic appearance of olfactory neuroblastoma diagnosed by needle aspiration biopsy has recently been reported.[74]

TUMORS OF BLOOD AND LYMPHATIC VESSELS

Lymphangioma

Lymphangioma may be capillary, cavernous or cystic. Cystic hygromas are usually multicystic and contain clear or straw-colored fluid. Most such lesions are diagnosed at birth or within the first two years of life.[75] The most common site of involvement is the neck[76] (Fig. 4.36). The typical presentation is a mass. Lyphangiomas also involve the skin, oral cavity and salivary glands.

HISTOLOGIC FEATURES. Histologic examination shows that such tumors are composed of small or large, irregular spaces lined by flattened endothelial cells (Fig. 4.37). The lumina usually contain pink, proteinaceous material and few lymphocytes. Red blood cells are also seen.

CYTOLOGIC FEATURES. Needle aspiration biopsy can be used to confirm the cystic nature of such lesions. The aspirated fluid is usually clear. Lymphocytes and a few histiocytes may coexist with erythrocytes (Fig. 4.37). Few endothelial lining cells are observed.

Hemangioma

Hemangioma is a not uncommon tumor of the skin of the face, head or neck, oral cavity, nasal or paranasal sinuses or soft tissues of the neck. Such tumors are common in infants and children and also occur in adults.

HISTOLOGIC FEATURES. Histologic study demonstrates capillary and cavernous patterns, with cuboidal or flattened endothelial cells lining small or large vascular spaces (Fig. 4.38). Needle aspiration biopsy usually yields one or more milliliters of blood admixed with a variable number of endothelial cells.

CYTOLOGIC FEATURES. In the capillary type, branching tufts of small capillaries appear as cohesive clusters of spindle-shaped cells that have indistinct cell borders and nuclei.[32] The chromatin is fine and nucleoli are usually not visible. In the cavernous type, the smears contain a few endothelial cells in small sheets or groupings[32] (Fig. 4.39). The cells have delicate cytoplasm and oval or spindle-shaped, uniform nuclei.

Hemangiopericytoma

Approximately 15 percent of hemangiopericytomas occur in the head or neck.[77] The most common sites of involvement are the nose, followed by the orbits, parotid glands and neck. Hemangiopericytomas may be benign or malignant, depending on the size of the lesion, its cellularity, the mitotic count and the degree of necrosis or hemorrhage. Tumors that have four or more mitoses per 10 high-power fields are regarded as malignant.[77] Local recurrence of tumors of the head or neck is common and metastases develop occasionally.

HISTOLOGIC FEATURES. Histologic study demonstrates that hemangiopericytomas are composed of small, round or oval, uniform cells surrounding small vascular spaces (Fig. 4.40). The stroma is sparse. Reticulin staining demonstrates tumor cells outside the vessel wall, with reticular fibers surrounding individual tumor cells.

CYTOLOGIC FEATURES. Nguyen and Neifer[78] have described the cytologic features of three cases of benign or malignant hemangiopericytoma. The tumor cells had round, oval or spindle-shaped nuclei and finely granular cytoplasm. The nucleoli were not prominent. Solitary tumor cells and groupings of such cells were observed (Figs. 4.41 and 4.42). Distinction between benign and malignant lesions was difficult, as was differentiation of hemangiopericytoma from other spindle cell mesenchymal tumors.

Nickels and Koivuniemi[18] have also described the cytologic features of five cases of malignant hemangiopericytoma.

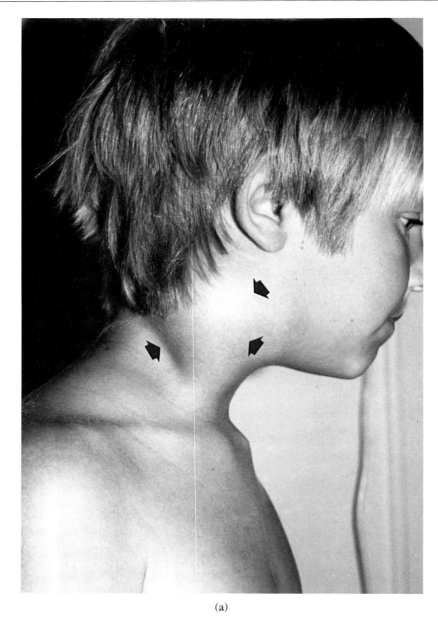

(a)

Fig. 4.36. (a) and (b) Large lymphangioma (cystic hygroma) in a young boy.

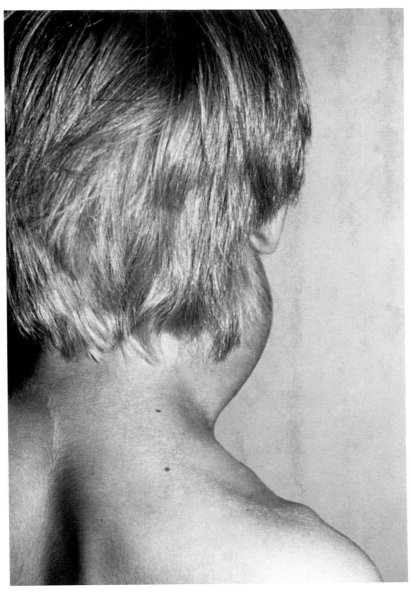

(b)

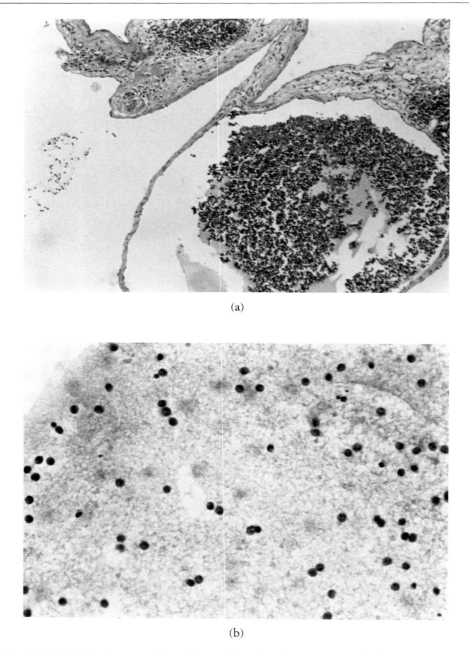

(a)

(b)

Fig. 4.37. (a) Histology specimen from a lymphangioma composed of numerous cystic spaces that contain proteinaceous material and lymphocytes. (b) Aspirate from a lymphangioma composed of lymphoid cells and amorphous, granular material in the background. Papanicolaou preparation. ×625.

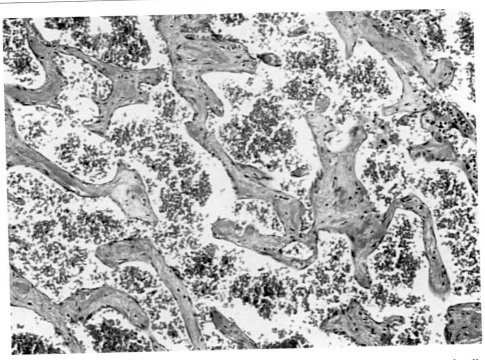

Fig. 4.38. Cavernous hemangioma. Note the large vascular spaces lined by flattened cells. Hematoxylin and eosin preparation. ×150.

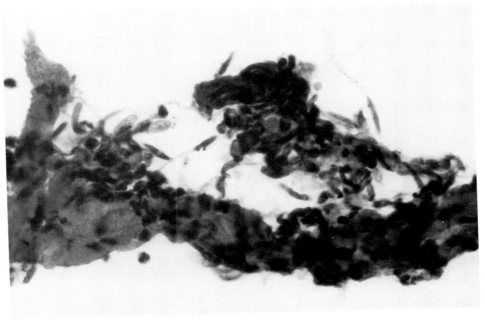

Fig. 4.39. Aspirate from the lesion shown in Figure 4.38. A few elongated endothelial cells in cohesive clusters. Papanicolaou preparation. ×625.

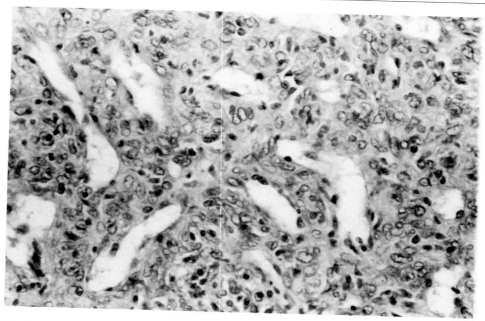

Fig. 4.40. Hemangiopericytoma. Note the uniform-appearing, round or oval cells surrounding small vascular spaces. Hematoxylin and eosin preparation. ×390. (Courtesy of Dr G.K.Nguyen.)

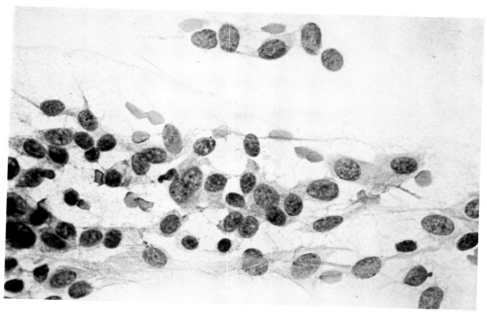

Fig. 4.41. Aspirate from the lesion shown in Figure 4.40. Note the solitary tumor cells that have round or oval nuclei. Papanicolaou preparation. ×625. (From Nguyen GK, Neifer R: *Diagn Cytopathol* 1:327–331, 1985, with permission.)

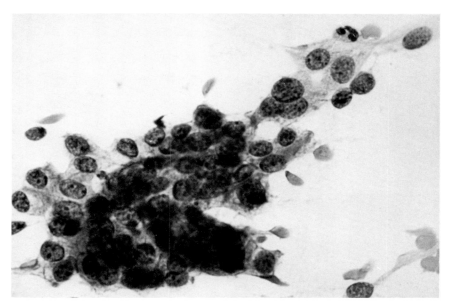

Fig. 4.42. Aspirate from the lesion shown in Figure 4.40. A cohesive cluster of tumor cells that have nuclear features similar to those seen in Figure 4.41. Papanicolaou preparation. ×625. (From Nguyen GK, Neifer R: *Diagn Cytopathol* 1:327–331, 1985, with permission.)

Angiosarcoma

Angiosarcoma is a rare malignant tumor of vascular origin. Tumors that arise from the endothelium of the lymphatic system are referred to as lymphangiosarcomas and those of blood vessel origin are called hemangiosarcomas. Angiosarcomas have been reported in a variety of sites. Lymphangiosarcomas usually occur in association with chronic lymphedema, the classical example being postmastectomy lymphangiosarcoma. Rare cases of lymphangiosarcoma have been reported in the scalp.[79] In this setting, such tumors are not usually associated with lymphedema. Hemangiosarcoma commonly occurs in the skin, liver or breasts. In cases of head or neck involvement, the tumor is usually found in the skin of the scalp or face or in the soft tissues of the neck.[80] Hemangiosarcomas are solitary or multifocal and may spread superficially or be nodular or ulcerative (Fig. 4.43). Hemangiosarcomas of the skin are blue and round or oval and have indistinct cell margins. They have also been reported in the nasal cavities and paranasal sinuses, where they are associated with pain, bleeding and obstructive symptoms.

HISTOLOGIC FEATURES. Microscopy shows that angiosarcomas are composed of small, proliferating vascular channels lined by large, abnormal endothelial cells (Fig. 4.44). Spindle-shaped and polygonal cells may also be observed. Differentiation of lymphangiosarcoma from hemangiosarcoma may be difficult on the basis of examination by light microscopy alone.

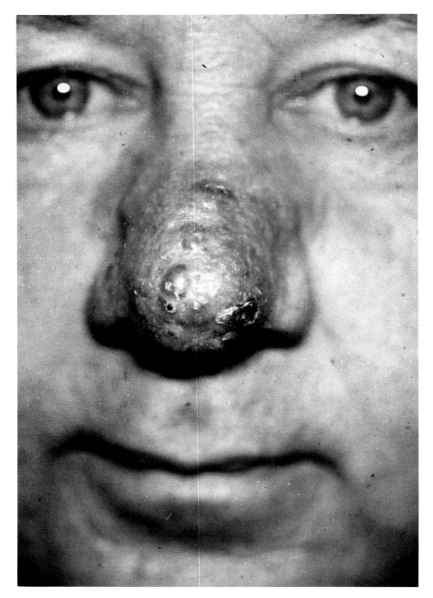

Fig. 4.43. Hemangiosarcoma of the nose before radiotherapy. Metastases subsequently developed in the upper part of the right side of the neck, as confirmed by needle aspiration biopsy. Shown in Figure 4.45.

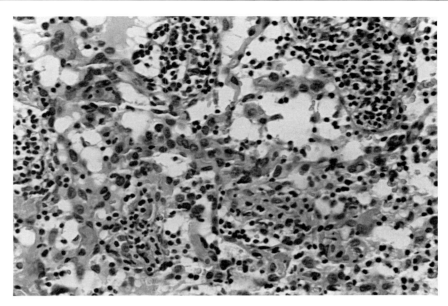

Fig. 4.44. Angiosarcoma. Note the small, proliferating vascular spaces lined by abnormal endothelial cells. Hematoxylin and eosin preparation. × 390.

CYTOLOGIC FEATURES. There have been few reports of the cytologic features of angiosarcoma.[2,32] The aspirates consist mostly of blood and a few cells in cohesive clusters. The tumor cell nuclei are round or oval and hyperchromatic and have longitudinal indentations.[2] Erythrophagocytosis may also be noted. The cytologic diagnosis is difficult, especially in cases of poorly differentiated angiosarcoma, in which the malignant nature of the lesion is evidenced by the cellular pleomorphism but the vascular nature may not be apparent. A diagnosis of small-cell sarcoma is justified in such cases. Figure 4.45 is from a case of hemangiosarcoma of the nose metastatic to the lymph nodes of the neck.

Jayaram[10] recently described the cytologic appearance of bilateral recurrent malignant hemangioendothelioma of the parotid region. The smears consisted of small, round cells in cohesive clusters and rosette-like or pseudoacinar structures. Solitary cells were also observed. The cytoplasm was scanty and the round or oval nuclei were only slightly pleomorphic. Small nucleoli were observed, as were mitoses.

DIFFERENTIAL DIAGNOSIS. The aspirates from vascular tumors are usually bloody and their cellularity·varies. Differentiation from other small-cell mesenchymal tumors may be difficult. The aspirates from carotid body tumors also may be bloody and contain few cells. However, the cells in such aspirates are larger and have more cytoplasm. The cytologic features of carotid body tumors are discussed in Chapter 6. Pseudoacinar or rosette-like structures may be seen in vascular tumors and differentiation from adenocarcinoma and neuroblastoma may be difficult. However, the nuclear abnormalities seen in angiosarcoma are not as severe as those encountered in epithelial cells. Moreover, the cytoplasm is more abundant in adenocarcinomas.

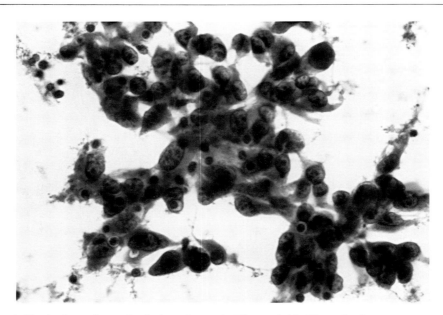

Fig. 4.45. Aspirate from the lesion shown in Figure 4.44. Note the loose groupings of malignant tumor cells surrounding small, irregular spaces. Papanicolaou preparation. ×625.

Rosette or pseudorosette-like structures are seen in neuroblastoma and, occasionally, in Ewing's sarcoma. However, the amorphous, fine, fibrillar material seen in smears from neuroblastomas is not observed in vascular lesions. Ewing's sarcoma is discussed on pages 254 and 255. A knowledge of the clinical history and appearance of the tumor, especially those of the skin and superficial tissues, are of considerable help in making the diagnosis.

TUMORS OF SYNOVIUM

Synovial Sarcoma

This uncommon tumor arises from the pluripotential mesenchyme and is capable of snyovial differentiation. Less than 50 percent of such tumors occur in the head or neck.[82,83] Common sites are the neck and hypopharynx. Most patients present with a painful mass; other signs and symptoms depend on the site of involvement and include dysphagia, hoarseness, dyspnea, hemorrhage and weight loss. Recurrence is a common feature of such tumors and less than 50 percent of patients survive more than five years from the time of diagnosis.[83] On gross inspection, such tumors usually are circumscribed, pink to gray masses.

HISTOLOGIC FEATURES. Histologic examination shows a biphasic pattern, consisting of spindle cells and epithelioid cells that form glandular structures. The relative proportions of the two components vary markedly and monomorphic forms that consist only of spindle cells have been described.

CYTOLOGIC FEATURES. The aspirates are usually appreciably cellular. There typically are groupings of small, oval or spindle-shaped cells coexisting with cuboidal or polygonal epithelioid cells.[31,32] The cells have scanty cytoplasm. The spindle cell nuclei are round or ovoid and uniform. The chromatin if finely granular and small nucleoli are observed. Some smears may consist only of spindle cells. In such cases, a definitive diagnosis of synovial sarcoma cannot be made.

DIFFERENTIAL DIAGNOSIS. If a biphasic pattern is observed in the needle aspirates, a definite diagnosis can be made. However, when only spindle cells are seen, differentiation from other spindle cell tumors is difficult.

MISCELLANEOUS TUMORS

Granular Cell Tumor

This uncommon tumor usually involves the striated muscle, skin or subcutaneous tissue, mucous membranes or underlying tissues of various organs, including the tongue, larynx, esophagus, gastrointestinal tract, bladder and breasts. Multiple tumors are not uncommon and malignant examples have been reported.[8,84,85] The histogenesis of this tumor remains unknown, although evidence points to a Schwann cell origin.[86] Patients are young or middle-aged and usually present with small, asymptomatic masses. On gross inspection, such tumors are firm and gray to white. They are not encapsulated.

HISTOLOGIC FEATURES. Histologic study shows large, polygonal cells that have an abundance of granular, eosinophilic cytoplasm and round or oval nuclei. The granules stain with periodic acid-Schiff and are resistant to the action of diastase.

CYTOLOGIC FEATURES. The smears consist of large, polygonal cells that have an abundance of granular cytoplasm. The nuclei are round or oval and uniform. The cytoplasm is eosinophilic with hematoxylin and eosin and cyanophilic with Papanicolaou stain. The chromatin is finely granular and a small nucleolus is usually visible. Bare nuclei may be seen in the background. Malignant tumors have been described by Betsill[85] and Geisinger and coworkers.[8] Nuclear atypia may be seen in malignant variants, but differentiation of benign from malignant tumors by aspiration biopsy cytology is exceedingly difficult. Strobel and associates[23] recently reported two cases of granular cell tumor studied by touch preparations. The granules in the tumor cell cytoplasm stained with periodic acid-Schiff and were resistant to the action of diastase; with the immunoperoxidase method, the granules were found to contain S-100 protein but not myoglobin.

Myxoma

This tumor occurs in all soft tissues but is most common in skeletal muscles of the limbs and shoulders. Lattes reviewed 205 cases of myxoma and was unable to document a single instance of metastasis; he thus believes that all myxomas are benign.[87] Malignant variants, however, have been reported by other investigators.[88] On gross inspection, such tumors are soft, circumscribed and gelatinous.

HISTOLOGIC FEATURES. Histologic study shows small, round or stellate cells in a matrix rich in acid mucopolysaccharides. Reticular fibers are observed, but the vascularity commonly seen in myxoid liposarcoma is lacking.

CYTOLOGIC FEATURES. The aspirates consist of a mucoid material that contains few cells.[32] The stellate and spindle-shaped cells have slender, bipolar processes. The tumor cell nuclei are oval and contain finely granular chromatin. The nucleoli are usually small or inconspicuous. The abundant mucoid substance in the background is best visualized with May-Grünwald-Giemsa stain.[32]

DIFFERENTIAL DIAGNOSIS. The differential diagnosis includes other spindle cell mesenchymal tumors and, in particular, myxoid variants of liposarcoma and malignant fibrous histiocytoma. Other myxoid tumors that may cause diagnostic difficulty are myxoid chondrosarcoma and chordoma.

Alveolar Soft-Part Sarcoma

This rare soft-tissue tumor commonly occurs in the limbs of young adults; such tumors occasionally develop in the head or neck. Women are more frequently affected than are men. The histogenesis of this tumor remains a subject of speculation, although its similarities to paraganglioma, granular cell myoblastoma and rhabdomyosarcoma have been pointed out. Recent evidence suggests a Schwann cell origin.[88] On gross inspection, such tumors are firm, circumscribed, gray to yellow masses that have areas of necrosis and hemorrhage.

HISTOLOGIC FEATURES. Histologic examination demonstrates a distinctive alveolar or organoid pattern in which large, polygonal tumor cells are separated by thin septa of connective tissue. The cytoplasm is finely granular, stains with periodic acid-Schiff and is resistant to diastase. Rhomboid, crystalline material that stains with periodic acid-Schiff can be demonstrated in the cytoplasm of the tumor cells.

CYTOLOGIC FEATURES. The aspirates usually consist of solitary tumor cells and small aggregates of such cells.[11,19] The tumor cells are large and polygonal or oval. The cytoplasm is granular and fragile, being easily fragmented. In well-preserved cells, it appears granular and is eosinophilic with hematoxylin and eosin and cyanophilic with Papanicolaou stain. A similar granular to flocculant material is seen outside the cells.[19] The tumor cell nuclei are round or oval and contain finely granular chromatin and prominent nucleoli. Mild variation in nuclear size is evident. Touch smears of alveolar soft-part sarcoma have shown that the granules within the cytoplasm stain with periodic acid-Schiff and are resistant to diastase.[89] Crystalloids may be seen in touch preparations but are difficult to demonstrate in needle aspirates.

DIFFERENTIAL DIAGNOSIS. Alveolar soft-part sarcoma may be difficult to differentiate from paraganglioma, metastatic follicular carcinoma of the thyroid, metastatic bronchoalveolar carcinoma, metastatic renal cell carcinoma or occasionally, malignant melanoma. The observation of an alveolar pattern of cells that have finely granular, periodic acid-Schiff-positive, diastase-resistant cytoplasmic granules suggests a diagnosis of alveolar soft-part sarcoma. Granular cell tumors have also similar periodic acid-Schiff-positive granules in the tumor cell cytoplasm. However, the cells in the latter tumor are solitary or in loose groupings and lack the alveolar arrangement seen in alveolar soft-part sarcoma. The history may be helpful in making the diagnosis, but histologic study of the excised tumor may be required for a definitive diagnosis.

Epithelioid Sarcoma

This uncommon tumor of obscure histogenesis characteristically occurs in young adults, more often in men than in women. Most such tumors involve the soft tissues of the hands, forearms or anterior tibial region.[90,91] Rare cases have been reported in the head or neck.[90,91] On gross inspection, such tumors are firm and grayish white and may have areas of necrosis.

HISTOLOGIC FEATURES. Histologic study shows that the tumor cells have a polygonal, epithelioid appearance with an abundance of eosinophilic cytoplasm and round or oval nuclei. Binucleated and spindle cell areas are also seen. Areas of central necrosis along with large, epithelioid cells at the periphery may suggest a granulomatous condition.

CYTOLOGIC FEATURES. The aspirates usually consist of solitary tumor cells and small loose groupings of such cells. The tumor cells are round to polygonal.[3] A few spindle cells may also be observed. The cytoplasm is abundant and homogeneous and the round or oval, hyperchromatic nuclei are located eccentrically. Nuclear pleomorphism is encountered. Most tumor cell nuclei contain a single large nucleolus. Binucleated and, occasionally, multinucleated cells are also seen. The differential diagnosis includes epithelioid tumors and, in particular, squamous cell carcinoma and malignant melanoma.

Extraskeletal Chondrosarcoma

This rare malignant cartilaginous tumor occurs in extraskeletal sites. Such tumors have been reported in deep and superficial soft tissues of adults and children. Two types have been described, myxoid chondrosarcoma and mesenchymal chondrosarcoma.[92] Although such tumors are most common in the limbs, they have also been reported in the head and neck.[93,94] The clinical findings depend on the site of involvement. Tumors of the orbits or craniospinal meninges are associated with headaches, visual disturbances and pressure symptoms. On gross inspection, such tumors are lobulated, soft and gray to yellow and have areas of necrosis and hemorrhage.

HISTOLOGIC FEATURES. Histologic examination shows that the myxoid variant is composed of small or elongated cells in nests or ribbons (Figs. 4.46 and 4.47). Areas of myxoid change are common and differentiation to cartilaginous tissue is noted. In

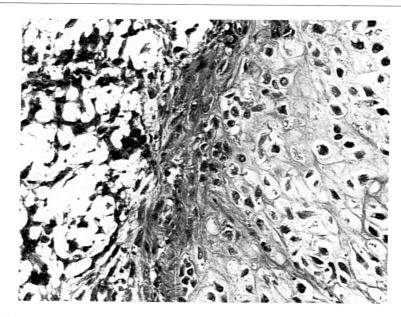

Fig. 4.46. Extraskeletal chondrosarcoma. Histology specimen contains myxoid and cartilaginous areas. Hematoxylin and eosin preparation. ×150. (From Tsang S, Nguyen GK: *Acta Cytol* 29:566–569, 1985, with permission.)

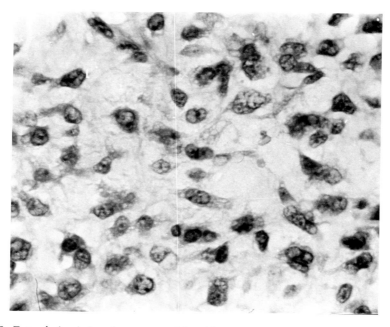

Fig. 4.47. Extraskeletal chondrosarcoma. Myxoid area. Hematoxylin and eosin preparation. ×390. (From Tsang S, Nguyen GK: *Acta Cytol* 29:566–569, 1985, with permission.)

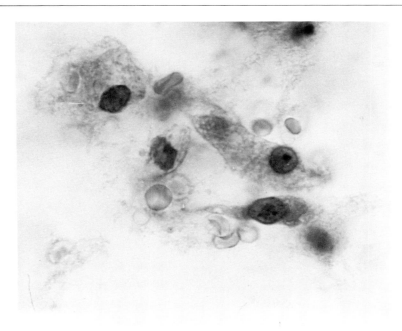

Fig. 4.48. Round to elongated mesenchymal cells with vacuolated, fibrillar cytoplasm. Papanicolaou preparation. ×400. (From Tsang S, Nguyen GK: *Acta Cytol* 29:566–569, 1985, with permission.)

mesenchymal chondrosarcoma, a primitive mesenchymal component that resembles hemangiopericytoma coexists with islands of cartilage.

CYTOLOGIC FEATURES. In the myxoid variant, needle aspirates usually consist of a drop of mucoid material that is composed of mesenchymal cells admixed with cartilaginous cells.[24,95] The mesenchymal cells are round, polygonal or spindle shaped and have vacuolated or fibrillar cytoplasm (Fig. 4.48). The nuclei are round or oval and contain prominent nucleoli. The cartilaginous cells have a small amount of vacuolated or homogeneous cytoplasm and round, hyperchromatic nuclei that contain prominent nucleoli. Small clusters of chrondroblasts that have a narrow rim of eosinophilic cytoplasm and pleomorphic nuclei are also seen (Fig. 4.49). The background material is amophous and mucoid. The aspirates from mesenchymal chondrosarcomas consist of small, round or oval, primitive mesenchymal cells. Cartilaginous cells may be encountered.

DIFFERENTIAL DIAGNOSIS. The differential diagnosis of myxoid chondrosarcoma includes myxoma, myxoid liposarcoma, the myoid variant of malignant fibrous histiocytoma and chordoma. This subject was discussed on page 223. When small, primitive mesenchymal cells as well as cartilaginous cells are found, mesenchymal chondrosarcoma can be diagnosed with certainty. If the two cell types are not observed, differentiation from other small-cell tumors is not possible.

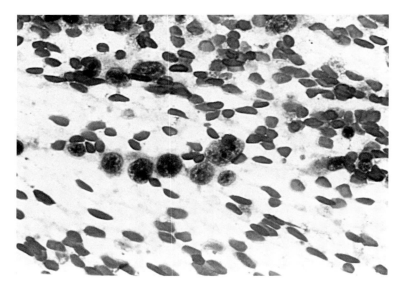

Fig. 4.49. A row of chondroblasts that have round nuclei and a scanty amount of eosinophilic cytoplasm. Papanicolaou preparation. × 400. (Courtesy Dr G.K.Nguyen.)

Extraskeletal Ewing's Sarcoma

Ewing's sarcoma is an undifferentiated neoplasm of mesenchymal origin that is composed of small, round cells and arises primarily in bone.[96] An extraskeletal variant also occurs.[97] Such tumors commonly involve the paravertebral tissues and legs, although occasional cases have been reported in the soft tissues of the cervical spine[97] and nasal fossa.[98] Most patients present with painful masses and symptoms of cord compression. On gross inspection, such tumors are soft and gray and have areas of necrosis and hemorrhage.

HISTOLOGIC FEATURES. Histologic examination shows that such tumors consist of small, round, uniform cells in compact masses or sheets (Fig. 4.50). The cytoplasm is scanty, poorly defined and vacuolated. Glycogen can be demonstrated in the cytoplasm of the tumor cells by use of periodic acid-Schiff reagent. The nuclei are round and larger than nuclei of lymphocytes. Perivascular palisading and neuroblastoma-like pseudorosettes are occasionally observed.

CYTOLOGIC FEATURES. The aspirates usually consist of numerous solitary tumor cells (Fig. 4.51) and small and large tissue fragments.[13] Cells arranged around elongated, stringlike capillaries, the so-called perivascular palisades, may also be seen.[13] Small groupings of cells arranged around a space that contains amorphous to fibrillar material, reminiscent of neuroblastoma, may also be observed (Fig. 4.52). The cells have a scant amount of ill-defined cytoplasm. Fine, reticular cytoplasmic wisps connecting the cells in thin monolayers may also be evident. The tumor cell nuclei are round or oval and about one and one-half to two times the size of a lymphocyte. The chromatin is finely granular and small nucleoli are visible. Pink, periodic acid-Schiff-

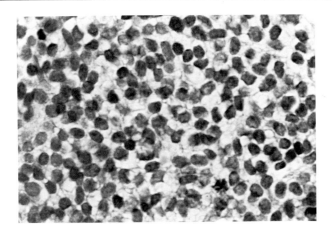

Fig. 4.50. Ewing's sarcoma. Note the small, round, uniform tumor cells. Hematoxylin and eosin preparation. ×625. (From Kontozoglou T, et al: *Acta Cytol* 30:513–518, 1986, with permission.)

positive granules that are digestible with diastase are seen in the cytoplasm of the tumor cells. The background is hemorrhagic and consists of granular, proteinaceous debris.

DIFFERENTIAL DIAGNOSIS. Other small-cell tumors that must be considered in the differential diagnosis include small-cell non-Hodgkin's lymphoma, embryonal rhab-domyosarcoma, neuroblastoma, oat cell carcinoma, carcinoid tumors and other apudomas, including Merkel cell carcinoma of the skin. Differentiation among these entities may be difficult. The history, age of the patient and site of the tumor should always be taken into account in making the diagnosis. A definitive diagnosis some-

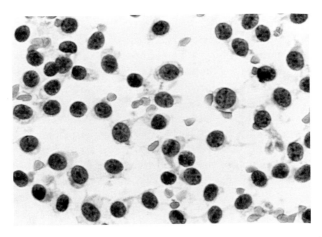

Fig. 4.51. Aspirate composed of solitary tumor cells that have scanty cytoplasm and round nuclei. Papanicolaou preparation. ×625. (From Kontozoglou T, et al: *Acta Cytol* 30:513–518, 1986, with permission.)

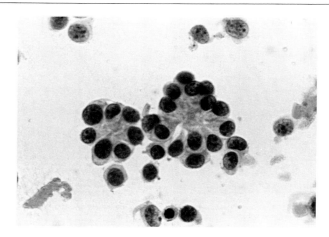

Fig. 4.52. Pseudorosette-like arrangement. Papanicolaou preparation. ×625.

times must await immunocytochemical study and examination by electron microscopy. The differential diagnosis of small-cell tumors is discussed in Chapter 3.

Chordoma

Chordoma is a rare neoplasm that is usually classified as a bone tumor. Such tumors occasionally arise in the head or neck.[1,2] The differential diagnosis of chordoma of the neck includes salivary gland neoplasms, lymphoma and metastatic carcinoma. Figure 4.53 shows a computed axial tomogram of a chordoma that presented as a mass in the suprasternal notch. Needle aspiration biopsy suggested the diagnosis. Most such tumors, however, are located in the sacrococcygeal or spheno-occipital region. They have an indolent biologic behavior, with a low potential for metastasis and a high incidence of local recurrence. On gross inspection, such tumors are soft, gray and lobulated and have a mucinous consistency.

HISTOLOGIC FEATURES. Histologic examination shows preservation of their lobulated nature. A variety of histologic patterns have been reported, but the typical appearance is that of a tumor composed of physaliphorous cells (Fig. 4.54). Small, epithelioid or spindle-shaped cells may also be encountered.

CYTOLOGIC FEATURES. The smears are usually hypercellular, consisting of sheets and clusters of large, vacuolated cells (Fig. 4.55) similar to the physaliphorous cells seen in histologic sections. Trabecular and cordlike arrangements may also be observed and signet-ring cells forming pearl-like clusters may be noted[99] (Fig 4.56). Small, nonvacuolated cells may also be encountered. The tumor cell nuclei are round or oval and are located centrally or eccentrically. A few elongated or spindle-shaped nuclei may also be seen in the smears. Multinucleation is occasionally noted. The chromatin is fine and the nucleoli are small. Mitoses are infrequently observed. The smears contain an abundance of extracellular material that stains bluish pink with the Papanicolaou method. The material has a fibrillar or myxoid appearance and stellate cells are embedded within it (Fig. 4.57).

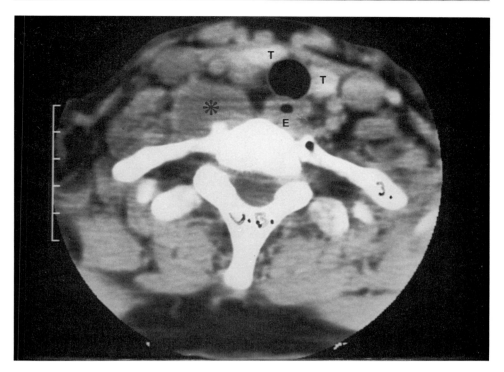

Fig. 4.53. Computed axial tomogram of a chordoma of the anterior aspect of T1, presenting as a mass in the suprasternal notch in a 48-year-old woman. *, Tumor mass; E, Esophagus; T, thyroid.

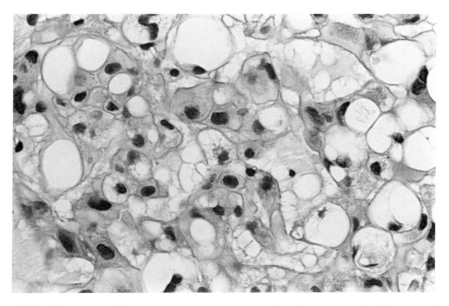

Fig. 4.54. Chordoma. Histology specimen contains physaliphorous cells. Hematoxylin and eosin preparation. ×390.

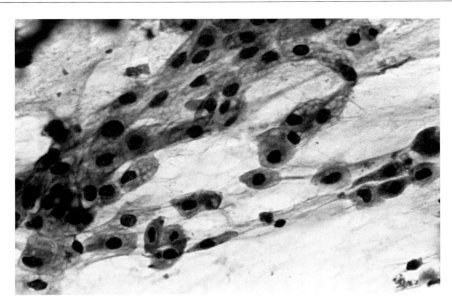

Fig. 4.55. Cytology specimen contains physaliphorous cells. Papanicolaou preparation. ×625.

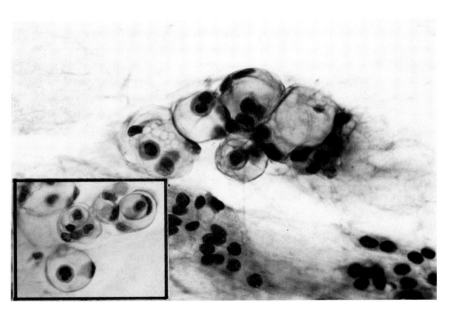

Fig. 4.56. Cytology specimen contains signet-ring-like cells. Papanicolaou preparation. ×625. (*Inset,* ×390.)

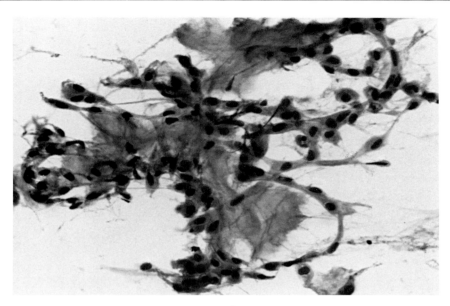

Fig. 4.57. Cytology specimen contains myxoid extracellular material and elongated or stellate cells. Papanicolaou preparation. × 390.

The differential diagnosis of chordoma includes metastatic adenocarcinoma (especially the clear-cell variants), chondrosarcoma, liposarcoma and myxopapillary ependymoma.

The abundant extracellular component occasionally causes diagnostic confusion with pleomorphic adenoma. Recent reports have suggested that the clinical radiologic, cytomorphologic, electron microscopic and cytochemical features should be taken into account before a diagnosis on needle aspirates is attempted.[99,100] Immunoperoxidase studies have shown that the tumor cells stain for neuron-specific enolase, S-100 protein, epithelial membrane antigen, keratin and vimentin.[99,100] These techniques are discussed and illustrated in Chapter 8.

REFERENCES

1. Rosenberg SA, Suite HD, Baker LH, et al: Sarcomas of the soft tissue and bone, in DeVita VT Jr, Hellman S, Rosenberg SA (eds): *Cancer. Principles and Practice of Oncology.* Philadelphia, Lippincott, 1982, pp 1036–1093.

2. Abele JS, Miller T: Cytology of well-differentiated hemangiosarcoma in fine needle aspirates. *Acta Cytol* 26:341–348, 1982.

3. Ahmed MN, Feldman M, Seemeyer TA: Cytology of epithelioid sarcoma. *Acta Cytol* 18:459–461, 1974.

4. Angervall L, Hagmer P, Kindblum LG, et al: Malignant giant cell tumor of soft tissues. A clinico-pathologic, cytologic, ultrastructural, angiographic and microangiographic study. *Cancer (Philadelphia)* 47:736–747, 1981.

5. Azua J, Arraiza A, Delgardo B, et al: Nodular fasciitis initially diagnosed by aspiration biopsy. *Acta Cytol* 29:562–565, 1985.

6. Franzen S, Stenkvist B: Diagnosis of granular cell myoblastoma by fine needle aspiration biopsy. *Acta Pathol Microbiol Scand* 72:391–395, 1968.

7. Fritsches HG, Miller EA: Pseudosarcomatous fasciitis of the breast. Cytologic and histologic features. *Acta Cytol* 27:73–75, 1983.

8. Geisinger KR, Kawamoto EH, Marshall RB, et al: Aspiration and exfoliative cytology including ultrastructure of a malignant granular-cell tumour. *Acta Cytol* 29:593–597, 1985.

9. Hood IC, Qizilbash AH, Young JEM, et al: Needle aspiration cytology of a benign and a malignant schwannoma. *Acta Cytol* 28:157–164, 1984.

10. Jayaram G: Cytology of hemangioendothelioma. *Acta Cytol* 28:153–156, 1984.

11. Kapila K, Chopra P, Verma K: Fine needle aspiration cytology of alveolar soft-part sarcoma. A case report. *Acta Cytol* 29:559–561, 1985.

12. Kim K, Goldblatt PJ: Malignant fibrous histiocytoma. Cytologic, light microscopic and ultrastructural studies. *Acta Cytol* 26:507–513, 1982.

13. Kontozoglou T, Krakauer K, Qizilbash A: Ewing's sarcoma, cytologic features in fine needle aspirates in two cases. *Acta Cytol* 30:513–518, 1986.

14. Kontozoglou T, Qizilbash A, Sianos J, et al: Chordoma: cytologic and immunocytochemical study of four cases. *Diagn Cytopathol* 2:55–61, 1986.

15. Miller TR, Bottles K, Abele JS, et al: Neuroblastoma diagnosed by fine needle aspiration biopsy. *Acta Cytol* 29:461–468, 1985.

16. Neifer R, Nguyen GK: Aspiration cytology of solitary schwannoma. *Acta Cytol* 29:12–14, 1985.

17. Nguyen GK, Jeannot A: Cytopathologic aspects of pulmonary metastasis of malignant fibrous histiocytoma, mixed variant. Fine needle aspiration biopsy of a case. *Acta Cytol* 26:349–353, 1982.

18. Nickels J, Koivuniemi A: Cytology of malignant hemangiopericytoma. *Acta Cytol* 23:119–125, 1979.

19. Nieberg RK: Fine needle aspiration cytology of alveolar soft-part sarcoma. *Acta Cytol* 28:198–202, 1984.

20. Popok SM, Zaib ZM: Fine needle aspiration biopsy of myositis ossificans. *Diagn Cytopathol* 1:236–240, 1985.

21. Ramsay I: Benign schwannoma. Demonstration of Verocay bodies using fine needle aspiration. *Acta Cytol* 21:316–319, 1977.

22. Silverman JF, Visa MD, Gardner N, et al: Aspiration biopsy cytology of malignant schwannoma metastatic to lung. *Acta Cytol* 29:15–18, 1985.

23. Strobel SL, Shah NT, Lucas JG, et al: Granular-cell tumor of the breast. A cytologic, immunohistochemical and ultrastructural study of two cases. *Acta Cytol* 59:598–601, 1985.

24. Tsang S, Nguyen GK: Aspiration biopsy cytology of metastatic extraskeletal myxoid chondrosarcoma and its cytologic differential diagnosis. *Acta Cytol* 29:566–569, 1985.

25. Layfield LJ, Anders KH, Glasgow BJ, et al: Fine needle aspiration of primary soft tissue lesions. *Arch Pathol Lab Med* 110:420–424, 1986.

26. Ackerman M, Idvall J, Rydholm A: Cytodiagnosis of soft tissue tumours and tumour-like conditions by means of fine needle aspiration biopsy. *Arch Orthop Trauma Surg* 96:61–67, 1980.

27. Cross BJH, Hoeg K, Hager B: Transthoracic fine needle aspiration of pulmonary and metastatic sarcomas. *Diagn Cytopathol* 1:221–227, 1985.

28. Dahl I, Hagmar B, Angervall L: Leiomyosarcoma of soft tissues. A corrective, cytological and histological study of eleven cases. *Acta Pathol Microbiol Scand Sect A* 89:285–291, 1981.

29. James AP: Cytopathology of mesenchymal repair. *Diagn Cytopathol* 1:91–104, 1985.

30. Frable WJ: *Fine Needle Aspiration Biopsy.* Philadelphia, Saunders, 1983, pp 304–324.

31. Koss LG, Woyke S, Szewski W: *Aspiration Biopsy. Cytologic Interpretation and Histologic Bases.* New York, Igaku-Shoin, 1984, pp 273–283.

32. Willems JS: Aspiration biopsy cytology of soft tissue tumours, in Linsk JA, Franzen S (eds): *Clinical Aspiration Cytology.* Philadelphia, Lippincott, 1983, pp 319–347.

33. Fu YS, Perzin KH: Non-epithelial tumours of nasal cavity, paranasal sinuses and nasopharynx. A clinicopathologic study. VIII. Adipose tissue tumours (lipoma and liposarcoma). *Cancer (Philadelphia)* 40:1314–1317, 1977.

34. Janecka IP, Conley J, Perzin KH, et al: Lipoma presenting as parotid tumours. *Laryngoscope* 87:1007–1010, 1977.

35. Shmookler BM, Enzinger FM: Pleomorphic lipoma: A benign tumour simulating liposarcoma. A clinicopathologic analysis of 48 cases. *Cancer (Philadelphia)* 47:126–133, 1981.

36. Enzinger FM, Harvey DA: Spindle cell lipoma. *Cancer (Philadelphia)* 46:1852–1859, 1975.

37. Chung EB, Enzinger FM: Benign lipoblastomatoses. An analysis of 35 cases. *Cancer (Philadelphia)* 32:482–492, 1973.

38. Lawson W, Biller HF: Cervical hibernoma. *Laryngoscope* 86:1258–1267, 1976.

39. Kindblom LG, Angervall L, Jarlstedt J: Liposarcoma of the neck. A clinicopathologic study of four cases. *Cancer (Philadelphia)* 42:774–780, 1978.

40. Saunders JR, Jacques DA, Casterline PF, et al: Liposarcoma of the head and neck: A review of the literature and addition of four cases. *Cancer (Philadelphia)* 43:162–168, 1979.

41. Enzinger FM, Letters R, Torloni H: Histologic typing of soft tissue tumours. International classification of tumours, #3, Geneva, World Health Organization, 1969.

42. Dahl I, Jarlstedt J: Nodular fasciitis in the head and neck. A clinico-pathological study of 18 cases. *Acta Oto-Laryngol* 90:152–159, 1980.

43. Dahl I, Akerman M: Nodular fasciitis. A correlative cytologic and histologic study of 13 cases. *Acta Cytol* 25:215–222, 1981.

44. Conley J, Healey WV, Stout AP: Fibromatosis of the head and neck. *Amer J Surg* 112:602–614, 1966.

45. Masson JK, Soule EH: Desmoid tumours of the head and neck. *Amer J Surg* 112:615–622, 1966.

46. Stout AP: Juvenile fibromatoses. *Cancer (Philadelphia)* 7:953–978, 1954.

47. Swain RE, Sessions DG, Ogura JH: Fibrosarcoma of the head and neck. A clinical analysis of 40 cases. *Ann Otol Rhinol Laryngol* 83:439–444, 1974.

48. Ozzello L, Stout AP, Murray MR: Culture characteristics of malignant histiocytomas and fibrous xanthomas. *Cancer (Philadelphia)* 16:331–344, 1963.

49. Fu YS, Gabbiani G, Kaye GI, et al: Malignant soft tissue tumours of probable histiocytic origin. (Malignant fibrous histiocytomas). *Cancer (Philadelphia)* 35:176–198, 1975.

50. Jakobiec SA, Howard GM, Jones IS, et al: Fibrous histiocytomas of the orbit. *Amer J Ophthalmol* 77:333–345, 1974.

51. Ogura JH, Toomey JM, Setzen M, et al: Malignant fibrous histiocytomas of the head and neck. *Laryngoscope* 90:1429–1440, 1980.

52. Perzin KH, Fu YS: Non-epithelial tumours of nasal cavity, paranasal sinuses and nasopharynx. A clinico-pathologic study. XI. Fibrous histiocytomas. *Cancer (Philadelphia)* 45:2616–2626, 1980.

53. Weiss SW, Enzinger FM: Malignant fibrous histiocytoma. An analysis of 200 cases. *Cancer (Philadelphia)* 41:2250–2256, 1978.

54. Weiss SW, Enzinger FM: Myxoid variant of malignant fibrous histiocytoma. *Cancer (Philadelphia)* 39:1672–1685, 1977.

55. Guccion JG, Enzinger FM: Malignant giant cell tumour of soft-parts. An analysis of 32 cases. *Cancer (Philadelphia)* 29:1518–1529, 1972.

56. Walas L, Angervall L, Hagmar B, et al: A correlative cytologic and histologic study of malignant fibrous histiocytoma: An analysis of 40 cases examined by fine needle aspiration cytology. *Diagn Cytopathol* 2:46–54, 1986.

57. Sermetis MJ, Lyons WS, DeGuzman VC, et al: Leiomyomata of the esophagus. An analysis of 838 cases. *Cancer (Philadelphia)* 38:2166–2177, 1976.

58. Cherrick HM, Dunlop DL, King OH Jr: Leiomyomas of the oral cavity. Review of the literature and clinico-pathologic study of 7 new cases. *Oral Surg* 25:54–66, 1973.

59. Fu YS, Perzin KH: Non-epithelial tumours of the nasal cavity, paranasal sinuses, and nasopharynx. A clinico-pathologic study. IV. V. Smooth muscle tumours (leiomyoma, leiomyosarcoma). *Cancer (Philadelphia)* 35:1300–1308, 1975.

60. Lavin P, Hajdu SI, Foot FW Jr: Gastric and extragastric leioblastomas. Clinico-pathologic study of 44 cases. *Cancer (Philadelphia)* 29:305–311, 1972.

61. Kakar PK, Puri ND, Lahari AK: Leiomyosarcoma of paranasal sinuses. *J Laryngol Otol* 92:333–336, 1978.

62. Fields JP, Helwig EB: Leiomyosarcoma of the skin and subcutaneous tissue. *Cancer (Philadelphia)* 47:156–169, 1981.

63. Rainer WG, Bruf R: Leiomyosarcoma of the esophagus: Review of the literature and report of three cases. *Surgery* 58:343–350, 1965.

64. Lattes R: Tumours of soft tissues. *Atlas of Tumor Pathology*. Series 2. Revised. Fascicle 1. Washington, DC, Armed Forces Institute of Pathology, 1982, pp 169–181.

65. Dito WR, Batsakis JG: Rhabdomyosarcoma of the head and neck. An appraisal of the histologic behaviour in 170 cases. *Arch Surg* 84:112–118, 1962.

66. Gupta PK, Myers TD, Baylin SB, et al: Improved antigenic detection in ethynol-fixed cytologic specimens. A modified avidin-biotin-peroxidase complex (ABC) method. *Diagn Cytopathol* 1:133–136, 1985.

67. Levitt S, Cheng L, Dupuis MA, et al: Fine needle aspiration diagnosis of malignant lymphoma with confirmation by immunoperoxidase staining. *Acta Cytol* 29:895–902, 1985.

68. Nadji M: The potential value of immunoperoxidase technique in diagnostic cytology. *Acta Cytol* 24:442–447, 1980.

69. Akhtar M, Ali MA, Sabbah R, et al: Fine needle aspiration biopsy diagnosis of round cell malignant tumours of childhood. A combined light and electron microscopic approach. *Cancer (Philadelphia)* 55:1805–1817, 1985.

70. Dasgupta TK, Braffield RD, Strong EW, et al: Benign solitary schwannomas (neurilem-momas). *Cancer (Philadelphia)* 24:355–366, 1969.

71. Gross RE, Farber S, Martin LW: Neuroblastoma sympatheticum: A study and report of 217 cases. *Pediatrics* 23:1179–1191, 1959.

72. Smyth NPD, Purna VP: Ganglioneuroma of the cervical autonomic nervous system. *Arch Surg* 77:39–46, 1958.

73. Todd GB, Brooks SEH: Ganglioneuroma of the vagus nerve. *J Laryngol Otol* 87:979–989, 1973.

74. Fagan MF, Rone R: Esthesioneuroblastoma: Cytologic features with differential diagnostic considerations. *Diagn Cytopathol* 1:322–326, 1985.

75. Bill AH Jr, Sumner DS: A unified concept of lymphangioma and cystic hygroma. *Surg Gynecol Obstet* 120:79–89, 1965.

76. Ninh TN, Ninh TX: Cystic hygroma in children. A report of 126 cases. *J Pediatr Surg* 9:191–195, 1974.

77. Enzinger FM, Smith BH: Hemangiopericytoma: An analysis of 106 cases. *Hum Pathol* 7:61–82, 1976.

78. Nguyen GK, Neifer R: The cells of benign and malignant hemangiopericytomas in aspiration biopsy. *Diagn Cytopathol* 1:327–331, 1985.

79. Reed RJ, Palomeque FE, Hairston MA III, et al: Lymphangiosarcoma of the scalp. *Arch Dermatol* 94:396–402, 1966.

80. Hodgkinson DJ, Soule EH, Woods JE: Cutaneous angiosarcoma of the head and neck. *Cancer (Philadelphia)* 44:1106–1113, 1979.

81. Bankacki M, Myers EN, Barnes L, et al: Angiosarcoma of the maxillary sinus: Literature review and case report. *Head Neck Surg* 1:274–280, 1979.

82. Cadman LN, Soule EH, Kelly PJ: Synovial sarcoma: An analysis of 134 tumours. *Cancer (Philadelphia)* 18:613–627, 1965.

83. Roth JA, Enzinger FM, Tennenbaum M: Synovial sarcoma of the neck: A follow-up study of 24 cases. *Cancer (Philadelphia)* 35:1243–1253, 1975.

84. Cadotte M: Malignant granular-cell myoblastoma. *Cancer (Philadelphia)* 33:1417–1422, 1974.

85. Betsill WL Jr: Cytomorphology of granular cell tumours. Description of 4 cases. *Acta Cytol* 26:734–735, 1982.

86. Fisher ER, Wechsler H: Granular cell myoblastoma: A misnomer: Electron microscopic and histochemical evidence concerning its Schwann cell derivation and nature (granular cell schwannoma). *Cancer (Philadelphia)* 15:936–954, 1962.

87. Lattes R: Tumours of soft tissue. *Atlas of Tumor Pathology.* Series 2. Revised. Fascicle 1. Washington, DC, Armed Forces Institute of Pathology, 1982, pp 32–36.

88. Sponscl KH, McDonald JR, Ghormley RK: Myxoma and myxosarcoma of the soft tissues of the extremities. *J Bone Joint Surg* 34:820–826, 1982.

89. Uehara H: Cytology of alveolar soft-part sarcoma. *Acta Cytol* 22:191–192, 1978.

90. Enzinger FM: Epithelioid sarcoma. A sarcoma simulating a granuloma or a carcinoma. *Cancer (Philadelphia)* 26:1029–1041, 1970.

91. Hajdu SI, Shiu MH, Fortner JG: Tendosynovial sarcoma: A clinico-pathologic study of 136 cases. *Cancer (Philadelphia)* 39:1201–1217, 1977.

92. Lattes R: Tumours of soft tissue. *Atlas of Tumor Pathology.* Series 2. Revised. Fascicle 1. Washington, DC, Armed Forces Institute of Pathology, 1982, pp 214–218.

93. Pittman MR, Keller EE: Mesenchymal chondrosarcoma. Report of a case. *J Oral Surg* 32:443–447, 1974.

94. Salvador AH, Beabout JW, Dahlin DC: Mesenchymal chondrosarcoma. Observations of 30 new cases. *Cancer (Philadelphia)* 28:605–615, 1971.

95. Calafati FA, Wright AC, Walowitz A, et al: Fine needle aspiration cytology of extra-skeletal chondrosarcoma. *Acta Cytol* 28:81–85, 1984.

96. Dahlin DC, Coventry MB, Scanlon PM: Ewing's sarcoma. A critical analysis of 165 cases. *J Bone Joint Surg* 43:185–192, 1961.

97. Angervall L, Enzinger FM: Extraskeletal neoplasm resembling Ewing's sarcoma. *Cancer (Philadelphia)* 36:240–251, 1975.

98. Pontius KI, Sebek BA: Extraskeletal Ewing's sarcoma in the nasal fossa. Light and electron microscopic observations. *Amer J Clin Pathol* 75:410–415, 1981.

99. Kontozoglou T, Qizilbash AH, Sianos J, et al: Chordoma: Cytologic and immunocy-tochemical study of four cases. *Diagn Cytopathol* 2:55–61, 1986.

100. Finley JL, Silverman JF, Dabbs DJ, et al: Chordoma: Diagnosis by fine-needle aspiration biopsy with histologic, immunocytochemical and ultrastructural confirmation. *Diagn Cytopathol* 2:330–337, 1986.

5

Congenital and Other Cystic Lesions of the Neck

INTRODUCTION

A number of cystic lesions occur in the head and neck (Table 5.1). In many cases, the diagnosis seems obvious because such lesions tend to occur in patients of certain age groups who have an appropriate history. However, the wide variety of conditions that can develop in the head and neck may be misdiagnosed, even the seemingly most obvious lesions, if only clinical judgment is used in their evaluation. Thus, although cysts of the midline of the upper part of the neck are usually of thyroglossal origin, such cysts are occasionally cystic metastases from primary papillary carcinoma of the thyroid. Moreover, cysts of the lateral neck that contain murky, yellow fluid may appear to be branchial cleft cysts; further assessment may, however, show that such cysts are liquefied matastases from squamous cell carcinoma. Branchial cleft cysts can be difficult to diagnose clinically or cytologically. For this reason, it is essential that the clinician gather information from all possible sources before contemplating surgical intervention, be it for a cystic lesion or any other abnormality of the head or neck.

THYROGLOSSAL DUCT CYSTS

Anomalies of the thyroglossal duct result from failure of the duct to involute and disappear during the sixth and seventh weeks of intrauterine life. Most such anomalies are cystic, but sinuses and fistulas have been reported infrequently. Most thyroglossal cysts develop in the midline (Fig. 5.1), but a few arise laterally, forming a tract that may extend upward to the middle portion of the hyoid bone. Most such lesions are encountered during childhood or adolescence, but occasionally cases have been described in adults.[1,2] Thyroglossal cysts may be soft or hard and often are found to contain clear yellow to slightly murky fluid on needle aspiration biopsy.

TABLE 5.1. Congenital Cysts

Thyroglossal duct cysts
Branchial cleft cysts
Thymic cysts
Dermoid and epidermoid cysts
Lymphoepithelial cysts
Mucoceles and related pseudocysts

Such cysts usually measure only a few centimeters in greatest dimension, but a few are much larger. They are lined by columnar or squamous epithelium (Fig. 5.2) unless infection has occurred, in which case the epithelial lining may be replaced by inflammatory cells and histiocytes. Thyroid tissue may be found in the wall of such cysts. Although carcinoma has been reported in cysts of the thyroglossal duct, the clinician should be aware that carcinoma metastatic to a pretracheal lymph node or a node of the middle of the neck is a much more common occurrence than is primary carcinoma in a thyroglossal cyst. Most carcinomas encountered in thyroglossal cysts are papillary carcinomas (Fig. 5.3), but follicular carcinoma and squamous cell carcinoma have been described. Approximately 50 cases of such lesions have been reported.[3]

BRANCHIAL CLEFT CYSTS

Most such cysts of the lateral aspects of the neck result from developmental anomalies of the branchial clefts, although Bhaskar and Bernier[4] have suggested that

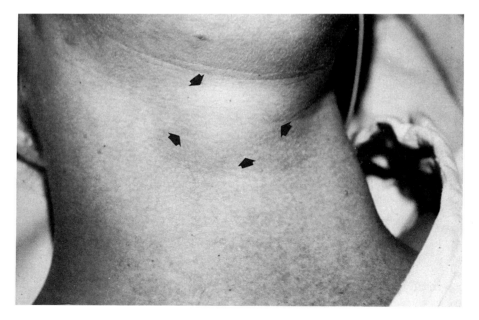

Fig. 5.1. Thyroglossal duct cyst (arrows) presenting as a mass in the midline of the neck.

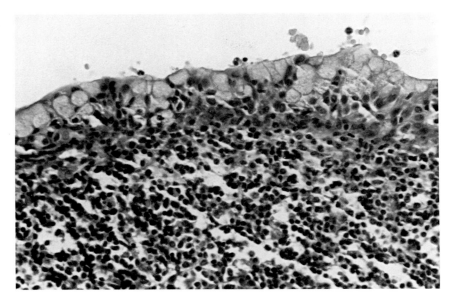

Fig. 5.2. Thyroglossal duct cyst. Note the columnar epithelial lining. Hematoxylin and eosin preparation. ×625.

branchial cleft cysts may derive from parotid inclusions within the cervical lymph nodes; these investigators have proposed the term lymphoepithelial cysts to describe such lesions. Most such anomalies occur in the second branchial cleft[5] and are manifested as cysts, sinuses or fistulas of the neck. They are usually situated along the anterior border of the sternocleidomastoid muscle (Fig. 5.4) but have been encountered in and around the parotid glands and ears. Occasionally, such cysts are bilateral. Although most patients are less than 30 years of age, such cysts have been reported after age 50.[1,5] There is no predilection for either sex. The cysts are soft to doughy and most of them are less than 5.0 centimeters in diameter and lined by squamous epithelium (Fig. 5.5). Occasionally, the lining cells are columnar. In cases with infection, the lining may be denuded and the walls of such cysts are composed of granulation tissue (Fig. 5.6). The characteristic feature of such cysts is an abundance of lymphoid tissue beneath the epithelial lining. Germinal centers may be observed (Fig. 5.7).

The development of squamous cell carcinoma in branchial cleft cysts is a subject of controversy. Many investigators believe that most such carcinomas are actually cystic metastases of the cervical lymph nodes and that a primary lesion elsewhere can be demonstrated on long-term follow-up.[6,7]

THYMIC CYSTS

Although most thymic cysts occur in the anterior mediastinum, occasional cases have been reported in the neck.[8] Most thymic cysts of the neck arise from remnants

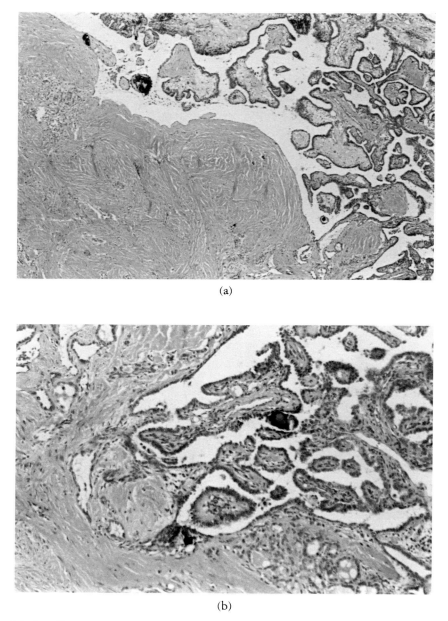

(a)

(b)

Fig. 5.3. Papillary carcinoma of the thyroid arising (a) in a thyroglossal duct cyst. Hematoxylin and eosin preparation. × 50. (b) High-power view of the tumor. × 150.

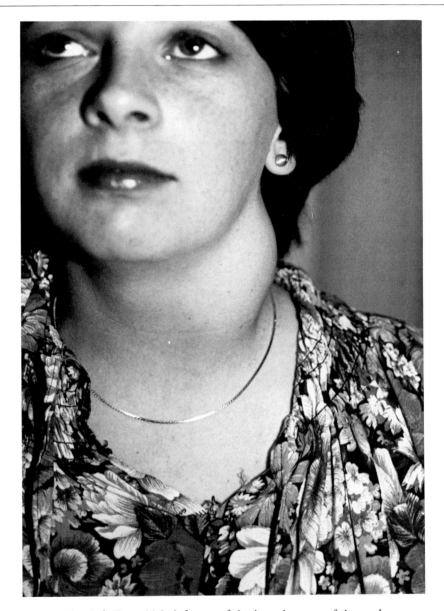

Fig. 5.4. Branchial cleft cyst of the lateral aspect of the neck.

of the thymopharyngeal duct that failed to involute. Because such cysts commonly arise in the anterior cervical triangle, they may be confused with branchial cleft cysts. Most thymic cysts of the neck occur in the first decade of life,[8] unlike branchial cleft cysts, which are usually encountered later in life. Histologic examination shows that such cysts are lined by columnar or squamous epithelium and have thymic tissue within their walls.

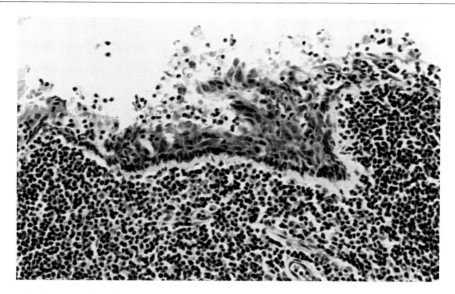

Fig. 5.5. Branchial cleft cyst. The lining is composed of squamous cells. Hematoxylin and eosin preparation. ×390.

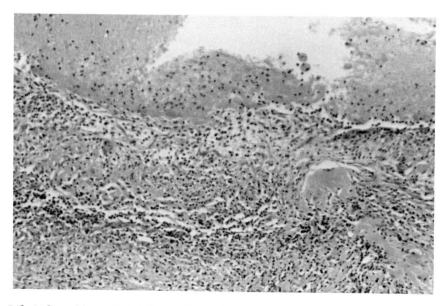

Fig. 5.6. Inflamed branchial cleft cyst. The epithelial lining has been destroyed by inflammation of the cyst wall. Hematoxylin and eosin preparation. ×150.

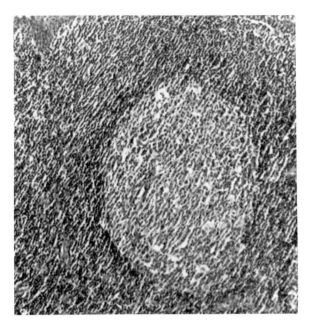

Fig. 5.7. Branchial cleft cyst. There is an abundance of lymphoid tissue within the cyst wall. Hematoxylin and eosin preparation. ×150.

DERMOID AND EPIDERMOID CYSTS

These cysts usually occur in the oral cavity but occasionally are manifested as masses in the neck. Most of them are situated in the midline (Fig. 5.8), but rare cases of lateral dermoid cysts present as masses in the submandibular triangle.[9] Dermoid and epidermoid cysts are doughy. Histologic examination demonstrates that dermoid cysts are lined by squamous epithelium with sebaceous and sweat glands in their walls. Respiratory epithelium may also be seen. Epidermoid cysts lack skin appendages and are lined by keratinized squamous epithelium.

CYTOLOGIC FEATURES

The contents of the cysts may be serous, mucoid or, if infected, purulent. Needle aspiration biopsy yields one or more milliliters of cystic material. The cytologic features of the various cysts are similar. The smears usually consist of solitary squamous cells (Fig. 5.9). The cells are large and polygonal and have small, round, pyknotic nuclei and delicate, pale-staining cytoplasm. Occasionally, atypical cells, some in a "pearl-like" configuration (Fig. 5.10), are observed coexisting with immature, parabasal-type squamous cells that have large, vesicular nuclei and dense cytoplasm. In the background, acellular squames, amorphous debris, lymphocytes, macrophages and neutrophils may be seen (Fig. 5.11). Columnar cells are encountered

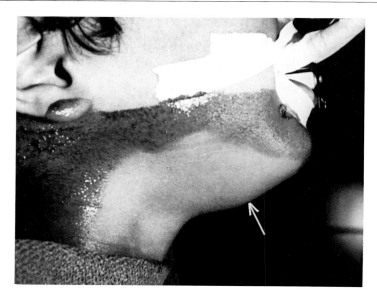

Fig. 5.8. Dermoid cyst (arrow) presenting as a swelling in the submental area in a young man.

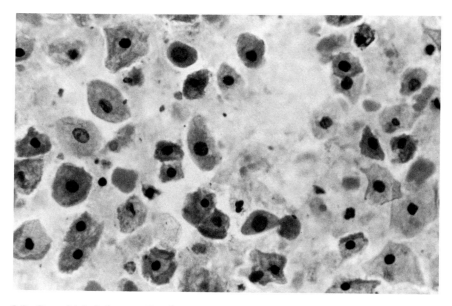

Fig. 5.9. Branchial cleft cyst. Cytology specimen contains large, polygonal squamous cells. Papanicolaou preparation. ×625.

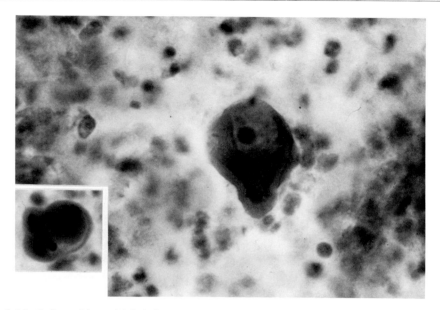

Fig. 5.10. Inflamed branchial cleft cyst. Cytology specimen contains markedly atypical squamous cells, leading to a misdiagnosis of metastatic squamous cell carcinoma. Papanicolaou preparation. × 1000. (*Inset*, × 625.)

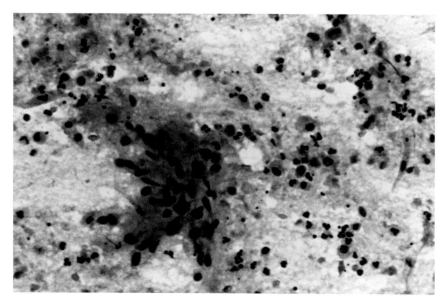

Fig. 5.11. Inflamed branchial cleft cyst. Cytology specimen contains cellular debris and inflammatory cells in the background. Papanicolaou preparation. × 390.

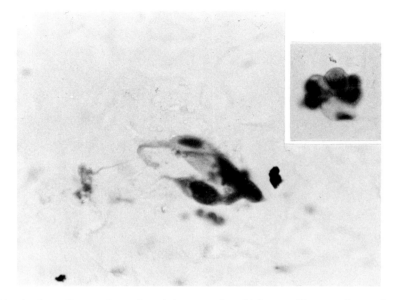

Fig. 5.12. Aspirate from a thyroglossal duct cyst in which a papillary carcinoma had arisen. Same patient as in Figure 5.3. Small groupings of markedly atypical cells suggested a malignant process. Papanicolaou preparation. ×625.

infrequently in branchial cleft and thyroglossal cysts. In some cases, the aspirates are devoid of cells or consist only of inflammatory cells. The diagnosis in such cases usually depends on the clinical findings unless the lesion is reaspirated. Papillary carcinomas may arise in thyroglossal cysts. In such cases, one expects to find sheets and small groupings of tumor cells admixed with inflammatory debris. Figure 5.12 shows the aspirate from the lesion illustrated in Figure 5.3. Even though the smear in this case was scanty, the nuclear atypia strongly suggested a malignant process.

In dermoid and epidermoid cysts, amorphous sebaceous material, sebaceous cells, squamous cells, anucleate squames and, in some cases, inflammatory cells may be observed (Fig. 5.13).

DIFFERENTIAL DIAGNOSIS

The differential diagnosis of cystic masses of the neck is summarized in Table 5.2. It is not possible to differentiate among thyroglossal, bronchial cleft and thymic cysts of the neck on the basis of cytologic study. Sebaceous cells are found in dermoid cysts but not in the other cyst types. Vascular tumors consist of oval or spindle-shaped endothelial cells in cohesive clusters, whereas congential cysts are composed of solitary squamous cells.

Cystic tumors of the salivary glands were discussed in Chapter 2.

Less than 1 percent of papillary carcinomas of the thyroid are manifested as cysts of the lateral aspects of the neck.[10] The cyst fluid is usually turbid, stained with

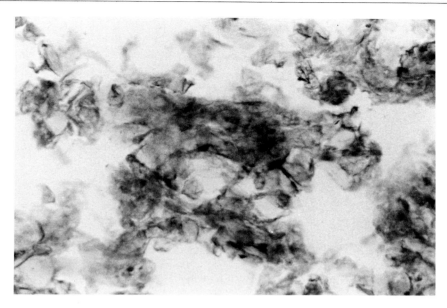

Fig. 5.13. Epidermoid cyst. Cytology specimen contains anucleate squames. Papanicolaou preparation. × 390.

blood and consists of inflammatory cells and hemosiderin-laden macrophages. If papillary fragments or monolayer sheets of epithelial cells are not found, a diagnosis of metastatic papillary carcinoma cannot be made. Betsill[10] has reported a primary papillary adenocarcinoma of the eyelid metastatic to the neck that presented as a cyst of the lateral aspect of the neck.

Metastatic keratinizing squamous cell carcinoma also can be manifested as a cyst of the lateral aspects of the neck.[1,11] In approximately 5 percent of such cases, only benign-appearing squamous cells are found and differentiation from branchial cleft

TABLE 5.2. Differential Diagnosis of Cystic Masses of the Neck

Thyroglossal duct cyst
Branchial cleft cyst
Thymic cyst
Dermoid or epidermoid cyst
Lymphangioma
Hemangioma
Cystic neoplasm of the salivary glands
Pleomorphic adenoma
Warthin's tumor
Low-grade mucoepidermoid carcinoma
Acinic cell carcinoma
Papillary cystic carcinoma
Cystic carcinoma metastatic to the cervical lymph nodes
Keratinizing squamous cell carcinoma
Papillary carcinoma of the thyroid

cysts may be difficult. Aspirates from inflamed branchial cleft cysts occasionally contain atypical squamous cells that resemble the cells of metastatic squamous cell carcinoma. As was discussed in Chapter 3, one of our cases of branchial cleft cyst contained such atypical cells, including "pearl-like" forms that had large, hyperchromatic nuclei, suggesting metastatic squamous cell carcinoma. No primary lesion was found and surgical excision of the mass in the lateral aspect of the neck revealed an inflamed branchial cleft cyst with atypical lining cells. The age of the patient may be helpful in differentiating branchial cleft cysts from metastatic squamous cell carcinomas.[1] Benign cysts usually occur before age 30, whereas metastatic squamous cell carcinomas tend to occur later in life.

PITFALLS

The major pitfall in needle aspiration biopsy of cystic lesions of the neck is that benign and malignant lesions of the salivary glands and thyroid, and keratinizing squamous cell carcinoma may be manifested as cysts of the lateral aspects of the neck. In most cases, differentiation of such lesions from congenital cysts is straightforward. If a residual mass persists after aspiration, the lesion should be reneedled and examined again. If the diagnosis is still in doubt or if there is clinical suspicion of a malignant process, the mass should be excised surgically and subjected to histologic study.

RESULTS

Our experience with congential cysts is similar to the experiences of other investigators. We have investigated 77 cysts of the neck by aspiration biopsy cytology. In 76 cases, a correct diagnosis was obtained; the exception was a branchial cleft cyst, the smears from which contained markedly atypical squamous cells and was regarded as malignant (Fig. 5.10). Carcinoma of a thyroglossal cyst was encountered in only one case. The smear was suspicious for a malignant process and papillary carcinoma was diagnosed on histopathologic examination. In the series reported by Engzell and Zajicek,[1] medial cysts were correctly diagnosed in 76 percent of cases and lateral cysts in 86 percent.

REFERENCES

1. Engzell U, Zajicek J: Aspiration biopsy of tumours of the neck. I. Aspiration biopsy and cytologic findings in 100 cases of congenital cysts. *Acta Cytol* 4:51–57, 1970.
2. Ward PH, Strahan RW, Acquarelli M, et al: The many faces of cysts of the thyroglossal duct. *Trans Amer Acad Ophthalmol Otolaryngol* 74:310–318, 1970.
3. Joseph TJ, Komorowski RA: Thyroglossal duct carcinoma. *Hum Pathol* 6:717–729, 1975.

4. Bhaskar SN, Bernier JL: Histogenesis of branchial cysts. A report of 468 cases. *Amer J Pathol* 35:407–423, 1959.

5. Simpson RA: Lateral cervical cysts and fistulas. *Laryngoscope* 79:30–59, 1969.

6. Compagno J, Hyams VJ, Safavian M: Does branchiogenic carcinoma really exist? *Arch Pathol Lab Med* 100:311–314, 1976.

7. Martin H, Morfit HM, Ehrlick H: A case of branchiogenic cancer (malignant branchioma). *Ann Surg* 132:867–888, 1950.

8. Fahmy S: Cervical thymic cysts: The pathogenesis and relationship to branchial cysts. *J Laryngol Otol* 88:47–60, 1974.

9. New GB, Erich JB: Dermoid cysts of the head and neck. *Surg Gynecol Obstet* 65:48–55, 1937.

10. Betsill WL Jr: False negative diagnosis in fine-needle aspiration cytology of head and neck cysts. American Society of Clinical Pathologists, check sample. *Cytopathology* C82-11 (C-113).

11. Micheau C, Cachin Y, Caillou B: Cystic metastasis in the neck revealing occult carcinoma of the tonsil. *Cancer (Philadelphia)* 33:228–233, 1974.

6

Carotid Body Tumors and Other Paragangliomas

INTRODUCTION

Paraganglion tissue arises from the neural crest and is distributed widely in the form of small nests, generally adjacent to autonomic nerves and their ganglia. A number of paraganglia are found in the head and neck and are closely associated with arterial vessels and cranial nerves of the ontogenetic gill-arches.[1] The branchiomeric, carotid body and intravagal paraganglia, for example, are histologically similar and are formed of lobules of compactly or loosely arranged cells separated by connective tissue elements (Fig. 6.1). The intercarotid paraganglia are the largest of the branchiomeric paraganglia, measuring approximately 3.0 by 1.5 by 1.5 millimeters and weighing between 5 and 20 milligrams each.[1] They are located along the medial aspect of the common carotid artery at its bifurcation and are regarded as chemoreceptor organs responsive to oxygen tension.[2] They are unusually vascular structures, with blood flow per unit of tissue greater than that of the heart or brain.

Hyperplasia of the carotid body occurs in persons living at high altitudes and in patients with chronic pulmonary or cardiovascular diseases. However, the enlargement is not of a magnitude to pose a clinical problem. Neoplasms of the carotid body and other paraganglia, although not frequent tumors of the head and neck, should always be considered in the differential diagnosis of any mass in the head or neck. Such tumors must be differentiated from metastatic carcinoma, reactive lymph node hyperplasia, lymphoma, nerve sheath tumors, aneurysms of the carotid arteries, branchial cleft cysts and tumors of the salivary glands. Vagal paragangliomas may present as a nasopharyngeal tumor and laryngeal paragangliomas must be differentiated from squamous cell carcinoma and other tumors that arise at that site.

Because of the close relationship of such lesions to the carotid arteries and cranial nerves and their extreme vascularity, it is important that the lesions be diagnosed preoperatively, so that preparations for surgical intervention can be made in advance and the diagnosis does not come as a surprise at the time of the operation. Mathews[3]

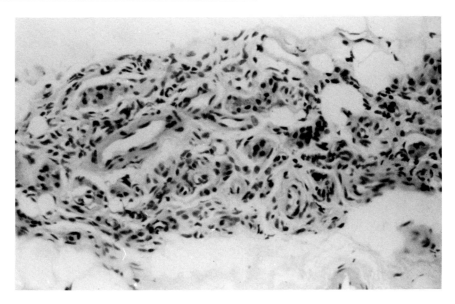

Fig. 6.1. Normal carotid body consists of small collections of cells separated by loose vascular connective tissue. Hematoxylin and eosin preparation. × 150.

in 1915 said of a tumor of the carotid body that "should one encounter it without having suspected the diagnosis the experience will not soon be forgotten." The extreme vascularity of such tumors has made carotid angiography the most useful diagnostic aid. Some clinicians are understandably reluctant to subject such tumors to needle aspiration biopsy, although there have been reports of needle aspiration biopsy of carotid body tumors.[1,4-8]

Of all the paragangliomas of the head and neck, carotid body tumors are the most common. Other less frequent paragangliomas are the jugulotympanic, vagal, laryngeal and orbital. The clinical features of such tumors differ according to the site of origin. However, the histologic and cytologic features of all paragangliomas are similar and will be described together.

CLINICAL FEATURES

Paragangliomas occur at all ages, but most patients are between 25 and 75 years of age.[1] Men and women are equally affected, although jugulotympanic and intravagale tumors are more common in women than in men.[1,7] The clinical signs and symptoms depend on the location of the tumor. Carotid body tumors usually are manifested as painless masses in the neck. They are situated deep to the sternocleidomastoid muscle at the level of the bifurcation of the carotid artery. A bruit may be heard over the mass.[1,4] The tumors are adherent to the adventitia of the carotid artery or may completely surround the vessel, necessitating carotid resection and arterial

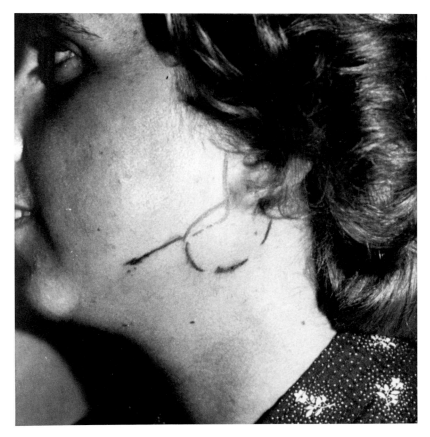

Fig. 6.2. Left parotid space mass in a young woman. The clinical diagnosis was parotid tumor. The diagnosis on aspiration biopsy cytology was consistent with paraganglioma.

reconstruction. Some carotid body tumors are manifested as hypopharyngeal masses and are associated with hoarseness. Compression of the vagal and hypoglossal nerves occasionally occurs with unusually large tumors.

Jugulotympanic paragangliomas may be associated with loss of hearing and, occasionally, neurologic symptoms.[1,9] Vagal paragangliomas usually are manifested as painless masses in the neck, behind and deep to the angle of the mandible (Fig. 6.2). Large vagal paragangliomas are sometimes manifested as retropharyngeal or nasopharyngeal tumors.[1,10] Compression of the cranial nerves may be associated with unilateral paralysis of the tongue, paralysis of the vocal cord and hoarseness. Laryngeal paragangliomas are usually associated with hoarseness and dysphagia.[1,5] Patients with orbital tumors may complain of throbbing pain and loss of vision.[1] Carotid body and other paragangliomas of the head or neck are usually nonfunctional, although functioning tumors have occasionally been reported.[1,6] Paragangliomas may be bilateral. From 2 to 23 percent of carotid body tumors are malignant.[1,11,12] Metastases usually occur in the regional lymph nodes, lungs and bones.

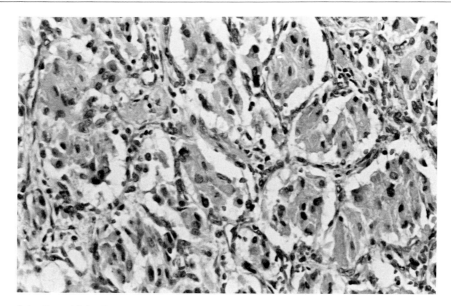

Fig. 6.3. Carotid body tumor. The organoid pattern is obvious. Hematoxylin and eosin preparation. ×350.

On gross inspection, such tumors are small and ovoid or lobulated and rarely measure more than 5.0 centimeters in diameter. They are firm to rubbery. Areas of hemorrhage are commonly observed.

HISTOLOGIC FEATURES

Histologic study shows that such tumors have a thin connective tissue capsule. Groups of neoplastic chief cells are surrounded by thin, fibrous septa that are rich in small blood vessels. The tumor cells are in an organoid or alveolar pattern (Fig. 6.3), also referred to as "Zellballen." This pattern is seen best with reticulin stain. The cells are oval or polygonal and have an abundance of pale to pink cytoplasm, which may be granular or have a dense, homogeneous quality (Fig. 6.4). Spindle-shaped cells may be seen in some tumors. The tumor cells infrequently have clear, vacuolated cytoplasm. The nuclei are large and pleomorphic and bizarre forms are occasionally observed. Mitoses are an uncommon feature. Dense bands of collagen may be observed, as may small collections of lymphocytes and plasma cells scattered throughout the tumor. In the cases we have studied, small areas of hemorrhage and localized deposits of hemosiderin were noted, possibly the result of needle aspiration biopsy. Grimelius stain demonstrates fine, black granules within the cytoplasm of the tumor cells. Electron microscopy shows electron-dense secretory granules that vary from 100 to 300 nanometers in diameter. Differentiation of benign from malignant paraganglioma is difficult on histologic examination. Hypercellularity, nuclear pleomorphism, necrosis and mitoses have been reported in malignant

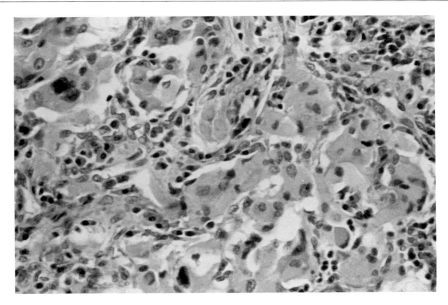

Fig. 6.4. Carotid body tumor. High-power view of a tumor composed of large, polygonal cells that have dense cytoplasm separated by thin, vascular septa. Hematoxylin and eosin preparation. ×625.

tumors, but the only reliable criterion of a malignant nature is metastasis to regional lymph nodes or distant viscera.[2] Figure 6.5 shows a malignant paraganglioma of the nasopharynx that had metastasized to a cervical lymph node.

CYTOLOGIC FEATURES

The aspirates from carotid body and other paragangliomas usually consist of one or two drops of bloody material. The smears contain large amounts of red blood cells. There are a few solitary tumor cells, but most tumor cells are in loose groupings. The tumor cells are large and polygonal and have an abundance of finely granular to dense cytoplasm (Fig. 6.6). Some cell groupings have elongated strands of cytoplasm, producing a lattice-like appearance (Fig. 6.7). With Papanicolaou stain, the cytoplasm appears pale greenish; with hematoxylin and eosin, it appears eosinophilic. The cytoplasm of some tumor cells appears dense and hyaline-like. No cytoplasmic granules are visualized with hematoxylin and eosin or Papanicolaou stain, although Engzell and colleagues[4] have observed red cytoplasmic granules with May-Grünwald-Giemsa stain. The nuclei are located centrally or eccentrically and vary greatly in size and shape (Fig. 6.8). The chromatin is fine to coarse and one or more nucleoli may be observed.

Differentiation of benign from malignant paraganglioma on aspiration biopsy cytology may be difficult because cellular atypia is seen in both tumor types. In a recent report of three cases of paraganglioma studied by aspiration biopsy cytology,

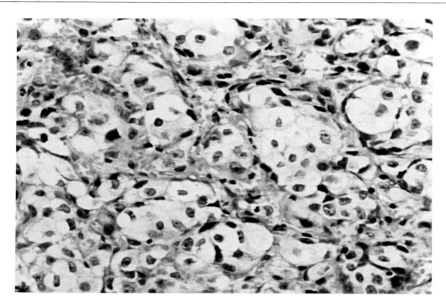

Fig. 6.5. Malignant paraganglioma. Note the small grouping of cells in an organoid pattern. Hematoxylin and eosin preparation. ×390. (From Hood IC, et al: *Acta Cytol* 27:651–657, 1983, with permission.)

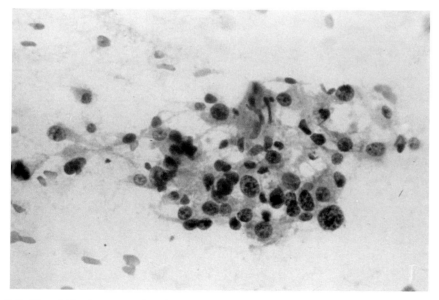

Fig. 6.6. Carotid body tumor. Cytology specimen contains loose groupings of cells that have granular cytoplasm. Nuclear atypia is evident. Papanicolaou preparation. ×625.

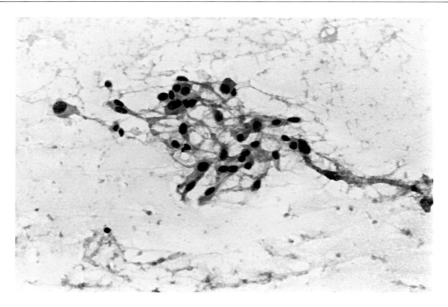

Fig. 6.7. Cytology specimen contains a loose grouping of cells that have elongated strands of cytoplasm. Hematoxylin and eosin preparation. × 390.

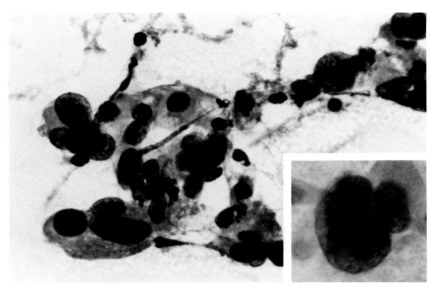

Fig. 6.8. Carotid body tumor. Cytology specimen contains tumor cells that have nuclear atypia, clumping of chromatin and small nucleoli. Hematoxylin and eosin preparation. × 1000. (*Inset*, × 1500.)

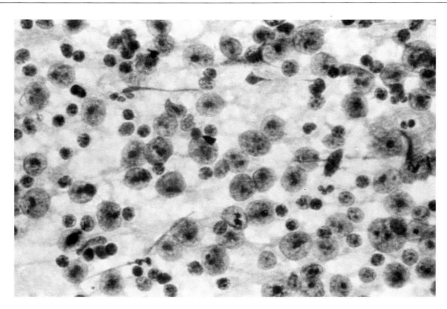

Fig. 6.9. Malignant paraganglioma. Cytology specimen contains tumor cells that have a scant amount of ill-defined cytoplasm, large, round or oval nuclei and one or more prominent nucleoli. A diagnosis of a malignant tumor can be made, but a definitive diagnosis would be difficult unless the history is known. Papanicolaou preparation. ×625.

tumor diathesis and mitoses were seen only in malignant variants.[8] The cells of malignant tumors had a scant amount of ill-defined, eosinophilic or clear cytoplasm and large, round, oval or spindle-shaped nuclei (Fig. 6.9). The chromatin was coarsely granular and nucleoli were prominent. The background consisted of proteinaceous, cellular debris and mitotic figures were frequently encountered. The cytologic features of carotid body tumors are summarized in Table 6.1.

DIFFERENTIAL DIAGNOSIS

Depending on the shape and arrangement of the cells, carotid body tumors and other paragangliomas may be mistaken for a variety of epithelial and mesenchymal neoplasms. The first carotid body tumor we studied cytologically was misinterpreted

TABLE 6.1. Carotid Body Tumors: Summary of Cytologic Features

Bloody aspirate that contains scanty cellular elements
Loose groupings and solitary cells
Large, ovoid or polygonal cells that have abundant cytoplasm. Slender cytoplasmic processes may be observed. Cytoplasm granular to dense. Nuclei pleomorphic, round to elongated. In malignant variants, tumor diathesis and mitoses noted.

as metastatic carcinoma. This misinterpretation resulted from the abundance of dense, eosinophilic cytoplasm and the large, pleomorphic nuclei of the tumor cells, which suggested squamous differentiation. Other investigators have also confused carotid body tumors with other neoplasms.[4] An acinar or follicle-like arrangement of the cells suggests follicular carcinoma of the thyroid and the oval or spindle-shaped nuclei may be misinterpreted as evidence of a neural tumor. With experience, misinterpretation occurs less frequently and a knowledge of the clinical findings, especially the location of the tumor and the presence or absence of a bruit, is essential. Moreover, the aspirates usually consist of a drop of blood with scanty cellular elements. The loose groupings of cells that have an abundance of granular to dense cytoplasm and pleomorphic nuclei are a clue to the diagnosis.

COMPLICATIONS

Because such tumors are extremely vascular, there is a theoretical risk of complication with aspiration.[3] Hemorrhage in such tumors is not uncommon and deposits of hemosiderin are usually found along the needle tract. However, this change does not interfere with subsequent histologic study. Hematomas may also form. Engzell and colleagues[4] reported one death due to carotid artery thrombosis and cerebral embolism after needle aspiration biopsy of a carotid body tumor. Because such tumors are known to invade the wall of the carotid artery, the thrombosis may not have been solely a result of the aspiration. We have not encountered any complication in the seven patients with paragangliomas we have investigated by needle aspiration biopsy and would not hesitate performing the procedure in a paraganglioma. However, Engzell and colleagues[4] have suggested that it is probably safer to perform carotid angiography in patients with a bruit and to reserve needle aspiration biopsy for cases in which the diagnosis is not obvious clinically and cases in which an angiogram is not diagnostic. Figures 6.10 and 6.11 are an angiogram and a computed axial tomogram, respectively, of the paraganglioma in the patient shown in Figure 6.2.

RESULTS

We have studied seven paragangliomas. Five of them were benign and two were malignant. Of the five benign lesions, one was a benign carotid body tumor and four were intravagal paragangliomas. The two malignant paragangliomas manifested as nasopharyngeal neoplasms. The malignant tumors had metastisized to the lymph nodes or lungs. The diagnosis of metastatic paraganglioma was not difficult in these cases because we had knowledge of the history and clinical findings. However, one benign tumor was misdiagnosed as metastatic carcinoma. Engzell and colleagues[4] have reported 13 cases of carotid body tumors subjected to needle aspiration biopsy; nine cases occurred during 1960–66 and four during 1967–68. Of the first nine cases, only three were diagnosed preoperatively; all four subsequent tumors were correctly diagnosed by aspiration biopsy cytology.

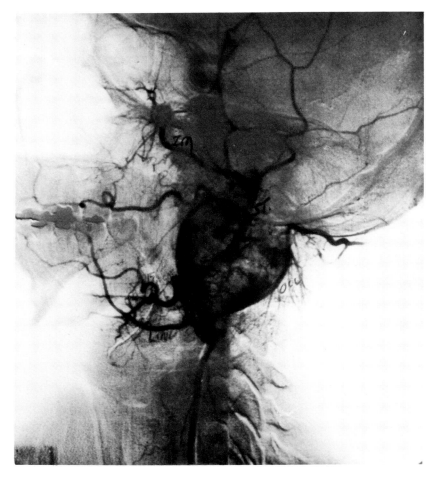

Fig. 6.10. Left carotid angiogram of a paraganglioma of the vagus nerve (glomus intravagale). Same patient as shown in Figure 6.2.

REFERENCES

1. Glenner GG, Grimley PM: Tumours of the extra-adrenal paraganglion system. (Including chemoreceptors.) *Atlas of Tumor Pathology.* Second series. Fascicle 9. Washington, DC, Armed Forces Institute of Pathology, 1974.

2. Briscoe TJ: Carotid body. Structure and function. *Physiol Rev* 51:437–495, 1971.

3. Mathews FS: Surgery of the neck, in Johnson AB (ed): *Operative Therapeusis.* New York, Appleton-Century-Crofts, 1915, vol 3, p 315.

4. Engzell U, Franzen S, Zajicek J: Aspiration biopsy of tumours of the neck. II. Cytologic findings in 13 cases of carotid body tumours. *Acta Cytol* 15:25–30, 1971.

5. Gallivan MVE, Chun B, Rowden G, et al: Laryngeal paraganglioma. *Amer J Surg Pathol* 3:85–92, 1979.

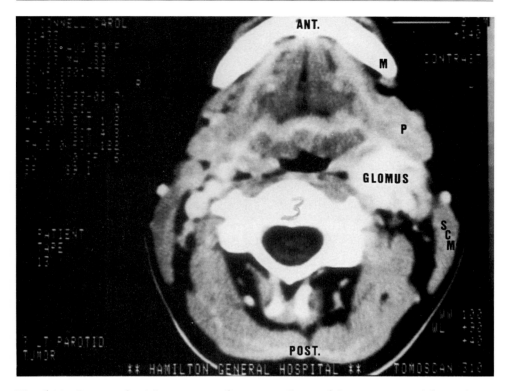

Fig. 6.11. Computed axial tomogram of a paraganglioma of the vagus nerve (glomus intravagale) that presented as a parotid space lesion. Same patient as shown in Figure 6.2. m, Mandible; p, parotid gland; scm, sternocleidomastoid muscle; ant, anterior; post, posterior.

6. Hamberger CA, Hamberger CB, Wersall J, et al: Malignant catecholamine-producing tumour of the carotid body. *Acta Pathol Microbial Scand* 69:489–492, 1967.

7. Hatfield PM, James AE, Schulz MD: Chemodectomas of the glomus jugulare. *Cancer (Philadelphia)* 30:1164–1168, 1972.

8. Hood IC, Qizilbash AH, Young JEM, et al: Fine needle aspiration biopsy cytology of paragangliomas. Cytologic, light microscopic and ultrastructural studies of three cases. *Acta Cytol* 27:651–657, 1983.

9. Cole JM: Glomus jugulare tumour. *Laryngoscope* 87:1244–1258, 1977.

10. House JM, Goodman ML, Gacek RR, et al: Chemodectomas of the nasopharynx. *Arch Otolaryngol* 96:138–141, 1972.

11. Shamblin WR, ReMine WH, Sheps SG, et al: Carotid body tumour (chemodectoma). *Amer J Surg* 122:732–739, 1971.

12. Statts ES, Brown RL, Smith RR: Carotid body tumors. Benign and malignant. *Laryngoscope* 76:907–916, 1966.

7

Miscellaneous Lesions

Needle aspiration biopsy of the head and neck is usually done on lesions that are easily visible and can be fixed between the fingers of one hand during aspiration. There are, however, various areas of the head and neck where lesions are less accessible but where needle aspiration biopsy is useful and can be easily performed.

SUPERFICIAL STRUCTURES

For a large number of skin or dermal lesions or deeper tumors that infiltrate the skin, needle aspiration biopsy permits rapid diagnosis. Obviously, most superficial basal cell or squamous cell carcinomas of the skin are easily sampled with a scalpel or punch biopsy instrument, but some plaquelike primary or metastatic lesions of the dermis or infiltrating the skin can be diagnosed just as easily or more easily by needle aspiration biopsy, although an inconclusive result may necessitate reaspiration or deeper open biopsy. Lesions that involve the underlying bone are more safely sampled by needle aspiration biopsy than by open biopsy technique because of the risk for bleeding or inducing infection into the bone (particularly the outer table of the skull).

A few lesions will be discussed in detail.

Merkel Cell Tumor

This small-cell undifferentiated carcinoma of the skin commonly occurs on the skin of the face and is easily mistaken for basal cell carcinoma or malignant melanoma. The tumor is a reddish, smooth-surfaced nodule that grows slowly (Fig. 7.1); a few such tumors are ulcerated, however. Histologic examination shows that such tumors are composed of small, uniform, undifferentiated cells in the dermis and underlying subcutaneous tissue.[1] Grimelius stain demonstrates granules in the cytoplasm of the tumor cells; electron microscopy reveals that these dense core granules are similar to the neurosecretory granules of the amine percursor uptake and decarboxylation

291

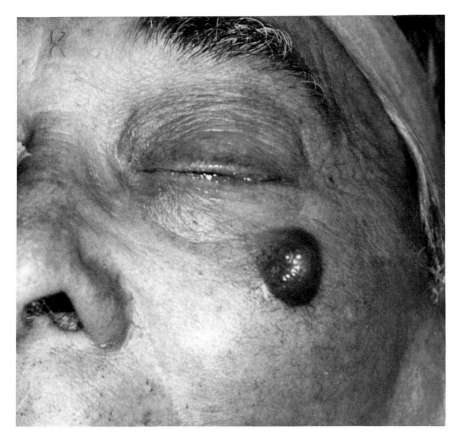

Fig. 7.1. Merkel cell tumor on the face of an elderly man. (Photograph courtesy of Dr. S. D. Archibald.)

(APUD) cell system. Metastases are common in the regional lymph nodes. The differential diagnosis includes small-cell tumors, namely, non-Hodgkin's lymphoma, small-cell undifferentiated carcinoma, islet cell tumor and others. This tumor was discussed in Chapter 3.

We have studied five patients with Merkel cell tumors. Most of the tumors had metastasized to the regional lymph nodes and the patients presented with masses in their necks (see Fig. 3.68). The history of a lesion on the face in combination with metastasis of small-cell tumor to a lymph node suggests Merkel cell tumor. Figures 3.69 and 3.70 illustrate the histologic and cytologic features of this neoplasm.

Malignant Melanoma

One-fourth of all malignant melanomas of the skin occur in the head or neck.[2] The most common sites are the skin of the face, ears, neck and scalp. Melanomas also arise in the mucosa of the oral cavity, nose, paranasal sinuses and orbits. Metastases in the lymph nodes of the neck are a frequent occurrence and enlargement of an involved lymph node is a common mode of presentation. Figure 7.2 shows an

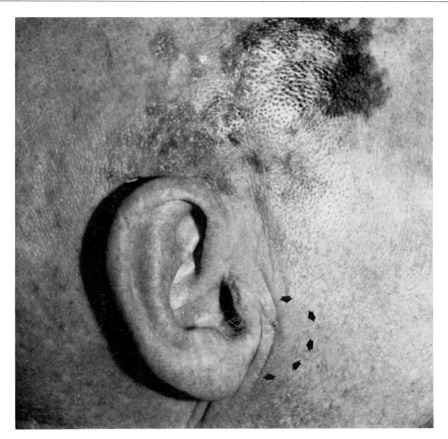

Fig. 7.2. Superficial spreading malignant melanoma with a small node in the superior lobe of the parotid gland (arrows) that was positive on needle aspiration biopsy.

elderly patient who presented with a superficial spreading melanoma over the skin of the temple. On careful examination, a small nodule in the superficial lobe of the parotid gland could be palpated. Aspiration biopsy cytology confirmed the diagnosis of malignant melanoma metastatic to an intraparotid lymph node. The cytologic features of malignant melanoma in aspirates were discussed in Chapter 3 and illustrated in Figures 3.73 to 3.77.

Tumors of the Epidermal Appendages

A variety of tumors of the skin appendages occur in the head and neck. Occasionally, such tumors have distinctive features and can be diagnosed on needle aspiration biopsy. In most cases, however, excision is required for a definitive diagnosis. The aspirates from pilar and epidermal inclusion cysts usually consist of amorphous material, anucleate squames or sebaceous cells. Inflammatory cells may be seen in the aspirates if rupture and secondary inflammation have occurred. A pilar cyst that mimicked malignant melanoma on clinical examination is shown in Figure 1.2.

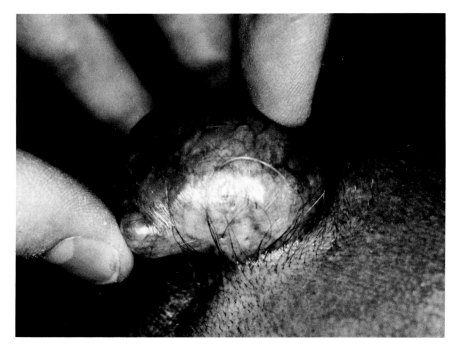

Fig. 7.3. Pedunculated tumor on the scalp of an elderly man with a history of cancer of the oropharynx. The cytologic diagnosis on needle aspiration biopsy was cylindroma, which was confirmed on excision.

A tumor that is distinctive clinically and cytologically is a cylindroma; an example of this tumor is shown in Figure 7.3. Cylindromas characteristically occur on the scalp as one or more dome-shaped nodules of variable size. Histologic study shows that such tumors have a distinctive appearance, consisting of islands, strands and trabeculae of basaloid epithelial cells surrounded by thin bands of eosinophilic hyaline. Small globules of hyaline can be seen between the epithelial cells within the islands of tumor cells. One also observes tubular lumina that contain amorphous material. The aspirate from the patient shown in Figure 7.3 consisted of numerous tissue fragments of small, basaloid cells and hyaline cylinders, similar to the appearance of aspirates from patients with adenoid cystic carcinoma (see Chapter 2).

Kaposi's Sarcoma

Kaposi's sarcoma typically involves the limbs, but there have been reports of head and neck involvement. Cutaneous and mucosal lesions occur. In the classical form, the patient is a middle-aged or elderly man of Jewish or Mediterranean origin.

Kaposi's sarcoma in patients with acquired immune deficiency syndrome (AIDS), however, differs from the classical form in that the patients are younger and the lesions are more widely distributed at the time of diagnosis and associated with a poor prognosis The pattern of involvement in AIDS also differs, with a high incidence of lesions of the viscera, lymph nodes and head and neck. Mucosal, cutaneous and lymphadenopathic forms are common and easily diagnosed by needle aspiration biopsy. Hales and colleagues[3] have recently reported their experience with fine-needle aspiration biopsy of Kaposi's sarcoma in 13 homosexual men. Seven lesions involved the oral cavity and appeared as flat or exophytic, reddish purple lesions. Five aspirates were obtained from enlarged lymph nodes and three were from soft-tissue masses.

The aspirates contained small tissue fragments composed of cohesive bundles of spindle-shaped cells. Loose grouping of such cells and solitary cells were also noted. Numerous bare nuclei were visible in the background. The chromatin appeared fine and small nucleoli were observed. Vascular spaces were not seen, although the large tissue fragments had irregular spaces, some of which contained red blood cells.

The differential diagnosis of Kaposi's sarcoma includes granulation tissue, mesenchymal repair, granulomatous inflammation and other soft-tissue sarcomas. If there is no history of homosexuality or AIDS, caution is advised in reporting needle aspiration biopsy specimens. Tissue biopsy should be requested for confirmation in such cases.

ORAL CAVITY

Most intraoral tumors are squamous cell lesions that arise from the epithelial lining of the mucosa. Accordingly, such lesions are most easily sampled by use of a biopsy forceps under direct vision. However, in a few squamous cell carcinomas, the overlying mucosa is intact; such lesions usually are deep-seated malignant tumors of the posterior part of the tongue. In cases in which the mucosa is intact, repeat superficial biopsy specimens may not be diagnostic and we have found that needle aspiration directly through the mucosa into the substance of the tumor is extremely accurate in this situation. In fact, this technique is more accurate than a Tru-cut needle biopsy, even when the latter is done under general anesthesia, because a Tru-cut needle can sample only one area at a time, whereas the former technique (easily done under local anesthesia or without anesthesia) allows one to sample several areas through the bulk of the tongue and yields diagnostic specimens in a high proportion of cases.

Tumors of the minor salivary glands occur throughout the oropharyngeal area. However, most such lesions are beneath the mucosa and in the hard palate are probably best sampled by use of the needle aspiration biopsy technique. This method is better tolerated by the patient than is deep biopsy, although, of course, the latter may be necessary if the aspirate is not diagnostic.

Lesions of the Minor Salivary Glands

As with the major salivary glands, enlargement of the minor salivary glands may be the result of inflammation or neoplasia (Figs. 7.4 and 7.5). The spectrum of such lesions is wide. This subject was discussed in detail in Chapter 2. The lesions that deserve reemphasis will be discussed again.

Ranula

A ranula is a mucous retention cyst that is usually manifested as a mass in the floor of the mouth; occasionally, such cysts extend deeply and are manifested as masses in the neck.[4] Ranulas are true cysts and are lined by columnar or squamous epithelium.

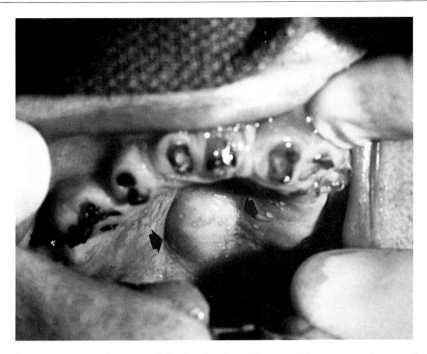

Fig. 7.4. Pleomorphic adenoma of the hard palate. The overlying mucosa is smooth. Such lesions are easily diagnosed by needle aspiration biopsy.

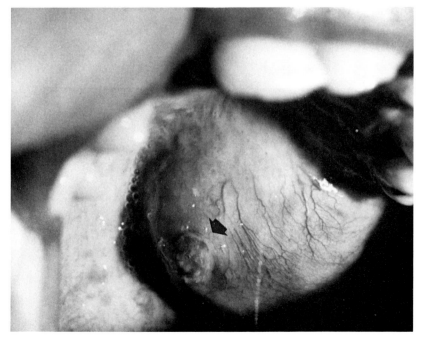

Fig. 7.5. Adenoid cystic carcinoma of the left side of the soft palate. The large tumor has ulcerated (arrow) through the overlying mucosa.

Differentiation from dermoid cyst, lipoma and salivary gland neoplasms may be difficult on the basis of clinical findings alone. The aspirates usually consist of thick, mucoid material. Epithelial lining cells may be seen in the smears coexisting with mucus and inflammatory cells.

Necrotizing Sialometaplasia

This painless, slightly raised, ulcerated or nonulcerated lesion usually involves the minor salivary glands in the hard palate.[5] Differentiation from squamous cell and mucoepidermoid carcinoma may pose a challenge. The aspirates consist of atypical squamous and glandular cells on a background of mucus and chronic inflammatory cells. This lesion was discussed in Chapter 2.

Polymorphous Low-Grade Adenocarcinoma

Another lesion that deserves brief mention is the so-called polymorphous low-grade adenocarcinoma of the minor salivary glands. This term was coined by Evans and Batsakis[6] to describe a distinctive tumor that has a predilection for the palate. This slowly growing, infiltrative neoplasm has a low potential for metastasis to the lymph nodes of the neck. Such tumors are characterized by cytologic uniformity and histologic diversity.[6] Few mitotic figures are observed and tumor necrosis is an uncommon feature. Solid, trabecular, tubular, papillary, cribriform and pseudoadenoid cystic patterns have been described. The stroma is mucinous or fibrotic. We recently studied one such case. The lesion was on the hard palate and the smears contained a few basaloid cells, some associated with mucous cylinders, a common feature of adenoid cystic carcinoma. On excision, however, the histologic pattern was more consistent with polymorphous low-grade adenocarcinoma than with adenoid cystic carcinoma.

Miscellaneous Polypoid Lesions

Irritational Fibroma

This sessile, nodular, reactive lesion is composed of fibrous tissue, most likely the result of mechanical irritation. Such tumors occur throughout the oral cavity but are most common on the buccal mucosa, palate and tongue. Needle aspiration biopsy usually yields scanty material because of the dense, fibrous nature of such lesions. For this reason, excisional biopsy is preferable to needle aspiration biopsy for such lesions.

Squamous Papilloma

Squamous papilloma is a common lesion of the mucosa of the oral cavity. Such lesions are easily recognized clinically and are managed by surgical excision.

Precancer

Leukoplakia is usually manifested as pale white to reddish, flat, plaquelike or nodular lesions. We usually do not aspirate such lesions and rely on surgical biopsy for the diagnosis.

Squamous Cell Carcinoma

Squamous cell carcinoma of the oral cavity commonly involves the lips, tongue, floor of the mouth, buccal mucosa and palate. Most such tumors are well or moderately differentiated. In most instances, the diagnosis can be easily made on a small surgical biopsy specimen. However, as was stated earlier, needle aspiration biopsy may be required for deep-seated lesions.

Carcinoma of the Tonsils

Approximately 80 to 90 percent of tumors of the tonsils are squamous cell carcinomas[7] and about 10 percent are lymphomas. Such tumors may be manifested as indurated, ulcerated masses. Fungating, polypoid lesions also occur. Needle aspiration biopsy is an easy method for making the diagnosis of such lesions and is highly accurate. Most epithelial tumors are moderately or poorly differentiated squamous cell carcinomas. The cytologic features of squamous cell carcinoma and lymphoma were discussed in Chapter 3 and will not be mentioned here.

Melanoma

This rare lesion presents as a small ulcer or a polypoid/nodular mass.[8] Most such lesions are pigmented. The diagnosis is usually suspected on the basis of clinical findings and can be confirmed by a small biopsy or needle aspiration biopsy. The histologic features of aspirates were discussed in Chapter 3. Cytologic study shows that the primary lesion and lymph node metastases have similar appearances. These tumors are aggressive and most patients are dead within two years of diagnosis.

Involvement of the regional lymph nodes is a common feature of carcinoma of the oral cavity and is the presenting sign in many cases. As was noted in Chapter 3, needle aspiration biopsy of lymph nodes can provide the diagnosis and direct further investigation and treatment without much loss of time and too much expense.

MAXILLARY ANTRUM

Malignant lesions of the maxillary antrum can be sampled by means of needle aspiration biopsy if they have broken through the anterior, medial, lateral, superior or inferior bony wall of the antrum. We have found that the most useful method is to aspirate through the superior alveolobuccal sulcus, entering the tumor in the area that would be exposed during a Caldwell-Luc operation. Tumors that have invaded directly through the skin of the face can be sampled directly by aspirating through the skin in that area. This technique is useful in patients who have undergone high-dose radiotherapy and who may have residual or recurrent disease. In this situation, needle aspiration through the area sampled previously may confirm the diagnosis of a malignant process and obviate surgical reopening of the Caldwell-Luc incision.

The usefulness of needle aspiration biopsy in the diagnosis of tumors of the maxillary antrum is illustrated in Figure 7.6. The tumor in this elderly man has broken through the bony wall, infiltrating the soft tissues and overlying skin and invading the left orbit. Needle aspiration biopsy through the skin provided the

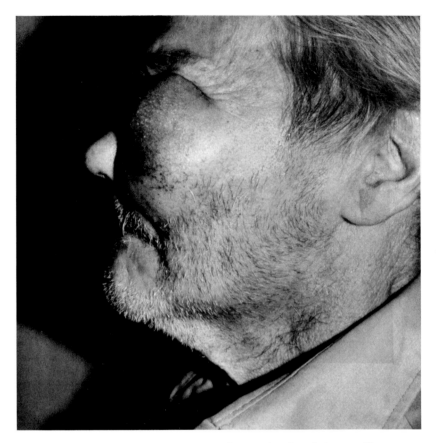

Fig. 7.6. Primary squamous cell carcinoma of the left side of the maxillary antrum. The tumor has invaded through the bone into the skin and orbit.

diagnosis of squamous cell carcinoma. No other primary tumor was found and the patient was treated with irradiation.

ORBITS AND PERIORBITAL REGION

Palpable periorbital lesions can be easily aspirated by the technique described in Chapter 1. Even if a lesion is in the posterior half of the orbit and causes proptosis without a palpable abnormality, aspiration biopsy can be performed blind by directing the needle toward the abnormality after a computed axial tomogram or sonogram has been reviewed. However, it is sometimes preferable to perform aspiration biopsy under direct guidance by computed tomography or sonography. Recent reports indicate that needle aspiration biopsy under the guidance of computed tomography is an effective technique for obtaining material for diagnosis.[9-11]

Zajdela and associates[12] have recently reported their experience with fine-needle

TABLE 7.1. Orbital and Periorbital Space-Occupying Lesions

Lesions of the Lacrimal Glands	Lymphoreticular Lesions
Lymphoepithelial lesion	Pseudolymphoma
Pseudolymphoma	Non-Hodgkin's
Granulomatous processes	Lymphoma
Non-Hodgkin's lymphoma	Leukemic infiltrates
Benign mixed tumor	Bony Lesions
Adenoid cystic carcinoma	Ossifying fibroma
Malignant mixed tumor	Fibrous dysplasia
Tumors of the Optic Nerves	Histiocytosis
Glioma	Ewing's sarcoma
Meningioma	Metastatic Neoplasms
Soft-Tissue Tumors	Neuroblastoma
Hemangioma	Carcinoma
Hemangiopericytoma	Malignant melanoma
Lymphangioma	Miscellaneous Lesions
Neurilemoma	Dermoid cyst
Neurofibroma	Mucocele
Rhabdomyosarcoma	
Malignant fibrous histiocytoma and other sarcomas	

biopsy of orbital and periorbital tumors without aspiration. They used a 25-gauge needle that was introduced into the lesion without a syringe and moved within the tumor mass in different directions. An air-filled syringe was attached to the needle after it had been removed from the lesion and the contents of the needle were expelled on a glass slide and smeared. No complications occurred with this technique. On the other hand, Kennerdell and coworkers[9] reported orbital hemorrhage in six of 50 patients who underwent needle aspiration biopsy. Both methods appear to be reliable, having an accuracy in excess of 90 percent.[9-12]

Lesions that are most often sampled by the needle aspiration biopsy technique are listed in Table 7.1. Loss of vision and proptosis are the most common clinical manifestations of such lesions.

Benign and malignant lesions of lacrimal gland origin have morphologic features similar to those of salivary gland origin. Common epithelial tumors include pleomorphic adenoma (benign mixed tumor), malignant mixed tumor and adenoid cystic carcinoma. Mucoepidermoid carcinoma of the lacrimal glands is a rare neoplasm and Warthin's tumor and acinic cell carcinoma do not occur in the lacrimal glands.[13] These entities were discussed in Chapter 2.

Astrocytomas and meningiomas may involve the optic nerves. Needle aspiration biopsy of gliomas and meningiomas has been reported. The aspirates from meningiomas consist of solitary polygonal or spindle-shaped cells or whorls of such cells.[10]

Differentiation of lymphoma from pseudolymphoma may be difficult on histologic or cytologic examination.[12,14] However, the diagnosis can be made if the smears are adequately prepared and cellular. The histologic and cytologic features and the differential diagnosis of lymphoma were discussed in Chapter 3.

Figure 7.7 is a computed axial tomogram from a patient who presented with right exophthalmos. The aspirate in this case contained few atypical lymphocytes. Although a definitive diagnosis of lymphoma could not be made, needle aspiration

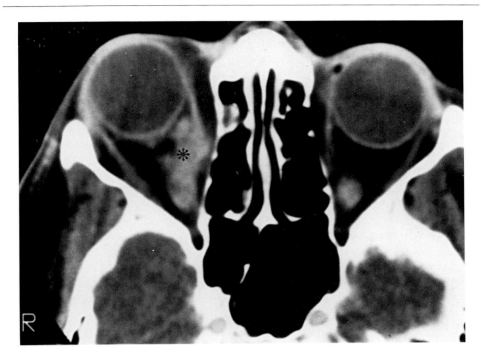

Fig. 7.7. Computed axial tomogram from a patient who presented with exophthalmos on the right. The asterisk indicates the lesion. The needle aspirate was nondiagnostic but ruled out a variety of lesions, including soft-tissue sarcoma. Open biopsy provided a diagnosis of non-Hodgkin's lymphoma.

biopsy ruled out metastatic carcinoma, soft-tissue sarcoma and other lesions. Open biopsy confirmed that the lesion was a small-cell non-Hodgkin's lymphoma.

Like lymphoma, rhabdomyosarcoma, malignant fibrous histiocytoma and other soft-tissue sarcomas may involve the orbits. In some cases, needle aspiration biopsy may provide a definitive diagnosis, but in other cases, histologic study is required for determining the tumor type.

Metastatic tumors not infrequently involve the orbits and periorbital tissues.[11] Carcinoma of the breast or lung, melanoma in adults and neuroblastoma in children are the usual causes. Needle aspiration biopsy can provide a definitive diagnosis in most cases and treatment can be instituted without delay. The histologic and cytologic features of metastatic tumors were discussed in Chapter 3. Orbital and periorbital tissues may also be involved by direct extension of a tumor arising in an adjacent structure. Figure 7.6 shows involvement of the left orbit by a squamous cell carcinoma of the maxillary antrum.

REFERENCES

1. Sidhu GS, Feiner H, Flotte TJ, et al: Merkel cell neoplasms. Histology, electron microscopy, biology and histogenesis. *Amer J Dermatopathol* 2:101–119, 1980.

2. Conley JJ, Pack GT: Melanoma of head and neck. *Surg Gynecol Obstet* 116:15–28, 1963.

3. Hales M, Bottles K, Miller T, et al: Diagnosis of Kaposi's sarcoma by fine-needle aspiration biopsy. *Amer J Clin Pathol* 88:20–25, 1987.

4. Quick CA, Lowell SH: Ranula and the sublingual salivary glands. *Arch Otolaryngol* 103:397–400, 1977.

5. Spark RP, Duncan BG: Necrotizing sialometaplasia. *Ann Otol Rhinol Laryngol* 87:409–411, 1978.

6. Evans HL, Batsakis JG: Polymorphous low-grade adenocarcinoma of minor salivary glands. A study of 14 cases of a distinctive neoplasm. *Cancer (Philadelphia)* 53:935–942, 1984.

7. Schulz MD, Linter DM, Sweeney L: Carcinoma of the palatine arch. *Amer J Roentgenol* 89:541–548, 1963.

8. Chaudhry AP, Hamperl A, Gorlin RJ: Primary malignant melanoma of the oral cavity. *Cancer (Philadelphia)* 11:923–928, 1958.

9. Kennerdell JS, Dekker A, Johnson BL: Orbital fine needle aspiration biopsy. The result of it in 50 patients. *Neuro-ophthalmol* 87:117–121, 1980.

10. Czerniak B, Woyke S, Daniel B, et al: Diagnosis of orbital tumours by aspiration biopsy guided by computerized tomography. *Cancer (Philadelphia)* 54:2385–2389, 1984.

11. Kennerdell JS, Slamovits TL, Dekker A, et al: Orbital fine needle aspiration biopsy. *Amer J Ophthalmol* 99:547–551, 1985.

12. Zajdela A, de Maublanc MA, Schlienger P: Cytologic diagnosis of orbital and periorbital palpable tumours using fine needle sampling without aspiration. *Diagn Cytopathol* 2:17–20, 1986.

13. Iwamoto T, Jakobiec FA: A comparative ultrastructural study of the normal lacrimal gland and its epithelial tumours. *Hum Pathol* 13:236–262, 1982.

14. Knowles DM, Jakobiec FA: Orbital neoplasms. A clinicopathological study of 60 patients. *Cancer (Philadelphia)* 46:576–589, 1980.

8

Ancillary Techniques

CYTOCHEMICAL METHODS

Specialized procedures similar to the ones used for histopathology are sometimes needed to determine the nature of cell products and to help identify the cell of origin of a tumor. Melanin pigmentation in tumor cells can be confirmed by using Masson-Fontana stain. (Plate II.1.) Similarly, mucin can be demonstrated in tumor cells by use of mucicarmine stain. Oil red O stain can be used to demonstrate neutral fat in cellular aspirates. (Plate II.2.) These cytochemical methods compliment use of the routine Papanicolaou and hematoxylin and eosin stains and are sometimes helpful in arriving at the diagnosis. Sachdeva and Kline[1] have emphasized the usefulness of cytochemical methods in the day to day operation of a cytology laboratory. Special stains can be applied to smears previously stained by the Papanicolaou method after decolorization. Rapid staining methods are described in detail in the article by these authors; the procedures take from five minutes to one hour. Similar cytochemical staining procedures are available in our laboratory and we have used them from time to time to supplement routine staining methods for diagnostic purposes.

IMMUNOPEROXIDASE METHODS

Tumors synthesize a wide variety of cell products, including oncofetal antigens, hormones and immunoglobulins. The identification of tumor markers plays an important part in diagnosis and in predicting the site of a primary tumor that has metastasized. The immunoperoxidase method is an immunocytochemical technique that demonstrates antigens in cells and tissues by making use of specific antibodies and the enzyme horseradish peroxidase. The commonly used substrate diaminobenzidine polymerizes in the presence of hydrogen peroxide and peroxidase to form an insoluble brown polymer that is deposited in the form of brown granules at the site of the antigen-antibody reaction. A number of immunoperoxidase techniques have been described in the literature; the most sensitive and most commonly used technique is the peroxidase-antiperoxidase method.[2] No attempt will be made to describe all the different techniques that are available and the reader is referred to a few standard textbooks on this subject.[3-5]

Specimen Preparation

Immunoperoxidase methods have been applied to histology and cytology preparations. Frozen and paraffin-embedded specimens are used in histology. In cytopathology, imprints, smears, cell suspensions, cytocentrifuge preparations and cell-block preparations have been used.

Direct-Smear Technique

Immunoperoxidase methods can be applied to direct smears made from needle aspirates. Extra smears can be prepared at the time of the aspiration procedure and fixed in 95 percent ethanol. If no extra unstained slides are available, smears previously stained by the Papanicolaou method can be used. Decolorization is not necessary. The advantage is the ability to apply the immunoperoxidase stains on older, previously stained smears when no other material is available. A disadvantage is the inability to use more than one stain because of the limited number of slides. Background staining is another drawback that seriously interferes with interpretation.

Cytocentrifuge Technique

The advantage of this technique is that a number of slides can be prepared from one aspirate for the application of more than one stain. The morphologic features of the cells are preserved unless the cytocentrifuge is used at high speed. A speed of 1500 revolutions per minute for five minutes is satisfactory. Background staining is not a problem. In this technique, the needle is rinsed in balanced electrolyte solution and the cells are concentrated by means of a cytocentrifuge. Rapid fixation is important once the cytocentrifuge comes to a stop. The smears can be fixed in 95 percent ethanol or by use of a spray fixative.

Cell-Block Technique

This technique is an excellent method for obtaining more than one section for immunostaining. The success of the technique depends on the presence in the aspirated material of small tissue fragments. After the direct smears are made, the needle is rinsed in balanced electrolyte solution. A second pass may be required if small tissue particles are not visible in the solution. The balanced electrolyte solution that contains the aspirated material is then centrifuged at 3000 revolutions per minute for approximately 10 minutes. The supernatant is discarded. If a cell button or pellet is formed at the bottom of the tube, it is removed and placed in a nylon cassette bag and fixed in 10 percent neutral formalin solution.

    If no cell button is obtained after centrifugation, eight drops of plasma are added to the mixture and stirred with a wooden applicator stick. Five drops of thrombin

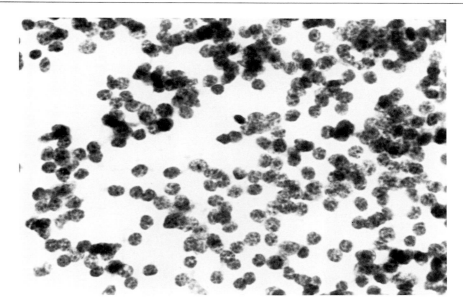

Fig. 8.1. Small-cell tumor, suggestive of a non-Hodgkin's lymphoma. Papanicolaou preparation. ×625.

are then added. The resultant clot, which forms in a few seconds, is then removed and placed in a nylon bag in 10 percent neutral formalin solution. After fixation, the clot is processed as a small biopsy specimen and embedded in paraffin. The advantage of this method is that more than one section can be cut from the cell block for special stains.

Many commercially produced antisera are readily available for immunoperoxidase staining. Tumor markers that are commonly studied include carcinoembryonic antigen, epithelial membrane antigen, cytokeratin, leukocyte common antigen, S-100 protein, vimentin, prostate-specific acid phosphatase, neuron-specific enolase and alpha-fetoprotein. The usefulness of immunocytochemistry in fine-needle aspiration biopsy is demonstrated by the following examples:

1. In the differential diagnosis of small-cell tumors. Figure 8.1 shows a smear from a mass in the neck of a 43-year-old man. The smear suggested a diagnosis of a small-cell neoplasm, probably a non-Hodgkin's lymphoma. Because there also was a mediastinal mass in this patient, the question of small-cell anaplastic carcinoma was raised. Immunoperoxidase staining for leukocyte common antigen, neuron-specific enolase and cytokeratins was performed on the cell block. The tumor cells were immunoreactive for leukocyte common antigen (Plate II.3.) and negative for neuron-specific enolase and cytokeratins, confirming the initial cytologic impression of non-Hodgkin's lymphoma.

2. In the further characterization of adenocarcinoma cells. Figure 8.2 shows a lymph node aspirate from a 75-year-old man with a history of adenocarcinoma of the rectum and prostate. A diagnosis of metastatic adenocarcinoma of the prostate was suggested on the basis of the Papanicolaou-stained smear. This impression was confirmed by staining with prostate-specific acid phosphatase. There was a

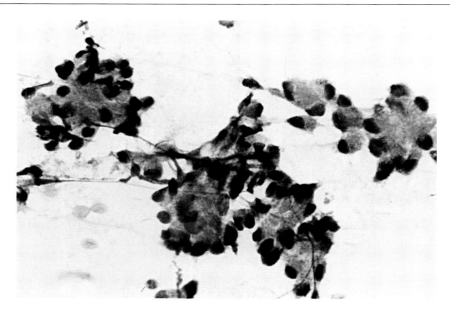

Fig. 8.2. Metastatic adenocarcinoma. Small acinar units are seen in the photomicrograph. Papanicolaou preparation. × 390.

positive reaction with this antibody. (Plate II.4.) Adenocarcinomas of the colon and rectum are negative with prostate-specific acid phosphatase and show a positive reaction with carcinoembryonic antigen.

3. In the separation of chordoma from other primary and metastatic neoplasms. In the head and neck, chordoma may present as a mass in the spheno-occipital region or in the lateral aspect of the neck, mimicking certain primary and metastatic neoplasms including clear-cell carcinoma, mucus-secreting adenocarcinoma, signet-ring cell adenocarcinoma, myxopapillary ependymoma, chondrosarcoma and liposarcoma. Figure 8.3 shows an aspirate from a mass in the neck of a 38-year-old man. The smear contains small clusters and sheets of cells. Many multivacuolated cells were seen, some having a signet-ring appearance. A review of the history revealed that the patient had been operated on six years earlier for a chordoma involving the C5 vertebral body. It was possible to render a diagnosis of recurrent chordoma on the basis of the results of the immunocytochemical studies. The tumor cells were positive for neuron-specific enolase, S-100 protein (Plate II.5.), epithelial membrane antigen and cytokeratins and was negative for carcinoembryonic antigen. In adenocarcinoma of the gastrointestinal tract, one would have expected positive staining for carcinoembryonic antigen and a negative reaction with neuron-specific enolase and S-100 protein.

ELECTRON MICROSCOPY

The usefulness of electron microscopy in the interpretation of fine-needle aspiration biopsy specimens has been the subject of a number of recent reports.[6-10] Although this modality is not routinely used because of the cost and time commitment, it is

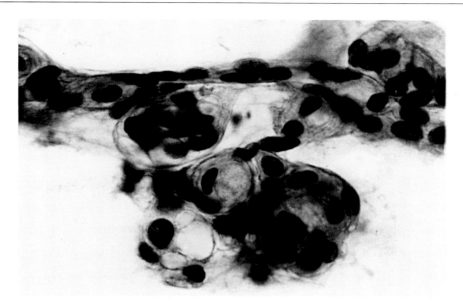

Fig. 8.3. Cohesive clusters of cells that have vacuolated cytoplasm, some suggestive of signet-ring cells. Papanicolaou preparation. ×625.

useful when a definitive diagnosis is not possible on light microscopy. It is thus especially useful in the investigation of undifferentiated or poorly differentiated tumors and soft-tissue sarcomas. A recent report has specifically demonstrated its utility in the diagnosis of round-cell malignant tumors of childhood.[10] No attempt will be made to cover this subject in great depth because it is well covered in the references cited.

Because the need for electron microscopy cannot be predicted at the time of biopsy, tissues should be properly fixed and readily available for subsequent study if necessary. The thrombin-clot technique can be used for ultrastructural studies, although some authors have recommended rinsing the needle in a 3 percent solution of glutaraldehyde (pH 7.2).[6,10] The sample is allowed to fix for at least one hour or overnight in a refrigerator and is then centrifuged at 1500 revolutions per minute for five minutes to obtain a pellet, which is then washed with cacodylate buffer and postfixed in 2 percent osmium tetroxide, dehydrated in graded acetones and embedded in a mixture of Epon and araldite. Akhtar and colleagues[11] have recently described an improved technique for processing aspiration biopsy material for electron microscopy. After fixation, the glutaraldehyde solution that contains the aspirated material is filtered by means of a nylon sieve that separates the red blood cells, which pass through the sieve, from the tumor cells, which are mostly held up in the sieve. The two samples are then processed by centrifuging as described earlier. Akhtar and colleagues have obtained a much higher cellular yield in the sample that is held up in the sieve by this method. The following examples illustrate the usefulness of electron microscopy for aspirated material:

1. Figure 8.4 shows a small-cell tumor demonstrated by light microscopy. The appearance on the Papanicolaou-stained smear was consistent with an undifferen-

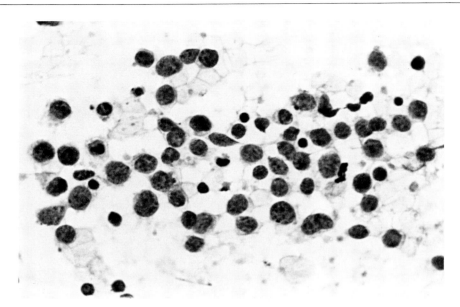

Fig. 8.4. Small-cell tumor, consistent with an undifferentiated carcinoma. Papanicolaou preparation. ×625.

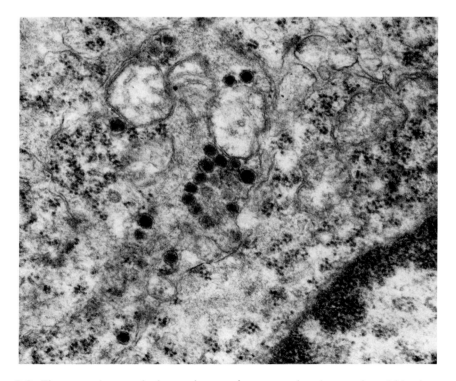

Fig. 8.5. Electron micrograph shows electron-dense cytoplasmic granules within the tumor cells. ×47,000.

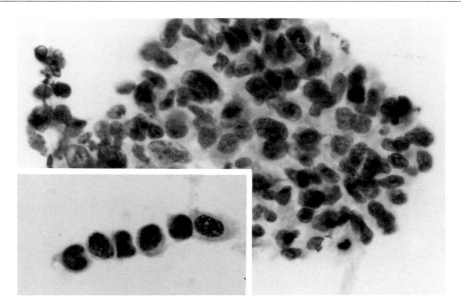

Fig. 8.6. Undifferentiated carcinoma, large-cell type. Papanicolaou preparation. ×625. (*Inset:* ×1000.)

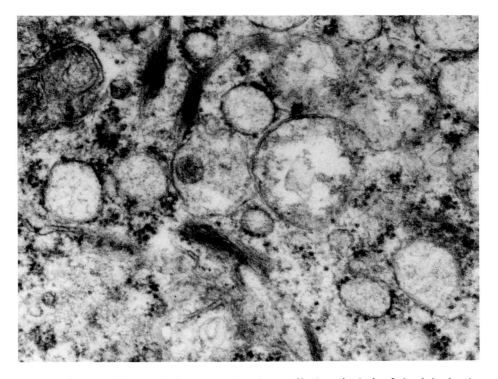

Fig. 8.7. Electron micrograph shows cytoplasmic tonofibrils and a lack of glandular lumina. ×63,750.

tiated carcinoma. Electron microscopy revealed many small cytoplasmic granules that had the typical appearance of neurosecretory granules, confirming the neuroendocrine nature of the tumor (Fig. 8.5).

2. This example demonstrates the usefulness of electron microscopy in delineating the nature of a mass as a second primary cancer rather than a metastasis from the original breast carcinoma. Light microscopy (Fig. 8.6) showed an appearance consistent with an undifferentiated large-cell carcinoma. Ultrastructural examination confirmed the squamous nature of the lesion by demonstrating desmosomes and tonofibrils and a lack of glandular lumina (Fig. 8.7).

REFERENCES

1. Sachdeva R, Kline TS: Aspiration biopsy cytology and special stains. *Acta Cytol* 25:678–683, 1981.

2. Sternberger LA, Hardy PH Jr, Cuculis JJ, et al: The unlabelled antibody enzyme method of immunohistochemistry. Preparation and properties of soluable antigen-antibody complex (horseradish peroxidase-antihorseradish peroxidase) and its use in identification of spirochetes. *J Histochem Cytochem* 18:315–333, 1970.

3. DeLellis RA: *Diagnostic Immunohistochemistry*. New York, Masson, 1981.

4. Sternberger LA: *Immunocytochemistry,* ed 2. New York, Wiley, 1979.

5. Nadji M, Morales AR: *Immunoperoxidase Techniques. A Practical Approach to Tumour Diagnosis*. Chicago, American Society of Clinical Pathology Press, 1986.

6. Akhtar M, Ali MA, Owen EW: Application of electron microscopy in interpretation of fine needle aspiration biopsies. *Cancer (Philadelphia)* 48:2458–2463, 1981.

7. Nordgren H, Akerman M: Electron microscopy of fine needle aspiration biopsy of soft tissue tumours. *Acta Cytol* 26:179–188, 1982.

8. Kindblom LG: Light and electron microscopic examination of embedded fine needle aspiration biopsy specimen in the preoperative diagnosis of soft tissue and bone tumours. *Cancer (Philadelphia)* 51:2264–2277, 1983.

9. Wills EJ, Carr S, Philips J: Electron microscopy in the diagnosis of percutaneous fine needle aspiration specimens. *Ultrastruct Pathol* 11:361–387, 1987.

10. Akhtar M, Ali MA, Sabbah R, et al: Fine needle aspiration biopsy diagnosis of round cell malignant tumours of childhood. A combined light and electron microscopic approach. *Cancer (Philadelphia)* 55:1805–1817, 1985.

11. Akhtar M, Bakry M, Nash JE: An improved technique for processing aspiration biopsy for electron microscopy. *Amer J Clin Pathol* 85:57–60, 1986.

Index

Page numbers in italics refer to illustrations

A

Abnormal swellings, in head or neck, 2–3
Acini of the salivary gland, 21, *22*
Acinic cell carcinoma, 86–92
  cystic variant, 86, *87, 88*, 90, *91*
  differential diagnosis, 90–92
  glandular configuration of, *87, 89*
  granulomatous inflammation in, *86, 88*
  histologic and cytologic features, 86–90
  vs. oncocytoma, 64
  vs. Warthin's tumor, 90–92
Acquired immune deficiency syndrome
     (AIDS), generalized persistent
     lymphadenopathy and, 134
Adenocarcinoma, 166–177
  cytologic features, 166–171
  differential diagnosis, 99, 171–177
  duct-like or glandular structures, *167–169*
  histologic and cytologic features, 98–99
  immunoperoxidase staining, 305–306,
    Plate II.4
  of kidneys, 166–167
  of lymph nodes, 166–167
  of salivary glands, 98–99
  well differentiated, *167–169*
Adenoid cystic carcinoma, 71–79
  basaloid cells in, *75, 76*
  branching pattern, *71, 74*
  cylindromatous type, *71, 73*
  differential diagnosis, 75–78
  histologic and cytologic features, 71–75
  metastatic vs. small-cell neoplasms, 78
  "mucous cylinders" in, *72, 74*
  of parotid gland, *Plate I.3*

  poorly differentiated, *75, 77*
  of soft palate, 295, *296*
  solid type, *71, 73*
  well differentiated, *75, 78*
Adenomas, pleomorphic and mono-
    morphic, 44–70
Adipose tissue tumors, 206–214
  lipoma and liposarcoma, 206–214
Air-dried staining, 10
Alveolar soft-part sarcoma, 250–251
Alveoli, 21–22
Ancillary techniques, 303–310
  electron microscopy, 306–310
Angioimmunoblastic lymphadenopathy,
    128
Angiosarcoma, of blood and lymph
    vessels, 245–248
Aspiration biopsy
  adipose tissue tumors, 206–214
  ancillary techniques, 303–310
  blood vessel tumors, 238–248
  carotid body tumors, 279–290
  clinical application, 2–3
  complications and results, 107–110
  congenital and cystic lesions, 265–277
  diagnostic pitfalls, 105–106
  early use, 4–5
  electron microscopy and, 150, 306–310
  fibrous histiocytic tumors, 219–223
  fibrous tissue tumors, 214–218
  fixation and staining, 10–11
  histology and cytology, 2–13
  indicators for, 117–118
  laboratory technique, 4–10
  lipoma and liposarcoma, 206–214

Aspiration biopsy (cont'd)
  of lymph nodes, 117–203
  lymphoma, 135–155
  lymph vessel tumors, 238–248
  metastatic neoplasms, 157–196
  miscellaneous lesions, 291–302
  non-Hodgkin's and Hodgkin's
    lymphomas, 135–155
  paragangliomas, 279–290
  pattern recognition in, 12
  peripheral nerve tumors, 230–235
  principles of interpretation, 11–12
  reporting method, 13
  results and complications, 198–199
  salivary glands, 15–116
  smooth muscle tumors, 223–225
  soft-tissue tumors, 205–264
  special studies, 118
  striated muscle tumors, 225–229
  of superficial structures, 291–295
  sympathetic nervous system tumors,
    235–238
  synovial tumors, 248–249
Autoimmune disorders, of salivary glands,
  16, 38–43

B
Bacterial infections, of salivary glands, 29
Basal cell adenoma, 64–70
  basosquamous whorling, 65, 68
  branching cords, 65, 68
  canalicular type, 65, 67, 69
  differential diagnosis, 65–70
  histologic and cytologic features, 65
  palisading at borders, 65, 66
  of salivary glands, 64–70
  sheets and clusters, 65, 67
Basaloid tumors, diagnostic pitfalls, 106
Benign lymphoepithelial lesion, 38–43
  differential diagnosis, 41
  histologic and cytologic features, 40–41
  and malignant melanoma, 41
  of salivary glands, 38–43
Benign mixed tumor, *see* Pleomorphic
  adenoma
Benign neoplasms
  basal cell and clear cell adenomas, 64–70
  diagnostic accuracy of selected reports,
    109
  oncocytoma, 60–64
  pleomorphic and monomorphic
    adenomas, 44–70
  results of cytology, 108
  of salivary glands, 16, 43–70
  sebaceous adenoma and lymphadenoma,
    70
  Warthin's tumor, 43–70

Biopsy, *see* Aspiration biopsy
Blood vessel tumors, 238–248
  angiosarcoma, 245–248
  hemangioma and hemangiopericytoma,
    239–245
Bone tumors, 256
Bony lesions, 300
Branchial cleft cysts, 27–30, 266–267
  pearl-like configuration, *271–273*
  squamous and inflamed, *270, 273*
  of sternocleidomastoid muscle, 267, 269
Breast cancer
  colloid type, 171, *175, Plate I.5*
  lymph node metastasis with, 158–160
  medullary, *11*
Burkitt's lymphoma, 140–142

C
Carcinoma ex pleomorphic adenoma,
  92–94
Carotid body tumors, 279–290
  clinical features, 280–282
  complications and results, 287
  differential diagnosis, 286–287
  granular and elongated cytoplasm, 283,
    284–285
  histologic and cytologic features, 282–
    286
  organoid pattern, 282
Cat-scratch fever, 32, 129, 134
Cell-block technique, 304–306
Cellular atypia, in cytology preparations,
  105–106
Centrifuge technique, 304
Cervical cytology, 12
Children
  acinic cell carcinoma in, 86
  mucoepidermoid carcinoma in, 79
Chondrosarcoma
  extraskeletal, 251–253
  myxoid and mesenchymal, 251, *252–*
    253
Chordoma, 256–259
  differential diagnosis, 259
  immunoperoxidase staining, 306, *Plate*
    II.5
  pysaliphorous cells, 256, *257–258*
  signet-like cells, 256, *258*
Chronic inflammatory disease
  diagnosis of, 118–119
  specific and nonspecific, 118–119
Chronic lymphadenitis, 36–37
Clear-cell adenoma, of salivary glands, 70
Clear-cell carcinoma
  differential diagnosis, 99–100
  histologic and cytologic features, 99
  of salivary glands, 99–100

Colloid carcinomas, 171, *175, Plate I.5*
Congenital and cystic lesions, 265–277
    branchial cleft, 266–267
    cytologic features, 271–274
    dermoid and epidermoid, 271, *272*
    diagnostic pitfalls, 276
    differential diagnosis, 274–276
    results of biopsy cytology, 276
    thryoglossal duct, 265–266
    thymic, 267–269
Cylindroma, 71
Cystic lesions, *see* Congenital and cystic
        lesions
Cysts, 5, 10; *see also* Congenital and cystic
        lesions
    cytologic features, 28
    neoplasms simulating, 105
    salivary gland, 16, 26–28
Cytochemical methods, 303
Cytology
    histology and, 2–13
    of salivary glands, 23–26
Cytopathologists, 1–2

D
Dermoid and epidermoid cysts, 271, *272*
    sebaceous cells in, 274–275
Diagnostic pitfalls
    basaloid and mucoepidermoid tumors,
        106
    cellular atypia, 105–106
    in congenital and cystic lesions, 276
    lymphocytes in smears, 106
    in lymphoma, 155–156
    in metastatic neoplasms, 196–198
    neoplasms simulate cysts, 105
    salivary glands, 105–106
Diffuse hyperplasia, 124–125
Direct-smear technique, 304
Dry eyes, *see* Keratoconjunctivitis
Dry mouth, *see* Xerostomia
Ductal cells, honeycomb appearance, 25

E
Electron microscopy, 306–310
Eosinophils, in lymph nodes, 123
Epidermal appendage tumors, 293–294
Epithelial cells, in true cysts, 28, *30*
Epithelioid histiocytes, scattered aggre-
        gates of, 129, *132*
Epithelioid sarcoma, 251
Ethanol, fixation with, 10
Ewing's sarcoma
    differential diagnosis, 255, *256*
    extraskeletal, 254–256
    pseudorosette cells, 254, 256

Exfoliate cytology, 12
Exophthalmos, with non-Hodgkin's lym-
        phoma, 300–301
Extraskeletal chondrosarcoma, 251–253

F
Facial paralysis, from adenoid cystic carci-
        noma, 71, *72*
Fat cells, 25
    lipomas in, 208–210
Fibromatosis, 215–216
    adult and juvenile variants, 215
    elongated fibroblasts in, 215, *216*
    histologic and cytologic features, 215–
        216
    spindle-shaped cells in, 216, *217*
Fibrosarcoma, 216–218
    differential diagnosis, 217
    histologic and cytologic features, 217
    spindle-shaped cells in, *217, 218*
Fibrous histiocytoma
    benign and malignant, 219–223
    differential diagnosis, 223
    giant-cell variant, 220, *222*
    myxoid type, 220, *221–222*
    storiform or pleomorphic, 219, *221–222*
Fibrous tissue tumors, 214–218
    fibromatosis, 215–216
    fibrosarcoma, 216–218
    nodular fasciitis, 214
Fixation and staining, 10–11
Floret cells, in pleomorphic lipoma, 208
Follicular carcinoma, 171, *172*
Follicular center cell lymphoma, 138, *139,*
        140, 143–144
Follicular hyperplasia, *124–126*
    of cervical lymph node, *11*

G
Ganglioneuroblastoma, 235–238
Ganglioneuroma, 235–238
Generalized persistent lymphadenopathy
        and AIDS, 134
Ghost cells, 162
Giant-cell carcinoma, 183–186
    differential diagnosis, 184–186
    pleomorphic nature of, 183, *186*
Granulomas
    caseous, 129, *131*
    classical epithelioid, 129, 132
    necrotizing, 132, *133*
Granulomatous lymphadenopathy, 129–
        134
    causes and patterns, 129
    histologic and cytologic features, 129–
        134

Granulomatous reaction
  cystic aeinic cell carcinoma, 86, 88
  in Hodgkin's disease, 132
  squamous cell carcinoma, 162, *163*

H
Head and neck
  adipose tissue tumors, 206–214
  ancillary techniques, 303–310
  aspiration biopsy of, 2–14
  blood vessel tumors, 238–248
  carotid body tumors, 279–290
  congenital and cystic lesions, 265–277
  fibrous histiocytic tumors, 219–223
  fibrous tissue tumors, 214–218
  lipoma and liposarcoma, 206–214
  lymph node aspiration biopsy, 117–203
  lymphoma of, 135–155
  lymph vessel tumors, 238–248
  malignant melanoma, 185–196
  metastatic neoplasms, 157–196
  miscellaneous lesions, 291–302
  paragangliomas, 279–290
  peripheral nerve tumors, 230–235
  smooth muscle tumors, 223–225
  soft-tissue tumors, 205–264
  striated muscle tumors, 225–229
  superficial structures, 291–295
  sympathetic nervous system tumors, 235–238
  synovial tumors, 248–249
  tumor incidence, 43
Heerfordt's syndrome, 32
Hemangioma, 239, *243*
Hemangiopericytoma, 239, *244*
Hemangiosarcoma, 245–248
  differential diagnosis, 247–248
  nasal ulcerative, 245, *246*
Hematoxylin-eosin staining, 10
Hibernomas, 207–208
  tumor cell vacuoles in, 208, *210*
Histiocytes, 123
  multinucleated giant, 132, *133*
Histiocytoma
  benign and malignant, 219–233
  fibrous, 219–223
Histology
  and cytology, 2–13
  of salivary glands, 21–23
Hodgkin's lymphoma, 150–155
  diagnosis of, 151, 155
  epithelioid granulomas in, 132
  histologic and cytologic features, 151–155
  Lukes-Butler classification, 150–151
  lymphocytic predominance and depletion, 152

mixed-cell type, 152, *153–154*
nodular sclerosis and mixed cellularity, 152
vs. reactive lymphoid hyperplasia, 127–128
Reed-Sternberg cells in, 150–155
Rye classification, 150–151
Hürthle cell carcinoma, 171, *173*
Hygroma, *see* Lymphangioma
Hyperplasia
  diffuse and mixed, 124–125
  of intraparotid lymph nodes, 36–37
  reactive lymphoid, 123–129

I
Immunoblastic sarcoma, cytologic features, 144, *145–147*
Immunoperoxidase methods, 303–306
  cell-block technique, 304–306
  direct-smear and centrifuge techniques, 304
  specimen preparation, 304
Implantation tumors, 4–5
Infectious mononucleosis, 125, *126*
  Reed-Sternberg cells in, 155
  transformed lymphocytes in, 127, *128*
Inflammatory lesions
  of salivary glands, 16–17, 28–37
  sialadenitis and lymphadenitis, 29–37
Intraparotid lymph nodes, hyperplasia of, 36–37
Irritational fibroma, 297

K
Kaposi's sarcoma, in superficial structures, 294–295
Keratoconjunctivitis (dry eyes), 38

L
Laboratory technique, aspiration biopsy, 4–10
Lacrimal glands
  autoimmune disorders, 38
  lesions of, 300
Large-cell carcinoma, 182, *183*
  differential diagnosis, 187
  electron microscopy, *309, 310*
Large-cell lymphoma, cytologic features, 140–148
Laryngeal paragangliomas, 279
Leiomyoma, 223
Leiomyosarcoma, 223–225
  cohesive clusters of elongated cells, 224, *225*
  cigar-shaped nuclei, *224*

Lennert's lymphoma, 135–136
Leprosy
 and granulomatous lymphadenopathy,
  130
 lepromatous, 130
 tuberculoid and lepromatous, 134
Lipoblastomas, 207–208
 multivacuolated, 211, 213
Lipomas, 206–210
 differential diagnosis, 208–210
 histologic and cytologic features, 207–
  208
 in mature fat cells, 208–210
Liposarcoma
 differential diagnosis, 214
 histologic and cytologic features, 211–
  214
 myxoid type, 211, 212–213
 round-cell type, 214
 well differentiated, 211–212
Lobulated lymphoma, 140, 142–143
Lymphadenitis, acute or chronic, 36–37,
  134
Lymphadenopathy, generalized persistent,
  134
Lymphangioma, 238, 240, 242
Lymphangiosarcoma, 245–248
 differential diagnosis, 247–248
Lymph nodes
 adenocarcinoma of, 166–177
 anatomic structures, 119, 198
 aspiration biopsy, 117–203
 benign enlargement of, 123–124
 cell types, 123
 cortical area, 119–120
 cytologic diagnosis, 198
 diagrammatic structure, 121
 giant-cell and spindle cell carcinomas,
  183–186
 histologic and cytologic features, 119–
  122
 indications for biopsy, 117–118
 locations in neck, 121
 metastatic neoplasms, 118, 157–196
 non-Hodgkin's lymphoma, 119
 normal, 119–123
 paracortex and medulla, 122
 in parotid glands, 36
 small-cell and large-cell carcinoma, 180–
  182
 results and complications, 198–199
 squamous cell carcinoma, 160–166
 undifferentiated carcinoma, 177–179
Lymphocytes, 122–123
 intermediate, 122
 predominance and depletion, 152
 small and large, 122–123
 in smears, 106

Lymphoepithelioma, 179, 180, 181
Lymphoglandular bodies, 123
Lymphogranuloma venereum, granulomas
  in, 129
Lymphoid hyperplasia, reactive, 123–129
Lymphoma, 135–155
 common types, 149
 diagnosis of, 135, 155–157
 lymphocytic, 17
 malignant, 102
 mixed-cell, 148–150
 necrosis and hyalinization, 156
 results of cytology, 156–157
 small-cell and large-cell, 138–148
 staging of, 118
Lymphoreticular lesions, 300
Lymph vessel tumors, 238–248
 lymphangioma, 238, 240–242

M
Macrophages, see Histiocytes
Malignant lymphoma
 diagnostic accuracy, 157
 cytologic classification, 135–138
 primary, 118
 of salivary glands, 102
 and Sjögren's syndrome, 102
Malignant melanoma, 3–4, 186–196
 cell types, 190, 191
 cytologic features, 190–195
 differential diagnosis, 195–196
 epithelioid type, 191, Plate I.6
 frequencies of cytologic features, 194
 giant-cell variant, 192, 193, 195
 Masson-Fontana stain, 303, Plate II.1
 of salivary glands, 103–104
 spindle cell type, 191, 192
 in superficial structures, 292–293
 undifferentiated type, 192, 193
Malignant tumors
 acinic cell carcinoma, 86–92
 adenocarcinoma, 98–99
 adenoid cystic carcinoma, 71–79
 carcinoma ex pleomorphic adenoma,
  92–94
 clear-cell carcinoma, 99–100
 diagnostic accuracy of selected reports,
  109
 lymphoma, 102
 mesenchymal, 103
 metastatic neoplasms, 103–104
 mixed, 94
 mucoepidermoid carcinoma, 79–86
 of salivary glands, 16, 71–104
 sebaceous carcinoma, 100–102
 squamous cell carcinoma, 94–96
 undifferentiated carcinoma, 96–98

Masson-Fontana staining, malignant
melanoma, 192, 195, 303, *Plate II.1*
Mast cells
in lymph nodes, 123
in Warthin's tumor, 59
Mature fat cells, lipomas in, 208–210
Maxillary antrum lesions, 298–299
Caldwell-Luc operation, 298
Melanin, Masson-Fontana staining, 192,
195
Melanoma, 3, *4; see also* Malignant
melanoma
of oral cavity, 298
Merkel cell tumor, 177, 182
cytologic features, 183, 185
of lips and face, 182, *184*
in superficial structures, 291–292
Mesenchymal tumors, *see also* Soft-tissue
tumors
of salivary glands, 103
vs. squamous cell carcinoma, 166
Metastatic neoplasms
adenocarcinoma, 166–167
of cervical lymph node, *11*
clinical and cytologic features, 157–160
diagnostic pitfalls, 196–198
giant-cell and spindle cell carcinomas,
183–186
in lymph nodes, 157–196
malignant melanoma, 103–104, 186–
196
Merkel cell tumor, 182–183
nasopharyngeal carcinoma, 179–180
results and complications, 108, 198–199
of salivary glands, 103–104
seminoma, 196
small-cell and large-cell carcinoma, 180–
182
squamous cell carcinoma, 104, 160–166
undifferentiated carcinoma, 177–179
Mikulicz's disease, 38–41
Miscellaneous lesions, 291–302
maxillary antrum, 298–299
of oral cavity, 295–298
orbital and periorbital, 299–301
of superficial structures, 291–295
Mixed-cell lymphoma, 148–150, 152
Mixed hyperplasia, 124–125
Monomorphic adenoma, 54–70
basal cell and clear-cell, 64–70
oncocytoma, 60–64
of salivary glands, 54–70
sebaceous, 70
Warthin's tumor, 55–60
WHO classification, 54
Mononucleosis, infectious, 125, *126*
Mucinous acini, 21, *22, 26*
Mucoceles, 26–28, *30*

Mucoepidermoid carcinoma, 79–86
vs. chronic sialadenitis, 83
diagnostic pitfalls, 106
differential diagnosis, 83–86
high-grade metastatic, 79, *81, 84*
histologic and cytologic features, 79–83
low grade vs. high grade, 85
monolayer sheet of intermediate cells,
80, *83*
mucus-secreting cells, 79, *81–82*
pearl formation in, 83, *84*
poorly differentiated, 80, *81*
of submandibular gland, *Plate 1.2*
Multivacuolated lipoblasts, 211, *213*
Myoepithelial cells, *23*
Myxoid liposarcoma, 211, *212–213*
Myxoma, 249–250

N
National Cancer Institute (NCI),
classification of non-Hodgkin's lymphoma, 136–137
Nasopharyngeal carcinoma, 179–180
Neck, *see* Head and neck
Needle biopsy, *see* Aspiration biopsy
Neoplasms, *see also* Benign neoplasms;
Malignant tumors
benign and malignant, 16
needle implantation, 4–5
of salivary glands, 16
simulating cysts, 105
Neurilemmoma, 230–231
spindle and myxoid areas, *232*
of vagus nerve, 230, *231*
Neuroblastoma, 235–238
olfactory, 238
rosette-like cells, 236, *237*
Neuroendocrine carcinoma, *see* Merkel cell
tumor, 182–184
Neurofibroma, 231–233
solitary or multiple, 231–232
Neurofibromatosis, 231, *233*
Neurofibrosarcoma, 233–235
multinucleated cells, 234, *235*
spindle cell variant, *234*
Neutrophils, in lymph nodes, 123
Nodular fasciitis, 214
Nodular sclerosis, 152
Noncaseating granulomas, 129, *131*
Nondiagnostic smears, 13
Non-Hodgkin's lymphoma, 135–150
exophthalmos with, 300–301
histologic and cytologic classification,
135–138
immunoperoxidase staining, 305, *Plate
II.3*
Lennert's classification, 135–136

Lukes-Collins classification, 135–136
mixed-cell, 148–150
NCL classification, 136–137
new classifications, 135–136
Rappaport's classification, 135–136
small-cell and large-cell, 138–148
Zajicek's classification, 137
Nonneoplastic cysts, cytologic features, 28, 31

O
Oil red O staining, sebaceous carcinoma, 303, *Plate II.2*
Olfactory neuroblastoma, 238
Oncocytic cells, 23, 26
mimicking malignancy, 61, *63*
in pleomorphic adenoma, 49, *52*
in Warthin's tumor, 56, *57–58*
Oncocytoma, 60–64
vs. acinic cell carcinoma, 64
binucleated forms, 61, *63*
dense eosinophilic cytoplasm, 61, *62*
differential diagnosis, 64
histologic and cytologic features, 61–64
polygonal cells, 61, *62*
salivary gland, 60–64
vs. Warthin's tumor, 59, 64
Open biopsy, *see* Surgical biopsy
Optic nerve tumors, 300
Oral cavity tumors, 295–298
Orbital and periorbital lesions, 299–301
Oxyphilic adenoma, *see* Oncocytoma

P
Papillary carcinoma, 167, *170*
of thyroid, 266, *268, 274*
Papillary cystadenoma lymphomatosum, *see* Warthin's tumor
Pap stain, for needle aspirates, 10, *11*
Paraganglioma, 19, *20,* 279–290; *see also* Carotid body tumors
angiogram and tomogram, *288–289*
clinical features, 280–282
complications and results, 287
differential diagnosis, 286–287
histologic and cytologic features, 282–286
jugulotympanic and vagal, 281
laryngeal, 281
malignant, 283, *284, 286*
of vagus nerve, 287, *288*
Parotid gland, 20, *21*
acinic cell carcinoma, 86–87
adenoid cystic carcinoma of, 78, *79, Plate I.3*
cysts, 26–28

pleomorphic adenoma of, *Plate I.1*
tumors of, 15–20
Pearl formations in mucoepidermoid carcinoma, 83, *84*
Pedunculated tumor, on scalp, *294*
Periorbital lesions, *see* Orbital and periorbital lesions
Peripheral nerve tumors, 230–235
neurilemmoma, 230–231
neurofibroma and neurofibrosarcoma, 231–235
Phagocytes, *see* Histiocytes
Plasma cells, in lymph nodes, 123
Pleomorphic adenoma, 44–54
cartilage-like area, 49, *54*
concentric laminated bodies in, 49, *52*
cystic degeneration, 49, *51*
differential diagnosis, 49–54
epithelial branching, 49, *50*
fibromyxoid stromal cells, 45, *47*
glandular and myxoid areas, 45, *46*
histologic and cytologic features, 45–49
incidence and ultrastructure, 44
massive type, 44, *45*
metaplastic and oncocytic changes, 45, *48*
myxoid elements, 45, *47, 53*
oval myoepithelial cells, 49, *51*
of salivary gland, *11,* 44–54, *Plate I.1*
Pleomorphic lipomas, 207–208
Polymorphous low-grade adenocarcinoma of oral cavity, 297
Polypoid lesions, 297–298
precancerous, 297
Postsurgical scarring, of submandibular gland, 31
Post-vaccinal lymphadenitis, 155

R
Ranula, 295–297
Reactive follicular hyperplasia, 36, *37*
Reactive lymphoid hyperplasia, 123–129
differential diagnosis, 127–129
histologic and cytologic features, 124–127
morphologic subtypes, 124
vs. non-Hodgkin's lymphoma, 127–128
Reed-Sternberg cells
high-power view, *153–154*
in Hodgkin's lymphoma, 150–151
in infectious mononucleosis, 127, *128*
Renal cell carcinoma, *178*
of lymph nodes, 166, *167*
Reporting method, cell differentiation, 13
Retention cysts, 26–28
Rhabdomyoma, 210, 225

Rhabdomyosarcoma, 226–228
  pleomorphic and embryonal, 227, *229*
  racket-shaped cells, 228, *229*
Round-cell malignant tumors, of children,
      150
Rye classification, of Hodgkin's lym-
      phoma, 150–151

S
Salivary glands, 15–116
  acinic cell carcinoma, 86–92
  adenocarcinoma of, 98–99
  anatomic structures, 20–21
  aspirates containing lymphocytes, 36, 39
  autoimmune disorders, 38–43
  basal cell and clear-cell adenomas, 64–
      70
  benign neoplasms, 43–70
  carcinoma ex pleomorphic adenoma,
      92–94
  clear-cell carcinoma, 99–100
  complications and results, 107–110
  cysts, 26–28
  diagnostic pitfalls, 105–106
  diagram of, *21*
  enlargement of, 15, 118
  histologic and cytologic features, 21–26
  inflammatory lesions of, 28–37
  major and minor, 20–21
  malignant lymphoma, 102
  malignant melanoma, 103–104
  malignant mixed tumor, 94
  malignant tumors of, 71–104
  mesenchymal tumors, 103
  metastatic tumors, 103–104
  Mikulicz's disease, 38–41
  minor lesions, 295–297
  mucoepidermoid carcinoma, 79–86
  normal, 20–26
  oncocytoma, 60–64
  pleomorphic and monomorphic
      adenomas, 44–70
  primary squamous cell carcinoma, 94–
      96
  sebaceous adenoma and carcinoma, 70,
      100–102
  Sjögren's syndrome, 38–41
  squamous cell carcinoma, 104
  undifferentiated carcinoma, 78, 96–98
  viral and bacterial infections, 29
  Warthin's tumor, 43–70
Sarcoidosis, 32
  granulomatous lymphadenopathy and,
      129, *131*, 134
Scalp tumors, 294
Schwannoma, *see* Neurilemmoma

Scirrhous carcinomas, 12
Sebaceous adenoma, of salivary glands, 70
Sebaceous carcinoma
  cytoplasmic vacuolation in, 100, *101*
  differential diagnosis, 101–102
  of eyelid, *11*
  histologic and cytologic features, 100–
      102
  of intraparotid lymph node, *102*
  oil red O staining, 303, *Plate II.2*
  of salivary glands, 100–102
Sebaceous lymphadenoma, of salivary
      glands, 70
Seminoma
  histologic appearance, *197*
  of lymph nodes, *196*
Serous acini, 23, *24, 25*
Sialadenitis
  acute and chronic, 29–32
  granulomatous, 32–36
Sialograms, for parotid lesions, 18–19
Sialolithiasis, 31
Sialometaplasia
  necrotizing, *84*
  in oral cavity, 297
Signet-ring carcinoma, 171, *174*
Signet-ring lipoblasts, 211
Signet-ring cells, immunoperoxidase
      staining, 306, *307*
Sinus histiocytosis, 124
Sjögren's syndrome, 38–41
Small-cell carcinoma, 180–182, 188–189
  undifferentiated, 96, 97
Small-cell lymphomas, cytologic features,
      138–140
Small-cell tumors
  adenoid cystic carcinoma versus, 78
  electron microscopy, 307, *308*
  immunoperoxidase staining, 305, *Plate
      II.3*
Smears
  lymphocytes in, 106
  nondiagnostic, 13
  quality of, 12
  well prepared examples, *11*
Smooth muscle tumors, 223–225
  leiomyoma and leiomyosarcoma, 223–
      225
Soft-tissue tumors, 205–264
  alveolar soft-part sarcoma, 250–251
  benign and malignant, 206–207
  blood and lymph vessels, 238–248
  chordoma, 256–259
  cytologic features, 206, 207
  diagnosis and management, 205–206
  epithelioid sarcoma, 251
  extraskeletal chondrosarcoma, 251–253

fibrous histiocytic, 219–223
granular cell, 249
myxoma, 249–250
nodular fasciitis, 214
pathologic classification, 206–207
peripheral nerve, 230–235
smooth muscle, 223–225
striated muscle, 225–229
sympathetic nervous system, 235–239
synovium, 248–249
Specimen preparation, 7–10
Spindle cell carcinoma, 183–186
Spindle cell lipomas, 207–208
Squamous cell carcinoma, 3, 160–166
anaplastic giant-cell, 162–166
cystic variant, 162
cytologic features, 160–164
differential diagnosis, 164–166
high-power view, 164
keratinizing and nonkeratinizing, 160,
    161, 162, Plate I.4
metastatic submandibular, 158
of oral cavity, 298
of parotid lymph node, 17, 19
poorly differentiated, 164
primary, 94–96
of salivary glands, 94–96, 104
spindle cell variants, 162, 164, 166
of submandibular gland, 11
well differentiated, 164
Squamous papilloma, 297
Staining
fixation and, 10–11
May-Grünwald Giesma technique, 10
Stensen's duct, adenocarcinoma in, 98
Striated muscle tumors, 225–228
rhabdomyoma and rhabdomyosarcoma,
    225–228
Sublingual gland, 20, 21
Submandibular gland, 20, 21
mucoepidermoid carcinoma of, Plate I.2
obstruction in immunocompromised pa-
    tient, 16, 17
squamous cell carcinoma of, 94, 95
Superficial structures, miscellaneous le-
    sions, 291–295
Surgical biopsy, 3, 12
Sympathetic nervous system tumors, 235–
    238
Synovial tumors, 248–249
Syphilis, granulomas in, 132
Syringe holders, 5

T
Tattooing, of aspiration tract, 16, 18
T-cell lymphoma, 144, 148

Thrombin-clot technique, for ultrastruc-
    ture studies, 307
Thymic cysts, 267–269
Thyroglossal lesions and cysts, 10, 265
Thyroid gland, 26
carcinomas, 158, 160
Tingible-body macrophages, 36, 37, 38
in follicular hyperplasia, 127
Tonofibrils, electron microscopy, 309, 310
Tonsils, carcinoma of, 298
Toxoplasmosis
granulomatous lymphadenopathy and,
    130, 134
Reed-Sternberg cells in, 155
Tru-cut biopsy, 2, 13
True histiocytic lymphoma, 144
Tuberculoid leprosy, 134
Tuberculosis, 32, 134
Tuberculous lymphadenitis, 120, 129
granulomatous inflammation in, 132,
    133
Tumor-like lesions, 206–207
of fibrous tissue, 214–218
Tumors, see Neoplasms

U
Ultrastructure studies, thrombin-clot tech-
    nique, 307
Undifferentiated carcinoma, 177–179
differential diagnosis, 98
electron microscopy, 307, 308
giant-cell and spindle cell, 183–186
histologic and cytologic features, 96
large-cell and small-cell, 187–189
of lungs and thyroid, 183–184
of lymph nodes, 177–179
of salivary glands, 96–98
small-cell and large-cell, 96–97, 180–
    182
Uveoparotid fever, 32

V
Vagal paragangliomas, 281
Viral infections, of parotid gland, 29
von Recklinghausen's disease, see
    Neurofibromatosis

W
Warthin's tumor, 41, 55–60
differential diagnosis, 59–60
epithelial lining in, 56, 57
histologic and cytologic features, 56–59
incidence and etiology, 55

Warthin's tumor (cont'd)
    malignant lymphoma in, 60
    multifocal involvement, 55
Wet-fixed smears, 10
World Health Organization (WHO)
        classification of monomorphic
        adenomas, 54

X
Xerostomia (dry mouth), 40

Z
Zellballen pattern, in carotid body tumors,
        282